The Moving Tablet of the Eye

The Moving Tablet of the Eye

The Origins of Modern Eye Movement Research

Nicholas J. Wade
and
Benjamin W. Tatler

Department of Psychology
University of Dundee
UK

OXFORD
UNIVERSITY PRESS

OXFORD
UNIVERSITY PRESS

Great Clarendon Street, Oxford OX2 6DP

Oxford University Press is a department of the University of Oxford.
It furthers the University's objective of excellence in research, scholarship, and education by publishing worldwide in

Oxford New York

Auckland Cape Town Dar es Salaam Hong Kong Karachi Kuala Lumpur Madrid Melbourne Mexico City Nairobi New Delhi Shanghai Taipei Toronto

With offices in

Argentina Austria Brazil Chile Czech Republic France Greece Guatemala Hungary Italy Japan Poland Portugal Singapore South Korea Switzerland Thailand Turkey Ukraine Vietnam

Oxford is a registered trade mark of Oxford University Press in the UK and in certain other countries

Published in the United States by Oxford University Press Inc., New York

First published 2005

British Library Cataloguing in Publication Data
Data available

Library of Congress Cataloging in Publication Data
Data available

Typeset by Newgen Imaging Systems (P) Ltd., Chennai, India
Printed in Great Britain
on acid-free paper by
Biddles Ltd, King's Lynn

ISBN 0–19–856616–6 (Hbk.) 978–0–19–856616–8
ISBN 0–19–856617–4 (Pbk.) 978–0–19–856617–5

Dedicated to the memory of
Dieter Heller

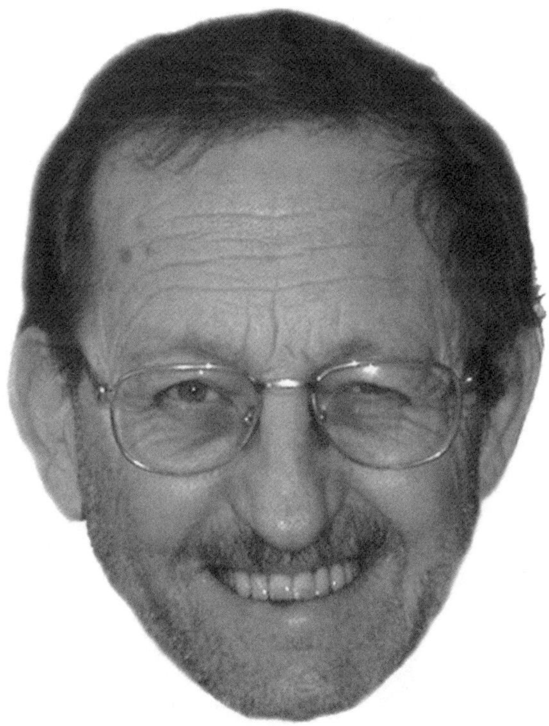

PREFACE

The importance of eye movements is implicitly acknowledged in our daily lives, both in terms of the inspections of our surroundings and the clues they provide to our interactions with other people. We judge not only where things are on the basis of our eye movements but also the moods and motives of those with whom we are communicating. These points are recognized in our language, which is replete with references to the eyes and their movements. Strangely, eye movements have not been accorded the same significance in historical terms. Whereas there are many histories of optics and ophthalmology, there are very few concerning eye movements. When they have been assayed historically, it has been in terms of their malfunction rather than their normal operation. Modern methods for examining eye movements have fuelled this flight from the past; most techniques now in use could not have been envisaged in the pre-computer era. Casual conversations with our colleagues reflected this veiled view of previous eye movement research and in so doing confirmed our desire to address the heritage of this important aspect of perception and communication. This is reflected in the title given to the book—*The moving tablet of the eye*—which is taken from a line in the poem *The temple of nature* by Erasmus Darwin (1731–1802). Darwin placed considerable theoretical importance on eye movements and examined them experimentally.

We do not wish to suggest that there have not been huge leaps in our knowledge of eye movements as a consequence of applying modern methods of measuring their characteristics. Indeed, we provide a survey of these methods and their applications. However, we do wish to counter the widespread view that all this knowledge derives from recent research. For most of the long observational history of eye movements, they have been considered to glide over scenes smoothly rather than proceed with a series of jerks interspersed with brief periods of fixation. The early modern period commenced with the establishment of such discontinuities in the ways the eyes moved. The flame that ignited the modern phase was that of a candle! William Charles Wells

(1757–1817) used a candle flame as a source for generating an afterimage and then compared its motion with that of real image marked on a wall or paper. By this simple procedure he was able to determine aspects of binocular eye movements and also the nystagmus that follows body rotation: the eyes moved smoothly in one direction and then engaged in a ballistic return that was accompanied by blindness. Thus, nystagmus was the initial class of eye movement that rocked the age-old belief in their smooth progress, and introduced the idea that we are not aware of the details of our own eye movements. It was followed, almost a century later, by the demonstration of discontinuous eye movements in the same direction when reading text. These short jerks became known as saccades, and it was the instrumental ingenuity of Raymond Dodge (1871–1942) that rendered them traceable photographically. Dodge used his technical prowess to demonstrate not only that eye movements were discontinuous, but also that vision was suppressed during them. The latter interest arose after Dodge fortuitously noticed that when looking in a mirror he could never see his own eyes moving; he could only ever see them stationary before or after the movement.

The depiction of such jerky eye movements astounded psychologists at the beginning of the twentieth century, and they were not confined to reading. Simple geometrical patterns gave the subjective impression of caressing the eyes around their contours but the reality was otherwise: the eyes engaged in a series of jerks and pauses that often bore little resemblance to the pattern perceived. This was established by George Malcolm Stratton (1865–1957), better known for his experiments on inverted vision. Such demonstrations posed problems for theories of visual illusions that were based on the pattern of eye movements. In this context, Stratton remarked that 'The mythology of the eye-muscles will someday make an interesting paragraph in the history of delusions in psychology'! We may be deluded by our subjective impressions of how the eyes move, but their manifold measurement in modern research is a welcome reality.

Stratton's 'interesting paragraph' has here expanded into a book, the origins of which owe much to Wells and Dodge. One of us had been pursuing Wells' research on nystagmus while the other had been mining the rich seam of Dodge's experiments on the saccade-and-fixate strategy. These represent two streams, the confluence of which has been rarely followed. One reflects the medical interest in eye movements and the other the psychological. We believe that considering the discontinuities involved in nystagmus and saccades has been neglected historically, and we hope that our attempt at uniting them will prove attractive to contemporary students of eye movements.

We have benefited from discussions with numerous people, only a few of whom we can mention. Hiroshi Ono has done much to broaden the appreciation of Wells' experiments on binocular visual direction as well as its relationship to that of Ewald Hering (1834–1918). Leo Hurvich directed us to a little known article by Hering, and without his helpful advice we might well have overlooked the prominence of Hering in the origins of eye movement research. Mike Land's interest and enthusiasm were catalysts to our early exploration of the origins of saccadic research and he has helped us to sustain momentum throughout the preparation of this book. Iain Gilchrist was the first to suggest writing up some of the historical material we had been discussing informally. They have all provided food for thought, and if it has been inappropriately digested the fault lies with us. We also wish to express our thanks to Martin Baum and Charlotte Owen of Oxford University Press for the assistance they have provided in preparing the book for publication.

Much of the nineteenth century research on eye movements was conducted in Germany, and some of the seminal works have been translated into English. This does not apply to all of them, however, and where we provide an English quotation from a German (or a French) work that is not attributed to a translator then the translation is ours. Dieter Heller was well-versed in the German literature and this book was planned with him as a joint author. He was one of the few researchers who retained an acute awareness of early enquiries into eye movements. His untimely death, in November 2003, deprived us of many insights that he would doubtless have contributed to this history. Accordingly, it is to the memory of Dieter that the book is dedicated. We thank Annalies Heller and her family for providing the portrait that accompanies the dedication, and for the hospitality they have offered over the years. The book could not have been completed without the succour and support of Christine and Victoria, to whom we express our heartfelt gratitude. In contrast to the pattern of our discontinuous and interrupted eye movements their encouragement has been continuous and constant.

Nicholas J. Wade
Benjamin W. Tatler

Dundee, April 2005

CONTENTS

1

Informing contemporary research

1.1 Introduction

Orpheus called the eyes, the looking glasses of nature: *Hesichius*, the doores for the Sunne to enter in by: *Alexander* the Peripatecian, the windowes of the mind, because that by the eyes we doe cleerely see what is in the same, we pearce into the deepe thoughts thereof, and enter into the privities of his secret chamber. (Du Laurens, 1596, from a translation in 1599, p. 19, original italics)

While the eyes may be windows to the mind, eye *movements* provide objective measures with which we can study a wide range of psychological and biological processes. The objectivity of eye movements arises because the manner of their operation is very unlike our introspection of them. We feel that our eyes wander smoothly over a scene, yet in reality their movements are discontinuous and extremely rapid. Even though the reality of eye movements is unavailable to the observer, it can be used to provide insights into the input to the visual system from which we can infer processes involved in vision and perception.

The quotation from André Du Laurens (1558–1609; Fig. 1.1, left), also known as Andreas Laurentius, reflects the symbolic significance attached to the eyes in antiquity. He was writing at the end of the sixteenth century, a few years before the study of vision was to be transformed by a better understanding of the optics of the eye and its gross anatomy. He was an anatomist of note, and his diagram of the base of the brain, showing the paths taken by the optic nerves is given in Fig. 1.1, right. Du Laurens came close to recognizing the optical function of the crystalline lens in the eye:

Finally, the eye is like vnto the looking glasse, and this receiueth all such shapes as are brought vnto it, without sending any thing of it owne vnto the object.

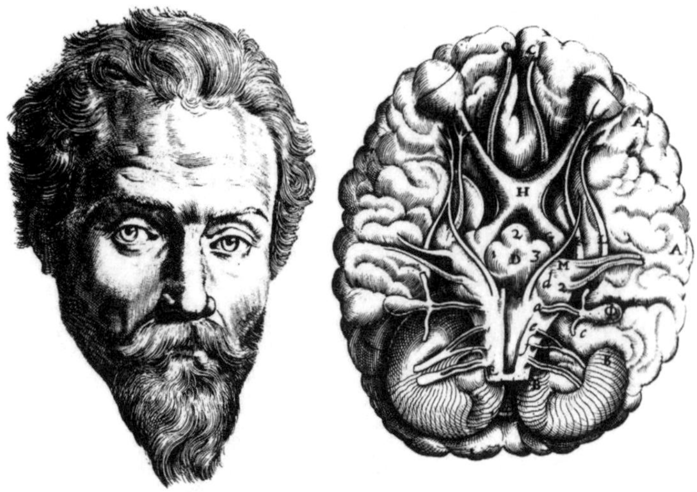

Figure 1.1
Left, André Du Laurens (1558–1609) after an engraving in Du Laurens (1613). Right, the diagram of the base of the brain from the same book.

They differ onely in this, that the looking glasse hath no power to recommend his formes and shapes vnto their judge, as the eye doth vnto the common sense by the nerue opticke. (Du Laurens, 1599, pp. 41–42)

The idea was developed with greater precision by Johannes Kepler (1571–1630; Fig. 1.2, left) who was led to the study of the eye because of his astronomical investigations: he described how the eye operated as an optical instrument, which focused light onto the retina to form an image. That is, the refractions of light through the cornea and crystalline lens were outlined with a novel degree of accuracy. Kepler (1604, 1611) concluded that the visual image is not 'caught' by the lens but 'painted' on the retina, the true sensitive element in the eye. He also correctly recognized that the retinal image must be inverted and reversed. However, it was with the image on the reddish-white concave surface of the retina that his optics ended. How the reversed and inverted image was perceived as upright was beyond the scope of his mathematical science, and he left the problem to natural philosophers.

On the analogy of the eye with the operation of a camera with a lens, Kepler was aware that the optical system could focus on objects at a particular distance. In order for a camera to focus on objects at different distances some change in the lens or the length of the camera was required. A similar problem operated for the eye, but its mechanism remained mysterious. Kepler did not determine how the lens may change shape to focus on near and

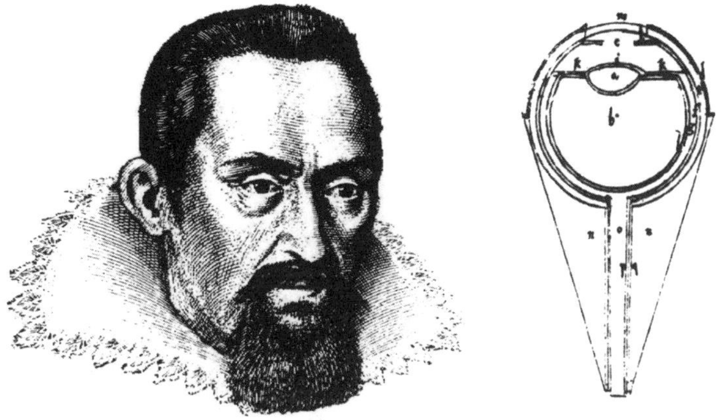

Figure 1.2
Left, Johannes Kepler (1571–1630), after a frontispiece engraving in Caspar (1938). Right, the diagram of the eye used by Kepler (1604); it was reproduced from Platter (1583).

distant objects. He did, however, shift the focus of vision from the lens to the retina. The recognition that the crystalline lens operated like a glass lens directed attention to both the image that was so formed and the surface upon which it was projected. The fact that objects at different distances could be brought to focus on the retina followed from his analysis, but it did not cast light on the manner in which this was achieved.

Kepler was concerned with the structure of the eye but he did not carry out any anatomical dissections to determine its features. He relied on those trained in anatomy, and for Kepler the reliance was on Felix Platter (1536–1614) of Basel. In 1583, Platter made a clear and strong statement about how the lens serves only to focus the rays of light converging on it. This was a significant turning point in visual science. For although Platter did not formulate a theory of the retinal image, understand the geometrical issues, or recognize the inverted nature of the image on the retina, he directed new attention to the role of the retina in photosensitivity at a time when most others were still regarding the lens as the sensitive organ. Platter recognized that the lens is not located in the centre of the eye, and in his drawings moved it closer to its correct location. Platter's anatomy, however, was not without fault. Among other things, his diagram of the eye (which was reproduced by Kepler, 1604; see Fig. 1.2, right) repeated the error of representing the optic nerve on the visual axis. The musculature for moving the eye was represented in a very schematic manner.

A few years after Kepler's analysis of the dioptrics of the eye, Christoph Scheiner (1571–1650; Fig. 1.3, left) provided a

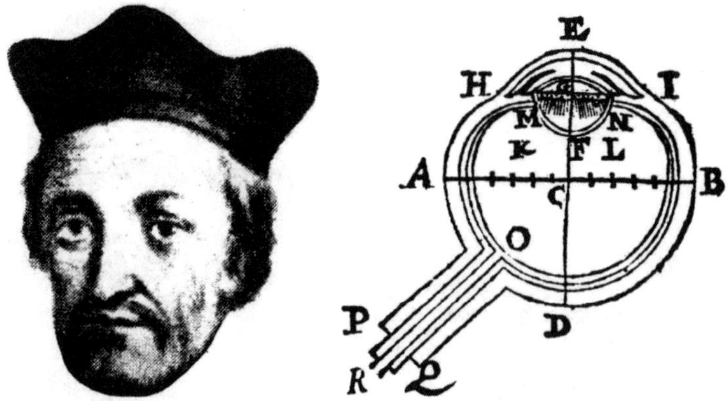

Figure 1.3
Left, Christoph Scheiner (1571–1650), after an illustration in Polyak (1957). Right, Scheiner's (1619) diagram of the vertebrate eye.

considerably more accurate illustration of the vertebrate eye (Fig. 1.3, right). Prior to Scheiner's diagram, the optic nerve was shown as aligned with the optic axis (as is the case in Platter's diagram in Fig. 1.2, right). Scheiner (1619) not only represented the front and rear curvatures of the lens correctly but he also placed the exit of the optic nerve in its correct nasal location. Scheiner (1630) made further comparisons between the eye and camera, and indicated the optical corrections that can be applied for long- and short-sightedness. The eye–camera analogy was bolstered by his demonstration of the image formed on the retina when an animal's eye is placed in the aperture of a *camera obscura*.

Scheiner's (1630) demonstration of image formation in an excised ox's eye was considered so valuable that it was repeated and illustrated seven years later by René Descartes (1596–1650; Fig. 1.4, left) in his book on dioptrics (Descartes, 1637/1902). His diagram (Fig. 1.4, right) of the cosmic observer viewing the inverted and reversed retinal image is perhaps one of the best-known illustrations in visual science. He described it in the following way:

> But you can be even more certain of this if, taking the eye of a newly deceased man, or, for want of that, of an ox or some other large animal, you carefully cut through the membranes which enclose it, in such a manner that a large part of the humor M which is there remains exposed without any of it spilling out because of this. Then, having covered it over with some white body thin enough to let daylight pass through it, as for example with a piece of paper or with an eggshell, RST, place this eye in the hole of a specially made window such as Z, in such a manner so that it has its front, BCD, turned toward some location where there are various objects, such as V, X, Y, illuminated by the sun; and the back of it, where the white body RST is located, toward the inside of the chamber P (where you will be), into which no light is allowed to enter except that which will be able to

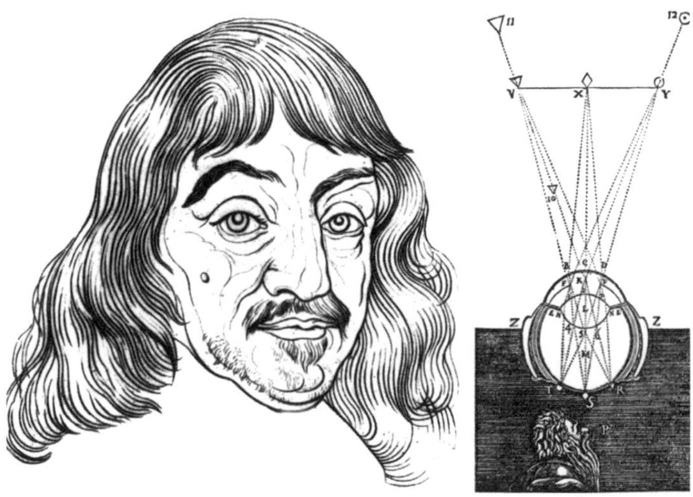

Figure 1.4
Left, René Descartes (1596–1650) after a portrait in Lavater (1799). Right, his figure of the cosmic observer viewing the inverted and reversed retinal image formed at the exposed back of an ox's eye placed in the aperture of a *camera obscura* (from Descartes, 1637/1902).

penetrate through the eye, all of whose parts, from C to S, you know to be transparent. For when this has been done, if you look at the white body *RST*, you will see there, not perhaps without admiration and pleasure, a picture which will represent in natural perspective all the objects which will be outside of it toward *VXY*. . . . Neither can we doubt that the images which we cause to appear on a white cloth in a dark chamber are formed there in the same way and for the same reasons as on the back of the eye. (Descartes, 1965. pp. 91–93 and 97, original italics)

Descartes refined Scheiner's model of the artificial eye by replacing the delicate retina with an eggshell. Thereafter artificial eyes became a standard feature of analyses of vision in texts on vision. With a better understanding of image formation in the eye and ocular anatomy, attention could be directed to the functions served by the structures of the eye—both internal and external. The initial problem addressed was an optical one: most visual scientists in the next three centuries examined the problem of accommodation—how the eye is able to focus on objects at different distances. The competing theories of accommodation tended to divert concern away from other aspects of vision, like how the eyes moved. Unlike Kepler and Scheiner, Descartes did have regard to the operation and representation of the extraocular muscles (see Chapter 2). In his *Treatise of man* Descartes (1662, 1664/1909) provided a speculative mechanistic account of how the paired muscles work by means of reciprocal action. Thereafter, interest in the structure of the extraocular muscles and of their mode of action took a more central role in analyses of vision.

One of the critical factors in the emergence of interest in how the eyes moved and what the consequences of such movements were for vision was the phenomenon of vertigo. Vertigo involves apparent rotation of the visual surroundings and of the body; it can be induced in many ways and it is often a symptom of disease. Nonetheless, vertigo can be induced with ease in the healthy—simply by rotating the body and stopping suddenly. Not only does the stationary body feel as though it is still moving, but the visual world appears to rotate as well. In the late eighteenth century, the question arose as to whether visual vertigo was a consequence of eye movements. The manner in which this was resolved was to capitalize on a long-known phenomenon—the afterimage. William Charles Wells (1757–1817) employed afterimages as stabilized retinal images, and was able to compare post-rotational movements of afterimages with those of real images. The importance of vertigo in uncovering the characteristics of eye movements will be described in Chapter 3. The afterimage became a valuable tool in the analysis of eye movements prior to the development of the modern devices to be described in Section 1.3. In the nineteenth century, Christian Ruete (1810–1867) used afterimages with great skill in order to determine torsion of the eye with oblique gaze. On the basis of his studies Ruete (1845, 1857) developed an instrument he called the ophthalmotrope (Fig. 1.5) to model the movements of both eyes. Hermann Helmholtz (1821–1894) wrote extensively about eye movements (see Chapter 4) and he provided a description of its operation:

> The two artificial eyeballs can turn around their centres on a ball pivot. On them are shown the equator, the cornea, and the vertical and horizontal meridians. Strong silk cords of various colours are fastened at those places where the muscles are attached. In order for the cords to maintain the directions of the muscles, four of them corresponding to the four recti are passed through four adjacent holes in the board *A* and made to hang vertically behind it by means of weights tied to them. Two of the cords, however, corresponding to the pair of oblique muscles in each eye, are passed around the little pulleys at the upper and lower ends of the vertical brass piece B, and then carried to the middle of the board *A*, where they also go through holes and are stretched by weights. The muscles in the two eyes with the same name are represented by cords of the same colour. To produce any desired rotation of one eye or of both of them, the cords are pulled, corresponding to the muscles which are stretched in a given movement of the eye, and which would therefore tend to resist the motion. On the other hand, those cords whose corresponding muscles in the eye tend to become shorter in

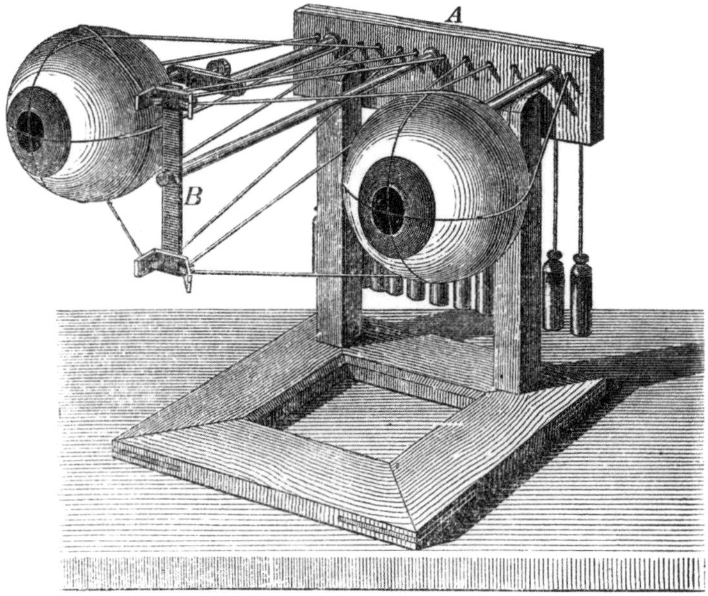

Figure 1.5
Ruete's (1857) ophthalmotrope as illustrated in Helmholtz (1867*a*).

the execution of the movement, will be relaxed, and so their weights will descend; and hence they are in the position to produce or reinforce motion. (Helmholtz, 1925/2000, pp. 118–119)

Ruete's ophthalmotrope, as well as the more complex one produced by Wilhelm Wundt (1832–1920) in 1862, displayed the understanding that had been achieved about the manner in which eye position was determined and also of the combined operation of the paired eye muscles. They were of considerable use in examining the pathology of eye movements and they emphasized the united activities of the two eyes. In addition, the ophthalmotropes indicated the importance that was placed on eye position following eye movements rather than the characteristics of the eye movements themselves. This concentration on eye position was, in part, due to the absence of methods of measuring eye movements. However, we hope to show that many insights regarding eye movements were derived before the more sophisticated recording devices to be described were available.

1.2 Scanning the way the eyes move

How do the eyes move and what influences the movements? There are many types of eye movements and one of the historical distinctions has been between those that occur within the eye itself and those that move the whole eyeball. The distinction was elegantly described by William Porterfield (ca. 1696–1771) in the first of two long essays on eye movements:

> The Motions of the Eye are either external or internal. I call *external*, those Motions performed by its four straight and two oblique Muscles, whereby the whole Globe of the Eye changes its Situation or Direction. And by its *internal* Motions, I understand those Motions which only happen to some of its internal Parts, such as the *Crystalline* and *Iris*, or to the whole Eye, when it changes its spherical Figure, and becomes oblong or flat. (Porterfield, 1737, p. 160, original italics)

The four straight muscles to which Porterfield was referring are the medial, lateral, superior and inferior recti and the oblique muscles are the superior and inferior. The six extraocular muscles are illustrated in Fig. 1.6. The muscles turn the eyeball around a centre of rotation indicated by the intersection of the superimposed axes of rotation in the figure. The axes of rotation can be considered as reflecting vertical (for the superior and inferior recti) and horizontal (medial and lateral recti) eye movements and those around the optic axes or torsional movements (superior and inferior obliques).

Landolt (1879, 1891) conducted detailed experimental studies of eye movements and their disorders, and described their functions succinctly: 'It is the office of the muscles of the eye to *direct the two eyes to the point of fixation in such a manner that the image of the object fixed shall fall simultaneously on the macula lutea of each eye*; or, in other

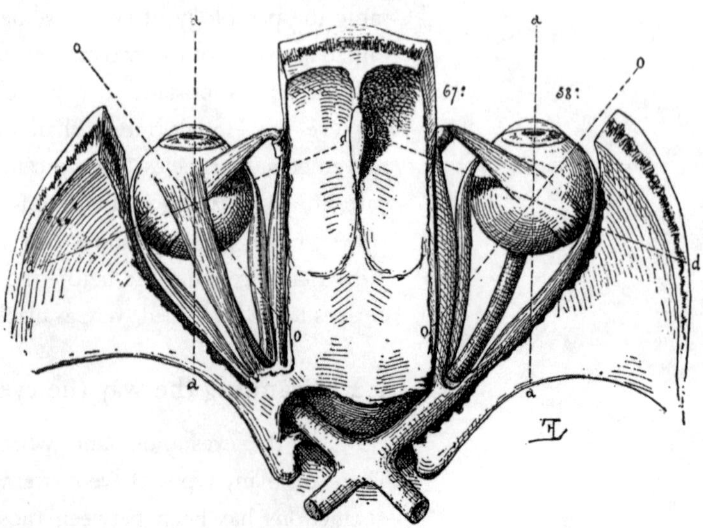

Figure 1.6
The extraocular muscles and the axes of rotation of the eyes, as illustrated by Landolt (1879).

words, to *secure single vision with the two eyes*' (1879, p. 40, original italics). That is, they serve binocular single vision and they enable extraction of spatial detail. Cones are not distributed evenly throughout the retina; rather their concentration is maximal in the *fovea* at the centre of the macula lutea or yellow spot, and they decrease rapidly with eccentricity into the periphery (Fig. 1.7). This distribution gives rise to distinct vision whereby only the centre of the visual field is resolved clearly and visual acuity decreases towards the periphery. Restriction of high acuity vision to the centre of the visual field necessitates movement of the eyes in order to bring this window of clear vision to bear on objects of interest. However, the cones do not react to light instantaneously, requiring in the region of 20 ms to respond; consequently, vision becomes blurred when the eyes move. This blurring can be quite severe even when the eye is moving at very slow velocities (see Carpenter, 1988). These restrictions—of distinct vision and cone physiology—have given rise to an exquisite range of types of eye movement, which operate to satisfy both the need for stability of the retinal image (to allow the cones time to respond) and the need to move the foveas of both eyes to regions or objects of interest.

When we fixate an object in the world, maintaining the image of that object on the visual axis is problematic due to two factors: movements in the environment and our own movements within

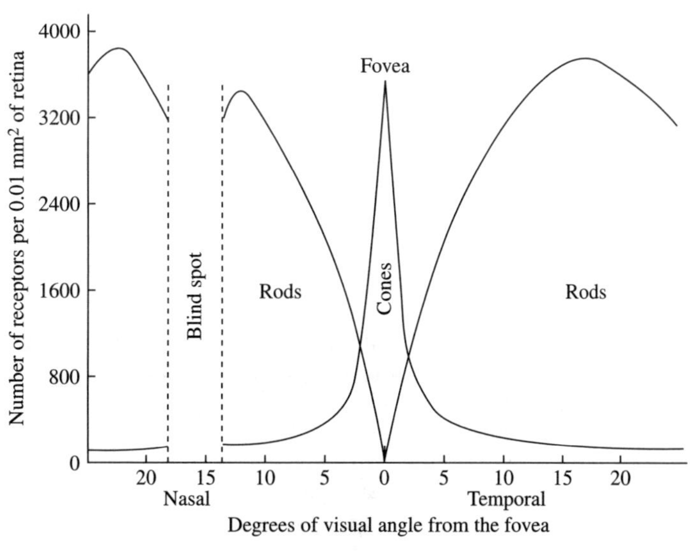

Figure 1.7

A schematic representation of the distribution of rods and cones over a horizontal region of the retina passing through the fovea and blind spot (after Wade and Swanston, 2001).

the environment. A characteristic pattern of eye movement known as opto-kinetic nystagmus (OKN) occurs when the whole visual scene moves. This happens when looking out of a window in a moving vehicle, and OKN was once known as railway nystagmus for this reason. OKN has two components, called the fast and slow phases. In the slow phase there is smooth pursuit of the moving field, which keeps the image on the same region of the retina. If the velocity of field movement increases above around $30^\circ\ s^{-1}$, the eyes lag progressively behind, and the maintenance of steady fixation on the object is less effective. The slow pursuit phase alternates with fast, saccadic eye movements that return the eyes to the straight-ahead position. OKN seems to be a primitive form of eye movement control, designed to prevent displacements of the retinal image during head movements.

Not only do the eyes but also the head and body move. Many eye rotations occur as a consequence of head movements, and their function is to maintain fixation on environmental stimuli despite the change in head position. Such compensatory eye movements result from stimulation of receptors in the vestibular system (see Howard, 1986), and they take place both quickly and with precision; they are referred to as vestibulo-ocular reflexes (VOR). Amongst these are the 'doll's eye reflexes'—when the head rotates upward and backward about a horizontal axis the eyes retain the same direction with respect to the environment. That is, they rotate in the opposite direction to the head, as occurs with many dolls that have movable eyes. There are similar compensatory eye rotations for the other rotations of the head in space.

Most rotations of the head are brief accelerations followed by decelerations. When the head rotates at a constant velocity for some seconds then the normal vestibular control mechanisms are disrupted. This can readily be experienced by rotating the body about a vertical axis for several revolutions and then stopping. The visual vertigo that follows is disturbing and is associated with feelings of nausea. Indeed, it was referred to as giddiness in previous centuries. Following rotation, the eyes undergo a particular pattern of movements: they rotate slowly in the direction opposite to previous body rotation and then rapidly return, repeating this cycle with decreasing amplitude. These are the slow and quick phases of nystagmus. The experimental origins of eye movement measurement are based on studies of postrotational nystagmus conducted in the eighteenth and nineteenth centuries, as will be detailed in Chapters 2 and 3.

The OKN and VOR operate to maintain a relatively stable image on the retina during fixation, but as we have already stated, the visual system must be able to move the eyes around the scene so that the objects of interest can be projected onto the fovea. In addition, a novel peripheral target or a moving one can elicit a fixation reflex, so that the target falls on the foveas. Such movements are accomplished by very rapid rotations of the eyes, known as saccades. During saccades, rotational velocities of up to $600° s^{-1}$ can be reached. Saccades are a family of ballistic eye movements with durations and peak velocities varying according to the amplitude of the rotation. For any particular amplitude of rotation, saccades show stereotyped position profiles, durations, and velocity profiles. The high velocities reached during saccades ensure that their duration is kept very short, ranging from approximately 30 ms for a 5° movement to 100 ms for a 40° saccade. In this way the period of visual disruption resultant from saccadic eye movements is minimized. During saccades the observer is effectively blind owing to limitations of photoreceptor response time course and to active suppression of the visual pathways during these eye movements. Thus, when we scan a visual scene, we do so primarily using this system of saccadic eye movements, punctuated by periods of fixation that typically last for around 300 ms. The origins of our current understanding of this strategy and its perceptual consequences will be discussed in Chapters 4 and 6.

While OKN and VOR work to maintain a relatively stable retinal image during fixation, stability is not absolute; small movements of the eyes do occur during fixation. They undergo high frequency, low amplitude tremors onto which are superimposed slow drifts and rapid flicks or microsaccades. Verheijen (1961) described how these can be observed by the simple expedient of generating an afterimage and then trying to maintain fixation. By fixating on the central white dot in Fig. 1.8 for long enough to generate an afterimage and then attempting to fixate on the black dot the minor involuntary movements of the eyes will be expressed in shifts of the negative (reversed contrast) afterimage. Such involuntary movements of the eyes are essential for maintaining the visibility of the targets that are fixated (see Chapter 6). When these minor

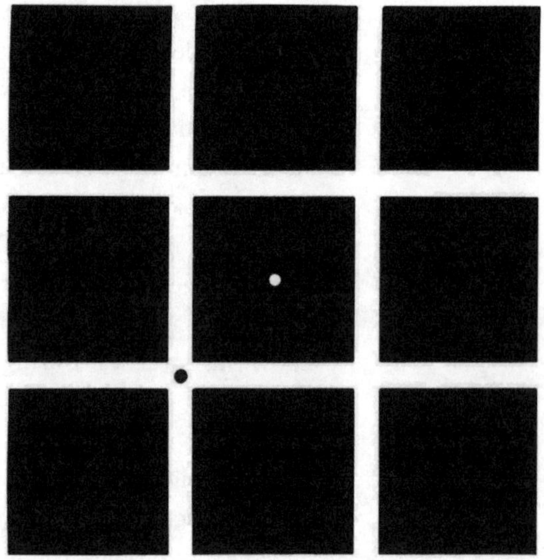

Figure 1.8
Fixate the central white dot for about 30 s, under good illumination, then look at the black one, you will be able to see the effects of small involuntary eye movements, in the form of rapid displacements of the afterimage squares (from Wade, 1982).

movements of light from a target over the retina are compensated for then vision ceases after a few seconds.

Motion over the retina can be a consequence of objects moving with respect to the eye or eye movements with respect to stationary objects. Under certain circumstances stationary objects appear to move. These are examples of visual motion illusions and they are very compelling. They were amongst the oldest illusions recorded and students of vision have puzzled over the reasons for their occurrence. One of the first interpretations of the illusions involved eye movements. If a stationary object appears to move, could this be a consequence of the eye moving so that the image moves over the retina? Such interpretations are examined in Chapter 5 for a variety of visual motion illusions and they typically appeal to pursuit rather than to saccadic eye movements.

As primates, we possess one further class of eye movements absent from many other animals; we can pursue a moving target so that light from that target remains on the fovea. If the eye rotates at the same velocity and in the same direction as a moving target then that target will be projected stably to the fovea and so remain clearly visible. While a pursuit eye movement is taking place, the image of the rest of the visual scene is displaced over the retina in the opposite direction to the eye movement. Pursuit eye movements vary in velocity according to that of the target, although there is an upper limit to target velocity of around $30^\circ\ s^{-1}$ if the eyes are to keep up with it.

Although the discussion so far has mentioned 'eyes' little has been said about their mutual movements. In smooth pursuit of an object at a constant distance from an observer, the two eyes move in the same direction and with the same velocity; these are version movements of the eyes. If the object approaches directly towards the observer then the eyes rotate in opposite directions—they converge, and retain convergence when the object stops. The object is then bifixated—fixated by both eyes. Vergence and version movements of the eyes occur to keep light from a target falling on the foveas of both eyes.

The patterns of eye movements described so far relate to those occurring in normal healthy observers. There are, however, systematic departures from these patterns, and the study of abnormal eye movements has been a cornerstone of medicine for centuries. The most common abnormality is in the lack of coordination between the two eyes so that bifixation is not possible. This occurs in strabismus or squint in which one eye deviates from the direction of the other. Strabismus can have early or late onset, and the visual consequences are greatly dependent upon this. For late onset there is initially double vision, but typically one eye is used in preference to the other to achieve singleness of vision. The misalignment of the eyes is very evident to anyone looking at a person so affected, and is probably one of the reasons why medical corrections for the condition have long been sought (see Chapter 2). Masks for correcting squint have been in use for many centuries. Studies of abnormal movements of the eyes have a similarly long history. The great classifier of medicine, François Boissier de Sauvages (1706–1767), called one condition 'nystagmus', and it involved the uncontrolled back and forth movements of the eyes. These conditions, and many more, are part of the ophthalmologist's repertoire (see Leigh and Zee, 1999; Noorden, 1996).

Eye movements are used extensively in a wide spectrum of research fields including psychology, biology, neuroscience, and medicine. A brief survey of the variety of applications of eye movements to the researcher now follows. Measures of the kinematics of eye movements reveal the characteristics of the various classes of eye movements; for example, the velocity and duration of saccades, both of which follow lawful relationships with the size of the eye movement (e.g. Carpenter, 1988; Westheimer, 1973). Similar approaches have allowed researchers to gain knowledge of the neural and muscular mechanisms involved in the generation of saccades and other types of eye movements (e.g. see Leigh and Zee, 1999). Inferences can be derived concerning the mechanisms and processes involved in programming eye movements, such as high- and low-level factors involved in selecting targets for fixation (e.g. Findlay and Walker, 1999; Itti and Koch, 2000; Karn and Hayhoe, 2000; Krieger et al., 2000; Rao et al., 1996; Reinagel and Zador, 1999), and competition between programmes for targets and distractors (e.g. Findlay, 1981; Theeuwes and Burger, 1998). Investigations of vision during eye movements have revealed the mechanisms responsible for the suppression of vision during saccades. Visual suppression during saccades raises questions about how our smooth and continuous perception arises from the disjointed input to the perceptual system that is a necessary consequence of our saccade-and-fixate behaviour. Explanations of visual stability across eye movements have become particularly prominent in recent years (Grimes, 1996; O'Regan and Noë, 2001; Rensink, 2002). Eye movements, their function and their implications have featured heavily throughout the history of research of the processes involved in reading (Erdmann and Dodge, 1898; Lamare, 1892; Rayner, 1998), scene viewing and perception (Buswell, 1935; Mackworth and Morandi, 1967; Rayner and Pollatsek, 1992; Yarbus, 1967) and certain aspects of visual memory (Hollingworth and Henderson, 2002; Irwin, 1992; Irwin and Zelinsky, 2002). Eye movements can allow insights into the neuropathology underlying disorders (Diefendorf and Dodge, 1908; Guitton et al., 1985). Common to all areas of research in which eye movements are studied, crucial insights into their normal functions and implications can be gained from eye movement dysfunction (see Carpenter, 1991; Duke-Elder and Wybar, 1973; Noorden, 1996). This chapter will now survey some of the wide variety of techniques that have been developed to measure eye movements for the above research fields and the historical origins of the devices that are used today.

1.3 Modern eye movement measuring techniques

The utility of eye movements in a wide range of disciplines is reflected in the range of devices and techniques that have been developed to measure them. Some of the most crucial advances in our understanding of eye movements came from the simplest and oldest of eye movement monitoring techniques: direct observation of a person's eyes. Although this is undoubtedly the oldest method it has not proved a particularly fruitful one for two reasons. First, the eyes move very rapidly so that the initial and final locations are the principal ones noted. Second, temporal resolution in vision is not very fine and so even with concentrated observation it is difficult to determine how the eyes have moved. An even simpler system is to feel the movements of the eyeball in the orbit itself. As we will see, this has often led to false conclusions regarding whether or how the eyes have moved. Movements of the eyes can be registered with a little more accuracy by placing the tip of the finger on the eyelid so that the rotations of the eyeball can be felt. Disatisfaction with these techniques has led to the search for more reliable ones. For example, Erdmann and Dodge (1898) used mirrors to observe people's eye movements during reading and also used this technique to examine vision during eye movements. The disadvantage of observation techniques is that only large eye movements can be identified. Various optical devices have been developed to reduce this limitation, such as magnifying lenses (Newhall, 1928) and telescopes (Ogle et al., 1949; Peckham, 1934).

One area that has benefited considerably from simply observing eye movements is the study of infant visual preferences. William James (1842–1910) remarked, from his armchair, that 'The baby, assailed by eyes, ears, nose, skin, and entrails at once feels it all as one great blooming, buzzing confusion' (1890, p. 488). The conclusion concerning infantile confusion was based on the observation of their seemingly random and chaotic movements. More detailed scrutiny indicated that some aspects of behaviour were systematic and could be used to determine what interests infants. For example, it was noted that infants spent different amounts of time fixating on visual patterns and so infant perceptual discrimination was inferred from the patterns of preferential fixation. Fantz (1961) presented babies with paired patterns and recorded how long they looked at each one by observing the infants' eyes through a peephole. Salapatek and Kessen (1966) recorded eye movements in infants only a few days old and showed that they were concentrated on contours or corners of simple patterns. Combinations of preferential looking and eye movement recording have been applied to determine the contrast sensitivities of infants (Hainline, 1998).

While direct observation techniques have been useful in research such as the infant work described above, these and many other studies (see Atkinson, 2000) have tended to use eye movements as tools for determining features of visual discrimination, rather than examining the eye movements themselves. As tools for examining the eye movements, direct observation techniques are limited and are prone to subjectivity on the part of the observer. In contemporary research direct observation is more usually used as a method for checking that eye movements do not occur during experiments where it is necessary to control fixation, rather than to study the characteristics of eye movements. The limitations of direct observation of a subject's eye movements have necessitated the development of objective techniques for measuring how the eyes move and where they move to. While many different eye tracking technologies exist they can be grouped according to the principle they employ to monitor eye position into afterimage techniques, attachment devices, optical devices, and electro-oculographic devices. For excellent reviews of eye tracking technologies, see Young and Sheena (1975*a*,*b*). As will be shown in the sections that follow, antecedents of many of the modern eye tracking technologies were being developed and used over a century ago. A good review of the range of eye tracking technologies being used early in the twentieth century can be found in Dodge (1916). However, as will be shown below, many more types of eye tracker were in use or had been attempted, than were reviewed in Dodge's article.

1.3.1 Afterimages

Afterimages can be seen following either brief, intense illumination of the eye or prolonged fixation on an illuminated stimulus. Thus, looking briefly at a bright light can result in its continued visibility when the eyes are closed, or directed away from the light to a uniform surface. Historically, they have been given several names, like ocular spectra and accidental colours, both of which refer to the coloured characteristics of the phenomenon. Characteristics of afterimages have been recorded for thousands of years, and they have thrown light on many aspects of vision.

Franz (1899) summarized this succinctly: 'In the history of afterimages we seem to have an epitome of the interrelations of physics, physiology, and psychology; and probably no other single phenomenon is so good an example of the growth of experiment and measurement in psychology' (p. 1). They have been applied to study involuntary eye movements (as is evident from Fig. 1.8), to determine eye position following eye movements, and to chart the course of nystagmus; they have also been enlisted to distinguish between the perceptual consequences of active and passive eye movements.

Despite this fruitful legacy, relatively little attention is paid to them in contemporary research. An exception is a study by Goltz et al. (2003); they used afterimages to evaluate current theories of motion perception. An afterimage was generated by asking participants to fixate a red dot on a white grid with a black background. The afterimage of the grid remained stable on the retina during subsequent eye movements, yet it was perceived to move when the observer tracked a moving target. The direction and magnitude of the perceived afterimage motion allowed the authors to reject standard explanations of motion perception (for reviews of standard motion perception theories see Carpenter, 1988; Ebenholtz, 2001; Shebilske, 1977).

1.3.2 Attachment devices

Amongst the most precise and accurate of modern eye trackers are those that use specially fitted contact lenses attached to the eye. The most commonly used contact lens eye tracker in recent years has been the scleral search coil (e.g. Collewijn et al., 1997; Findlay, 1997; McConkie and Loschky, 2002; Steinman and Collewijn, 1980; Fig. 1.9). Two perpendicular wire coils are embedded in the contact lens and the experimental participant is situated within two large perpendicular electromagnetic coils. The potential difference in each coil varies as the eye moves and is independent of head movements. By measuring changes in the potential difference, eye position can be measured to a very high degree of precision.

While the first search coil eye trackers were introduced by Robinson in 1963, they are descendants of a family of eye trackers based upon the notion that eye movements can be recorded by monitoring the movement of an object attached to the surface of

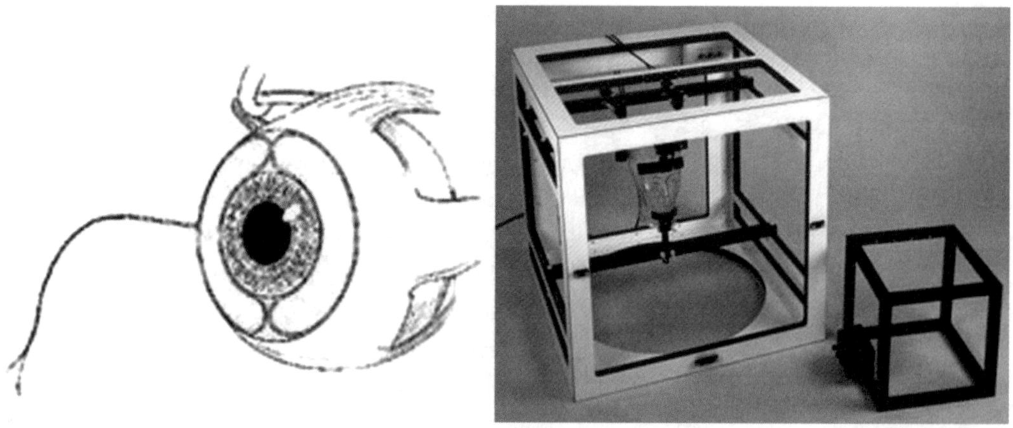

Figure 1.9

A scleral search coil eye tracker. Left, a diagram of the wires embedded within the silicone rubber contact lens worn on the eye. Right, cages containing magnetic coils to generate the magnetic fields needed to calculate eye position. The glass head indicates the position of the participant's head during experiments. Eye position is calculated by the relative movement of the two wires embedded in the contact lens within the magnetic fields generated in the cage. Images reproduced by kind permission of Skalar Medical BV.

the eye. The earliest incarnations of attachment eye trackers registered when eye movements occurred but did not monitor their magnitude. They were introduced towards the end of the nineteenth century, and used a variety of attachments to the eye (see Chapter 4). The majority of attachment eye trackers attempt to allow the researcher to measure the characteristics of eye movements by registering them on a recording surface. Early version of such eye trackers recorded eye movements mechanically, using a lever or similar device to translate the movement of the eye onto a recording surface. One of the problems associated with the early mechanical attachment eye trackers was the additional force that was applied to the eye which added to its inertia.

Variants of the attachment eye trackers were developed soon after these early mechanical devices, which avoided some of the limitations associated with the lever systems. One was the idea of using reflected light from an attachment on the eye's surface, rather than a lever system. Orschansky (1899) developed the first successful version of this eye tracker. He attached a small mirror to an aluminium eye-cup and recorded the reflection of a beam of light from the mirror in order to monitor eye position; similar eye trackers were used by Marx and Trendelenburg (1911) and Dohlman (1925), although the latter used a rubber eye-cup rather than an aluminium one.

Several variants of eye trackers that monitored light reflected from a mirror attached to the eye were developed during the twentieth century and were used for some of the key eye movement studies of this period. Ditchburn and Ginsborg (1952) used a reflection-based contact lens method for their landmark study of the visual consequences of viewing a stabilized retinal image. In their experiments, 'The subject wears a contact lens which is specially made to fit his eye tightly and on which a small optical flat has been worked. The flat is covered (by vacuum evaporation) with a highly reflecting opaque film of rhodium' (p. 36). The reflections from this 'mirror' were then used to move an image precisely in register with the small eye movements (drift and microsaccades) that occur within fixations (e.g. Adler and Fliegelman, 1934; Lord and Wright, 1948; for a review see Carpenter, 1988), such that the image on the retina could be stabilized. Using this technique, Ditchburn and Ginsborg were able to show that when an image is perfectly stabilized on the retina, it disappears, presumably due to adaptation.

Yarbus' (1967) studies of eye movements during picture viewing are now considered key developments in our understanding of the active nature of eye movements and how high level factors such as an active task, can influence where we look. These studies used records of light reflected from a mirror affixed to a rubber suction cap attached to the eye. Yarbus developed a number of variants of these caps, which either attached at or near to the cornea. Fig. 1.10 shows two of the rubber caps developed and used by Yarbus, together with the apparatus used for recording the light reflected from the caps.

The vast majority of attachment eye trackers used contact lenses, however some eye tracking techniques have involved the attachment of mirrors or reflecting media directly upon the surface of the eye. Judd et al. (1905) placed a small spot of Chinese white on the cornea and took a series of photographs of the eye and part of the head, at about 9 frames per second. Adler and Fliegelman (1934) affixed a mirror directly onto the sclera. Barlow (1952) placed a small drop of mercury on the cornea and another drop on the forehead. The movements of these two drops of mercury were recorded onto photographic film and used to derive both head and eye movements.

While eye tracking devices that measure reflected light from an attachment on the eye dominated much of the twentieth century,

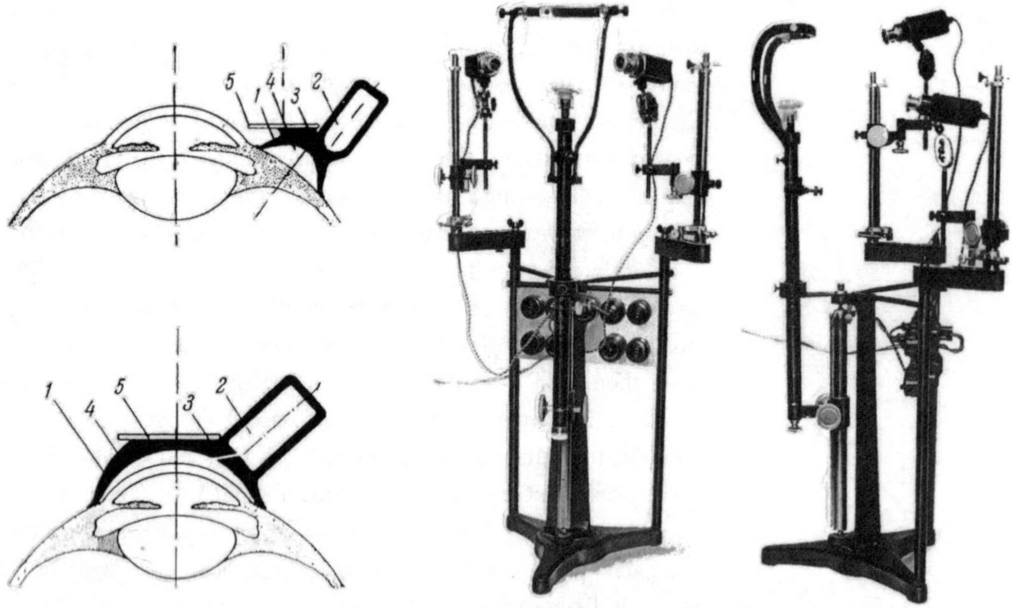

Figure 1.10
Left, two of the rubber eye cups designed and used by Yarbus to record eye movements. Several variants of eye cup were used by Yarbus, each with advantages in particular experimental settings. Eye movements were measured by recording light reflected from mirrors attached to the rubber eye cups. Right, the apparatus used to illuminate the eye and record the light reflected from the mirrors (All images after Yarbus, 1967).

the most common contact lens in recent years has become the scleral coil described at the head of this section.

1.3.3 Optical devices

An alternative to devices that measure light reflected from a mirror attached to the eye is to measure light reflected directly from the surface of the eye. A number of variants of optical eye trackers exist in which the wavelength of light, the light source and the medium for recording the reflection varies. These optical eye trackers are by far the most common form of eye tracker available today. Dodge and Cline (1901) were the first to attempt to photograph the eye itself, recording images of the eye onto a falling photographic plate. However, they found that the eye needed to be illuminated with an intense light source and that the margin between the iris and the pupil was hard to define in the photographic records. While attempting to develop this photographic technique Dodge and Cline found that:

Satisfactory results were first obtained when, after considerable experimentation, we hit upon the plan of utilizing the eccentric surface of the cornea as a reflector. Instead of photographing the eye directly, we photographed the movement of a bright vertical line as it was reflected from the surface of the cornea. Such lines give clean-cut records permitting considerable magnification in reading, while the amount of light needed is comparatively small. (1901, pp. 148–149)

Following this discovery, Dodge and Cline developed the 'Dodge Photochronograph', depicted in Fig. 1.11. This device was extremely effective for recording the characteristic of eye movements and was used extensively by Dodge and his colleagues, providing key insights into the details of eye movements (e.g. Diefendorf and Dodge, 1908; Dodge, 1903, 1904; Dodge and Cline, 1901). The Dodge Photochronograph represents a key turning point in the development of eye tracking technologies and it inspired a proliferation of eye tracking devices. Corneal reflection devices have become widely used since their inception by Dodge and Cline. Buswell (1935) used a corneal reflection eye tracker to study eye movements of observers as they viewed pictures and geometric patterns. Buswell's device is shown in

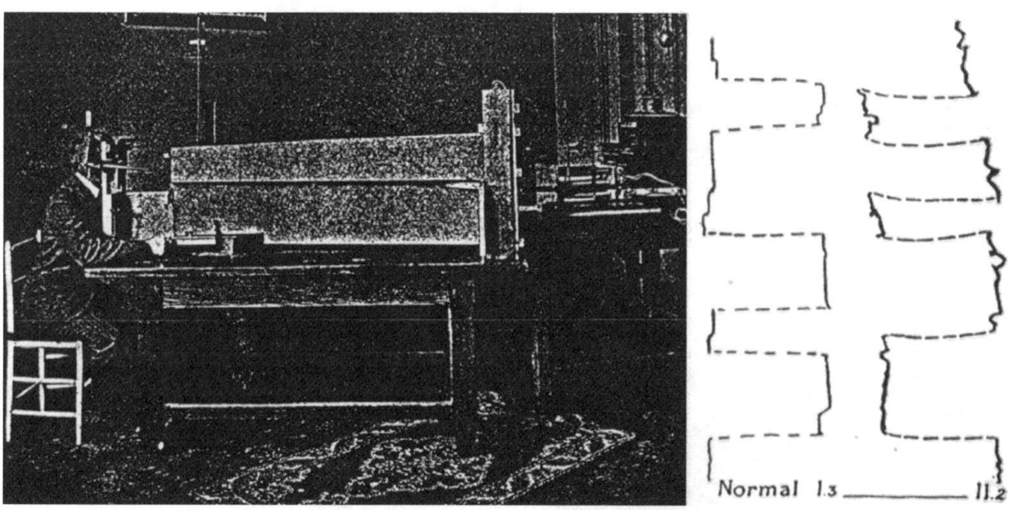

Figure 1.11

Left, the Dodge Photochronograph, which recorded light reflected from the cornea onto a falling photographic plate (figure 1 from Diefendorf and Dodge 1908). Right, an example eye movement record reproduced from one of the photographic plates (part of plate I from Diefendorf and Dodge 1908). Time proceeds from bottom to top in the trace and saccades can be seen as horizontal displacements. In order to reproduce the eye movement trace 'The records were projected by lantern and drawn from the projected image on a much enlarged scale. The resulting lines reproduce the original records very well, save that the dashes are relatively fainter grey in the records. The exact shape of each dash is not accurately reproduced . . . the photographic plate was moving so slowly that the dots run together in the vertical lines, appearing as dashes only during eye-movement. The dashes represent flashes of light succeeding each other every 0.01 second.' (Diefendorf and Dodge, 1908, p. 462).

Fig. 1.12. The camera recording the light reflected from the surface of the cornea was positioned at right angles to the subject so that they had a clear field of view for observing text or images placed in front of them. Head movements were also recorded using this device; this was to correct the eye position record for any slight movements of the subject's head during viewing. Head movements were measured by recording the reflection of light from a chromium bead placed on a pair of glasses worn by the observer. In his experiments using this eye tracking device, Buswell found that eye movements cluster around regions of interest in pictures and that there was greater consistency between observers early in viewing than after several minutes of viewing the same picture. Contemporary eye trackers still use the method of tracking the light reflected from the cornea; for example, the Applied Science Laboratories, ISCAN, and SR Research eye trackers use a combination of corneal reflection and pupil tracking (see below) and are now commonly used (e.g. Canosa et al., 2003; Pelz and Canosa, 2001; Smeets et al., 1996).

The outside surface of the cornea is not the only surface from which light is reflected in the eye. Light projected onto the eye reflects from the external surface of the cornea, the internal

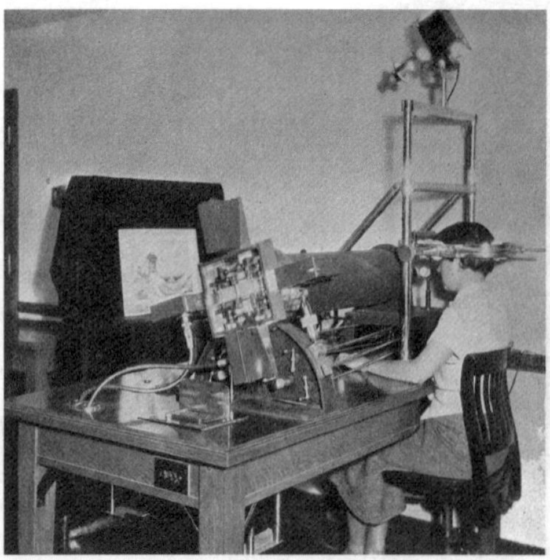

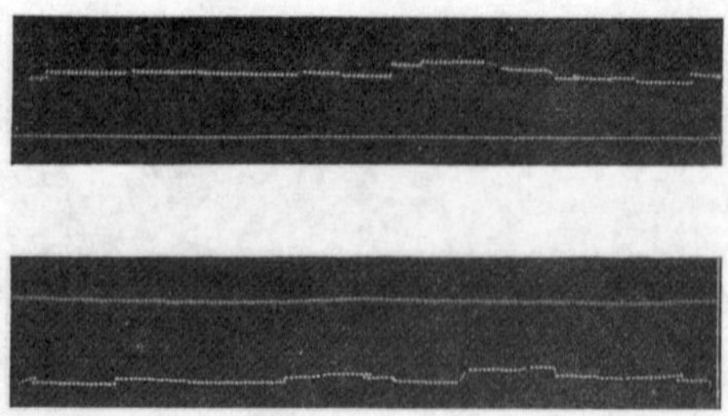

Figure 1.12

Left, a subject seated at Buswell's eye tracker. Eye movements were recorded by measuring the light reflected from the surface of the eye. The light illuminating the eye was projected from underneath the table, and the reflection was recorded, via a series of lenses and mirrors by the recording equipment positioned to the side of the subject; this arrangement left the subject's forward field of view free to observe experimental stimuli ahead of them. Right, example records from the Buswell eye tracker. The upper record shows horizontal movements of the eye and head; the lower record shows vertical movements of the eye and head. Each dot represents one thirtieth of a second. (After Buswell, 1935.)

surface of the cornea, the external surface of the lens, and the internal surface of the lens. These reflections are known as Purkinje images. Purkinje images can be used to track eye position with greater accuracy than eye trackers that monitor only the reflection of from the external surface of the cornea. Cornsweet and Crane (1973) developed an eye tracker that used the relative motion of the first (external surface of the cornea) and fourth (internal surface of the lens) Purkinje images in order to provide very accurate eye movement measures. This modern variant of the simple corneal reflection technique is widely used in contemporary research (e.g. Ballard et al., 1995; Currie et al., 2000; Hayhoe et al., 1998; Pollatsek and Rayner, 2002; Zelinsky et al., 1997; Fig. 1.13). A more thorough treatment of modern corneal reflection eye trackers can be found in Duchowski (2003).

While the use of reflections from the surfaces of the cornea or lens has been widespread, alternative optical eye tracking techniques have been developed. Higgins and Stultz (1953) magnified and recorded an image of a blood vessel in the sclera perpendicular to the recording apparatus, illuminated with ultraviolet light. The blood vessel functioned equivalently to an attachment such as a mirror on the surface of the eye: a fixed marker whose movement can be tracked to infer the movement of the eyeball. Dirschel and Lange (1956) developed an eye tracker

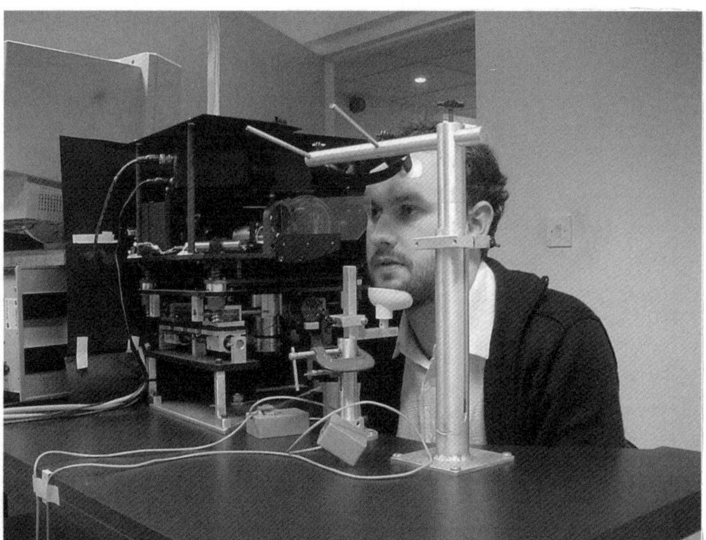

Figure 1.13
A dual Purkinje image eye tracker.

that measured the movements of the limbus (the border between the iris and the sclera). A narrow band of light was projected into the eye such that half fell onto the sclera and half onto the iris. Eye movements were registered by recording the amount of light reflected back from the eye; the sclera reflects more light than the iris, so movements of the eye change the amount of light reflected. Rather than record the movements onto photographic media, movements were recorded as the current from the photoelectric cell used to record the reflection from the eye. Photoelectric rather than photographic recording media were first used by Dohlman (1935) but this technique has become increasingly common since the middle of the twentieth century. Indeed the earliest versions of the limbus trackers described above used photoelectric arrays to record the movement of the limbus (Smith and Warter, 1960; Torok et al., 1951). Modern limbus eye trackers commonly use infrared rather than visible light to illuminate the eye and eye movements are registered photoelectrically. Modifications of the limbus technique have been to include a measurement of the border between the pupil and the iris (e.g. Wheeless et al., 1966) or to use reflections from the pupil. Pupil and limbus reflection eye trackers are used extensively in modern research (e.g. Carpenter, 2001; Gilchrist and Harvey, 2000; Hodgson et al., 2000; Johansson et al., 2001; Parkhurst and Niebur, 2003; Tatler, Gilchrist et al., 2005; Walker et al., 2000).

Curthoys, Moore, and colleagues have developed a variant of optical eye tracker in which eye position is calculated from a video record using image processing techniques (Moore et al., 1991, 1996). The development of this technique has been chronicled by MacDougall (2003): it tracks the position of striations in the iris and derives torsional eye position to an accuracy of 0.1°. Thus, this video-based system offers spatial accuracy comparable with techniques such as the scleral search coil, without the discomfort and disruption to participants that is associated with search coils. One limitation of the iral striations technique is that it requires that the iris is constricted using Pilocarpine eye drops. In order to avoid the need to constrict the pupil, and so increase the utility of the method, the group is currently developing a technique based upon tracking scleral markers. This approach has been used successfully in guinea pigs, using 3 mm diameter circles applied with a permanent marker (Kim, 2004; Fig. 1.14).

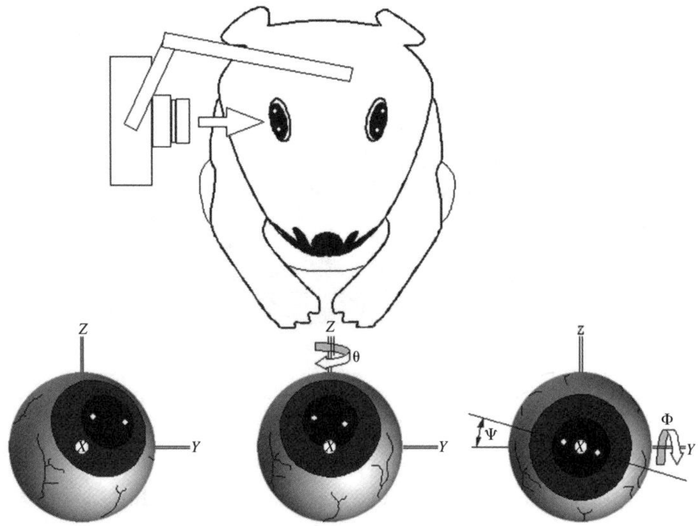

Figure 1.14

Top, diagram of the experimental setup for recording the eye movements of guinea pigs in Kim (2004). The camera is positioned to point at the centre of the eye at rest, essentially of the eye at the mid-orbital position. The two white dots on the eye indicate the position of the markers used to calculate eye position. Bottom, diagrams to show the three-dimensional positions of the two scleral markers and how their positions change as the eye moves. The change between the left and middle panels represents the change in markers associated with a rotation around the *z*-axis. The change between the middle and right panels indicates the change in the position of the markers associated with a rotation around the *y*-axis. The angle Ψ indicates the angle of torsion between the position of the eye (as indicated by the two markers) and the *y*-axis of the eye. These diagrams are all re-drawn from Kim (2004).

Using scleral markers to track eye movements in this way represents somewhat of a return to the earlier techniques discussed above, such as those of Higgins and Stultz (1953) who tracked scleral blood vessels, and even techniques where reflections from markers on the eye were recorded (e.g. Adler and Fliegelman, 1934; Barlow, 1952; Judd et al., 1905).

1.3.4 Remote devices

In many of the early optical eye trackers, the recording device and source of illumination were situated very close to the eye, mounted on a headrest and required that the participant's eye was kept close to the recording or illumination device. As a result it was necessary to restrain the head of participants throughout experiments. One modern variant of such optical eye trackers is commonly known as a remote eye tracker (Fig. 1.15). In these

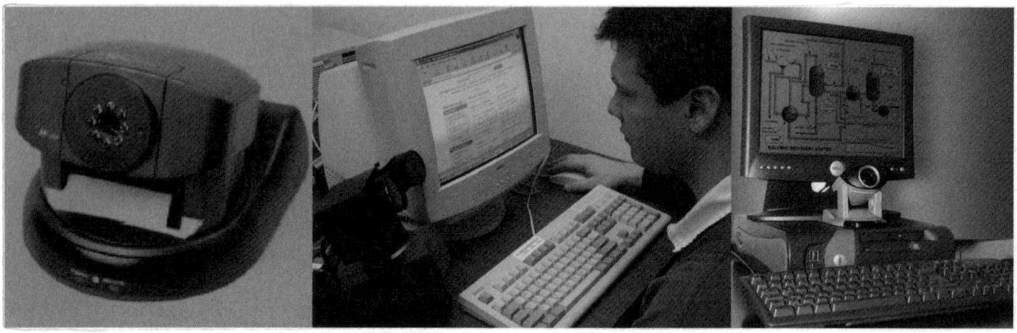

Figure 1.15
A selection of commercially available remote eye trackers. Images reproduced by kind permissions of Applied Science Laboratories (left), ISCAN (middle) and SensoMotoric Instruments (right).

eye trackers, the recording device is removed to a location further from the participant's eye and it is only required that the participant places their chin on a rest, rather than requiring full restraint of the head. The principles employed in tracking eye movements are the same as in other optical devices, using either corneal reflection, pupil tracking, or both. By reducing the necessity to fully restrain the head of a participant and by removing the optics to a location further from the participant, the range of applications and participant groups with which eye tracking experiments can be conducted with ease is much increased. Such remote systems have been used in a wide range of situations including infant studies (e.g. Johnson et al., 2003; McMurray et al., 2000), human–computer interaction (e.g. Adjouadi et al., 2004; Farid et al., 2002), driving (e.g. Wilkie and Wann, 2003), and to record eye movements within an fMRI scanner (e.g. Fink et al., 2001; Gitelman et al., 2000).

As computing technologies improve so do the possibilities for more sophisticated tracking of eye movements and techniques for compensating for head movements and varying levels of illumination. One such recent development of remote eye tracking technology has been developed by Seeing Machines (Fig. 1.16). With this eye tracker, no head restraint is necessary and software is able to determine gaze direction for a freely behaving participant as long as their eyes remain within the recording camera's field of view. While this does not allow for completely free and natural movement by the participant in all real world settings, it allows unconstrained eye tracking in

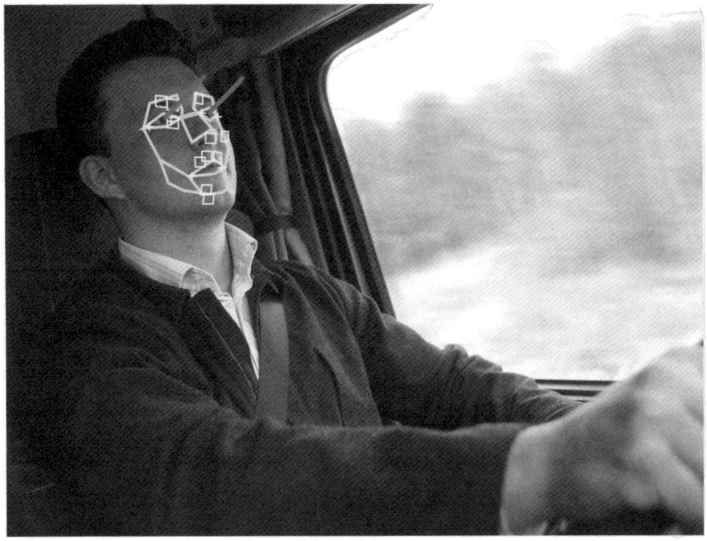

Figure 1.16
An image showing the direction of gaze calculated using faceLAB software for a participant when driving a car. Image reproduced by permission of Seeing Machines.

situations such as driving and aviation and might improve the ease of eye tracking experiments with participant groups such as children.

1.3.5 Electro-oculographic devices

Eye movements can be measured electrically because potential differences exist between the inner and outer surfaces of the retina and the cornea and sclera (Mowrer et al., 1936). These potential differences form the corneoretinal potential and can be used to monitor eye position. Skin electrodes placed near the eyes can detect the rotations of the electrostatic dipole and these can be used to infer eye position information. Schott (1922), Meyers (1929), and Jacobson (1930*a*,*b*) first used this type of eye tracker. Ford et al. (1959) refined electro-oculographic techniques so that horizontal and vertical eye movements could be recorded simultaneously. Variations of this technique have since been used frequently (e.g. Ilg and Hoffmann, 1993; Jeannerod et al., 1966; Rosander and von Hofsten, 2004; Toglia, 1973; Uenoyama et al., 1964).

One advantage of electro-oculographic recording is that it can register movements of the closed eyes. The technique has been applied widely in clinical studies of eye movements and during sleep, but it does not have the same accuracy and precision as other recording devices.

1.3.6 Portable eye tracking techniques

While the above categories describe the principles employed to measure eye movements, an important recent development in eye tracking technology has been to produce devices that are portable and thus can be worn under less constrained experimental conditions than most eye trackers. The first head mounted eye tracker was developed by Hartridge and Thompson (1948). This innovation heralded the birth of greater freedom during eye tracking experiments. Shackel (1960) and Mackworth and Thomas (1962) refined the design of head mounted eye trackers to allow greater freedom for the participant. Thomas (1968) used a head mounted eye tracker that comprised a single camera on a helmet that recorded both the scene in front of the wearer's head and (via a series of prisms and lenses) the corneal reflections from a light source positioned just below the eye (Fig. 1.17).

More recently Land (1993; Land and Lee, 1994) developed a portable eye tracker that used a head mounted camera to record simultaneously the scene and the eyeball onto a video (Fig. 1.18). Gaze direction could then be calculated and superimposed onto the picture of the scene for each frame. This eye tracker allowed experiments to be conducted under relatively unconstrained conditions and has provided some of the first explorations of eye movements in the real world, during activities such as tea

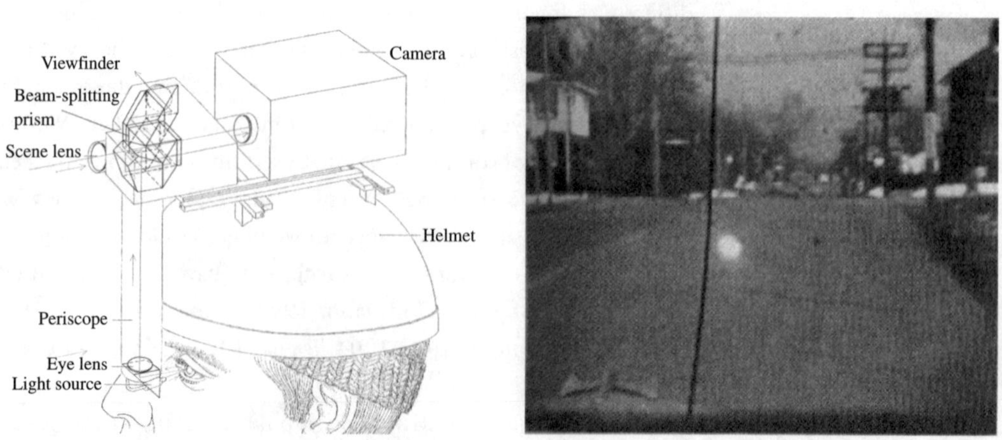

Figure 1.17

Left, a schematic of the portable, head-mounted eye tracker used by Thomas to monitor eye movements in real world settings. Right, a frame from a video sequence of a subject seated inside a moving car. The bright spot on the image indicates the position of the subject's fovea. In this example the subject is looking at the surface of the road (after Thomas, 1968).

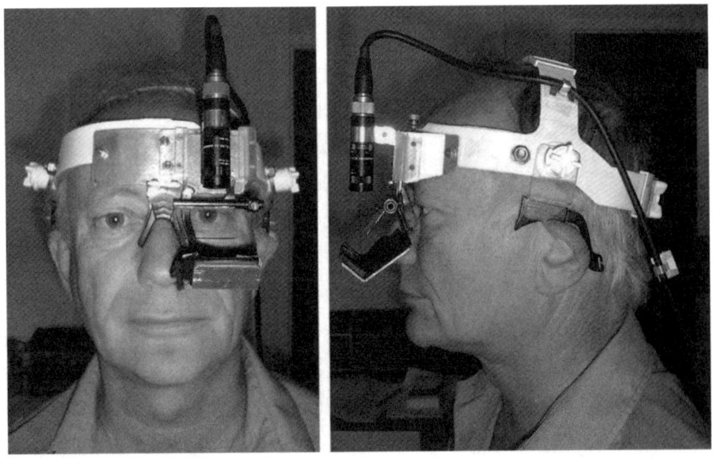

Figure 1.18
The portable eye tracker developed (and here worn) by Land to record eye movements as participants carry our real world tasks. Recording equipment is fully portable and worn in a backpack.

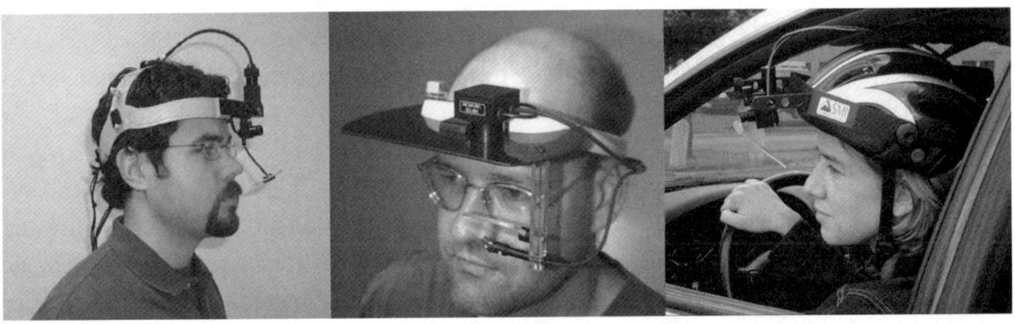

Figure 1.19
A selection of commercially available portable eye trackers. Images are reproduced by kind permissions of Applied Science Laboratories (left), ISCAN (middle) and SensoMotoric Instruments (right).

making (Land et al., 1999), driving (Land and Lee, 1994) and cricket (Land and McLeod, 2000).

Commercial versions of portable eye trackers are now available widely and are used extensively in modern research (e.g. Canosa et al., 2003; Pelz and Canosa, 2001; Schnell et al., 2004; Smeets et al., 1996; Fig. 1.19). These commercial portable eye trackers typically use pupil tracking (some additionally use corneal reflection tracking) to monitor eye movements.

Portable eye trackers allow eye movement research to extend outside the laboratory and for the researcher to investigate the role of eye movements in real world activities. This real world experimentation represents a crucial component of the advancement of our understanding of vision in everyday life.

1.4 The moving tablet of the eye

The principal reason for the development of all the devices described above is because eye movements lie at the heart of contemporary studies of vision. Accordingly, understanding their dynamics is essential for any adequate theory of reading and recognition, and abnormalities of eye movements provide clues to aspects of medical malfunction. If eye movements are so important, it might be assumed that their measurement has a long history. Such is not, however, the case. A good example relates to the discontinuities of eye movements—they engage in saccades interspersed with brief intervals of fixation. This dynamic sequence has only been known about for a little over two centuries. One of the reasons often given for the late descriptions of the kinematics of the eye is that its study is dependent upon suitable sophisticated instruments, which are of modern invention. This, also, is not the case. One of the most widely studied visual phenomena—afterimages—was enlisted to make the initial studies of eye movements in the late eighteenth century, as will be detailed in Chapters 2 and 3.

Our aim in this book is the draw attention to the experimental studies of eye movements that were conducted before systematic equipment was available, and to integrate this with contemporary research. This period has been neglected in the many excellent books that are concerned with eye movements. Our aim has informed not only the content of the book but also its title. The title is taken from a line in the second section of Canto 3 of *The temple of nature* by Erasmus Darwin (1731–1802), whose portrait is shown in Fig. 1.20. The verse (lines 55–64) in which it occurs is:

> FIRST the new actions of the excited sense,
> Urged by appulses from without, commence;
> With these exertions pain, or pleasure, springs,
> And forms perceptions of external things.
> Thus, when illuminated by the solar beams,
> Yon waving woods, green lawns, and sparkling streams,
> In one bright point by rays converging lie
> Plann'd on the moving tablet of the eye;
> The mind obeys the silver goads of light,
> And IRRITATION moves the nerves of sight.

The poem was published in 1803, the year after Darwin's death, and it contains within it much that is attributed to his

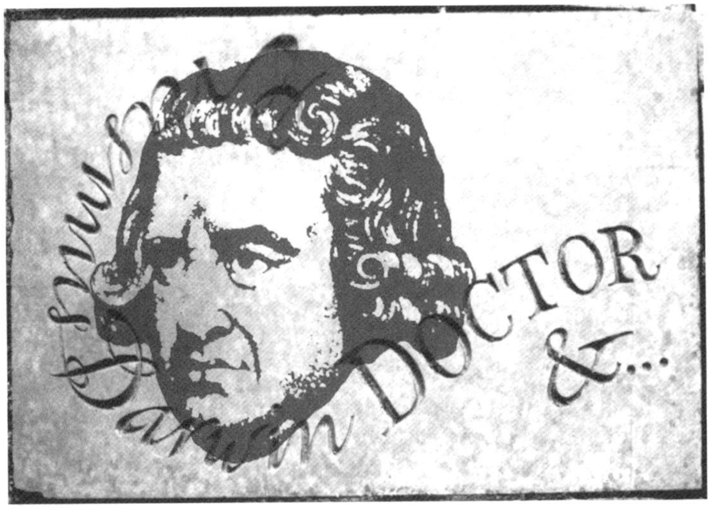

Figure 1.20
Portrait of Erasmus Darwin (1731–1802) superimposed on one of the paving stones in the garden at Erasmus Darwin House, Lichfield. Other paving stones mark his contributions as a scientist, inventor, evolutionist, humanitarian, and poet.

grandson, Charles Robert Darwin (1809–1882), concerning the principle, but not the mechanism, of evolution. It also demonstrates the importance in which eye movements have been held, even before their detailed properties were appreciated. In his notes to this verse Darwin elaborates on the meaning of the last line:

> Irritation is an exertion or change of some extreme part of the sensorium residing in the muscles or organs of sense in consequence of the appulses of external bodies. The word perception includes both the action of the organ of sense in consequence of the impact of external objects and our attention to that action. (Darwin, 1803, p. 87)

Erasmus Darwin's major work on physiology and psychology was *Zoonomia* the first volume of which was published in 1794. His interests in eye movements were more than poetic and, as is evident from the verse reproduced above, his poetry reflected his science. Perception was considered to be intimately involved with action, and in the context of vision the representatives of that action were muscular motions of the eyes. Darwin conducted experiments on eye movements, using afterimages as a means of determining their characteristics. Moreover, he devoted a chapter of his *Zoonomia* to describing phenomena that are related to eye movements.

Thus, it is our intention to draw attention to the early origins of studies of eye movements. The selection of our title from an eighteenth century poem is not arbitrary. Much of our contemporary knowledge is built upon the experimental enquiries that were conducted in the late eighteenth and early nineteenth centuries. This will provide the leitmotif that informs much of the historical discussion that follows.

2

Origins of eye movement research

2.1 Introduction

The origins of any area of scientific endeavour are often difficult to divine. This is certainly the case for the study of eye movements, which are an integral part of deriving information about our surroundings and upon which our actions are based (see Heller, 1988). As Du Laurens (1596) so eloquently indicated, eye movements can provide windows to the mind, but it is not this aspect of their actions that has excited researchers. After all, such a statement does not address the question of how the windows move. Eye movements have also been enlisted as a theoretical tool in support of empiricist philosophy. George Berkeley (1685–1753) proposed that muscular action, including eye movements, was essential in learning the third dimension of visual space.

The less arbitrary starting points that have been sought relate to measurements of the ways the eyes move and the positions they adopt after a movement. On this basis, the origins of eye movement research have been accorded to a number of researchers. Boring (1942) suggested that the monograph by Johannes Müller (1801–1858; Fig. 2.1, right) published in 1826 marked the onset of systematic studies. Carmichael (1926), on the other hand, argued that the article by Charles Bell (1774–1842; Fig. 2.1, left) in 1823 was a more appropriate starting point. Bell (1823) described the muscle sense (or proprioception as Sherrington later called it) and distinguished by experiment the consequences of active and passive eye movements on visual direction. Because of his work linking the senses and their muscular attachments to

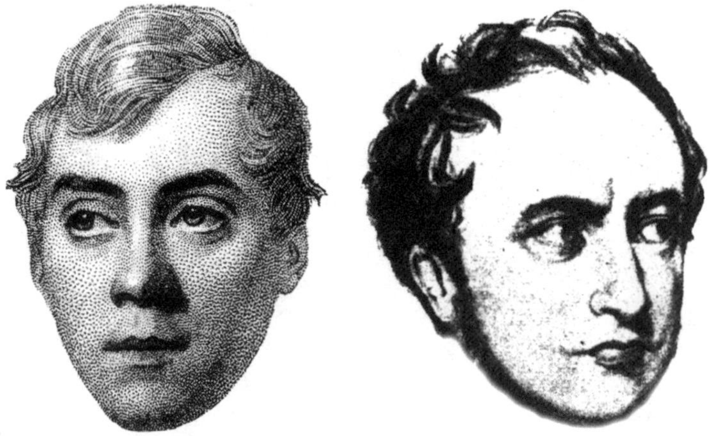

Figure 2.1

Left, Charles Bell (1774–1842) after a frontispiece engraving in Bell (1870). Right, Johannes Müller (1801–1858) after a portrait in Hirsch (1929).

brain function, Bell has been called the father of physiological psychology.

Müller published two books on vision in 1826: one (Müller, 1826*a*) was on comparative physiology in which he gave detailed descriptions of eye position following eye movements; the other (Müller, 1826*b*) was on subjective visual phenomena. In the latter, Müller elaborated on some of the phenomena that had been investigated by Jan Evangelista Purkinje or Purkyně (1787–1869). Eye movements were one of the many topics examined by Purkinje in his first book (Purkinje, 1823*a*; translated in Wade and Brožek, 2001) and he discussed them in the context of vertigo and strabismus in his second book (Purkinje, 1825). A decade later, Müller provided a more extensive survey of vision in his *Handbuch der menschlichen Physiologie*; this book was translated into English as *Elements of physiology* (Müller, 1840, 1843) and it has recently been reprinted (Müller, 2003). Müller's interests in eye movements were aroused by Purkinje's (1823*a*) deliberations on the ways the eyes moved over different patterns. Müller was concerned with relating binocular eye movements to binocular single vision, and to the breakdown of the latter in squinting or strabismus. These topics will be surveyed in Section 2.2.

While it is obvious that eye movements had been commented upon long before Müller and Bell provided more precise methods of determining some of their characteristics, many of these comments were based on careful observation. Moreover, the experimental examination of eye movements had been undertaken previously by some workers (see Tatler and Wade, 2003). Perhaps the most distinctive feature of eye movements is their binocularity—they tend to move together. It is, therefore, perhaps unsurprising that some of the earliest examinations of eye movements considered binocular eye movements and the consequences of disruptions to binocular single vision in conditions such as strabismus.

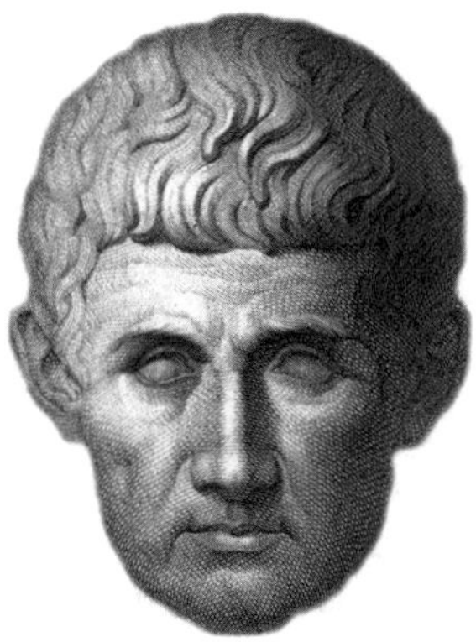

Figure 2.2
Aristotle (ca. 384–322 BC) after an engraving in Wood (1880).

2.2 Binocular eye movements

The eye movements that are both easier to observe in others and to produce oneself are voluntary. We can direct our eyes to objects of interest at will, and when we do this we are usually aware of the rotations of the eyes in the orbits. The ability to introspect upon one's own voluntary eye movements has allowed this class of eye movements to be commented on since antiquity. Much of the early commentary considered the observation that when the two eyes are directed from one location to another they tend to move together. For example, Aristotle (ca. 384–322 BC; Fig. 2.2) remarked: 'So when one eye moves, the common source of sight is also set in motion; and when this moves, the other eye moves also' (Ross, 1927, p. 957b). This statement is important because it is based on the assumption that the eyes move as a unit. Such conjoint motion of the eyes is not always in the same direction, as Aristotle noted in his distinction between version (movements in the same direction) and convergence eye movements. He also commented that there were certain movements that were not possible, namely, divergence beyond the straight-ahead, and movements of one eye upward and the other downward:

> Why is it that we can turn the gaze of both eyes simultaneously towards the right and the left and in the direction of the nose, and that of one eye to the left or to the right, but cannot direct them simultaneously one to the right and the other to the left? Similarly, we can direct them downwards and upwards; for we can turn them simultaneously in the same direction, but not separately. Is it because the eyes, though two, are connected at one point, and under such conditions, when one extremity moves, the other must follow in the same direction, for one extremity becomes the source of movement to the other extremity. (Ross, 1927, pp. 957b–958a)

Virtually the same statement was made over two thousand years later by that towering figure of visual science,

Hermann Helmholtz (1864), in the Croonian Lecture delivered to the Royal Society of London: 'We cannot turn one eye up, the other down; we cannot move both eyes at the same time to the outer angle' (p. 192). The difference between Aristotle and Helmholtz was that the latter could support the statement by experiment, using afterimages.

Thus, the initial descriptions of how the eyes move were made in the context of binocular vision. Indeed, this is one of the first areas of vision that received experimental attention. Claudius Ptolemy (ca. 100–170; Fig. 2.3, left) appreciated that monocular and binocular visual directions were not necessarily the same. In order to confirm this empirically, he constructed a board on which he could place vertical rods at different distances in the midline (Fig. 2.3, right). There followed a description of one of the most commonly used examples of crossed and uncrossed visual directions: with fixation on the far rod, the nearer one appeared double, and to the left with the right eye and to the right with the left eye; the reverse occurred with fixation on the nearer rod. Essentially the same demonstration is now more frequently made with two fingers, rather than rods, held at different distances from the eyes. Ptolemy stated that singleness of vision with two eyes occurred when the two visual directions corresponded, thus introducing the concept of correspondence into binocular vision. He modified his board to take three rods and found that objects appeared single to two eyes when they were in the same plane as the fixation point. These facts were interpreted

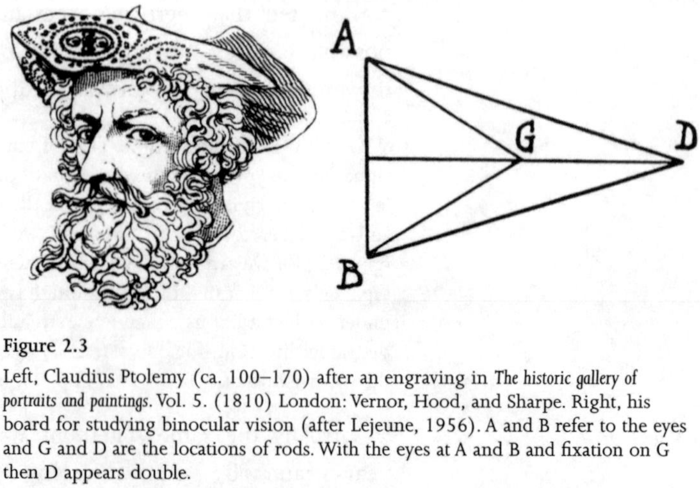

Figure 2.3

Left, Claudius Ptolemy (ca. 100–170) after an engraving in *The historic gallery of portraits and paintings*. Vol. 5. (1810) London: Vernor, Hood, and Sharpe. Right, his board for studying binocular vision (after Lejeune, 1956). A and B refer to the eyes and G and D are the locations of rods. With the eyes at A and B and fixation on G then D appears double.

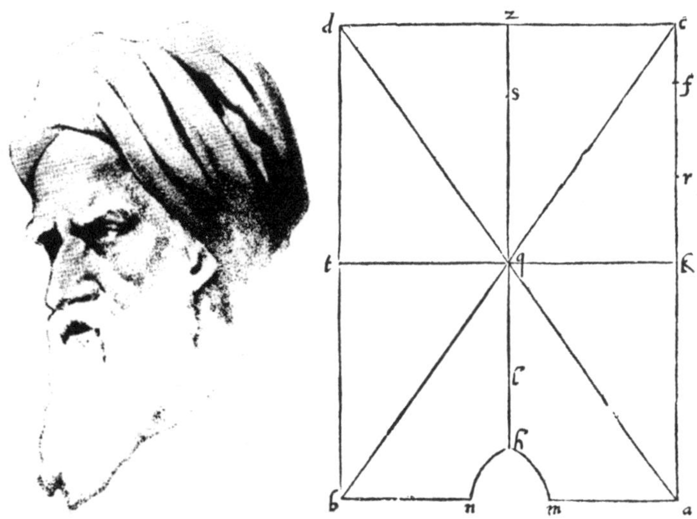

Figure 2.4
Left, Alhazen or Ibn al-Haytham (ca. 965–1039) after an illustration in Duke-Elder and Abrams (1970). Right, Alhazen's board for viewing cylinders with both eyes (after Alhazen, 1572). The eyes were located at *a* and *b* with fixation on a wax cylinder at *q*; cylinders at *t* and *k* were seen double.

in terms of the visual axes and the common axis (see Howard, 2002; Howard and Wade, 1996; Lejeune, 1956; Smith, 1996).

A similar board was made by Ibn Al-Haytham or Alhazen (ca. 965–1039; Fig. 2.4), and he also conducted experiments with it on binocular vision (see Howard, 1996; Sabra, 1989). Ptolemy gave a similar description of eye movements to that attributed to Aristotle, but he did appreciate the function eye movements served: they resulted in corresponding visual pyramids for the two eyes, thereby assisting binocular vision:

> These phenomena [of binocular combination] occur only by virtue of the horizontal separation of the eyes since the height and the depth of the eyes are the same. Both visual axes turn until the bases of the pyramids coincide on the object. It is possible for the eyes to turn in opposite directions left and right, but not up and down. They retain their vertical position, but can converge horizontally. (Lejeune, 1956, p. 34)

The translation of Alhazen's book on optics into Latin in the thirteenth century awakened medieval Western scholars to the physics of light, its mathematical treatment, and its application to vision. Alhazen integrated his analysis of binocular vision with that of the conjoint movements of the eyes:

> We say, then, that when a beholder looks at a visible object, each of his eyes will regard that object; when he gazes at the object, both of his eyes will equally and similarly gaze at it; when he contemplates the object, both of his eyes will equally contemplate it; and when sight moves over the object in order to contemplate it, both eyes will move over it and contemplate it.

When the beholder fixes his sight on an object, the axes of both eyes will converge on the object, meeting at a point on its surface. When he contemplates the object, the two axes will move together over the surface of the object and together pass over all its parts. And, in general, the two eyes are identical in all their conditions, and the sensitive power is the same in both of them, and their actions and affections are severally always identical. When one eye moves for the purpose of vision, the other moves for the same purpose and with the same motion; and when one of them comes to rest, the other [likewise] is at rest... When both eyes are observed as they perceive visible objects, and their actions and movements are examined, their respective actions and movements will be found to be always identical. (Sabra, 1989, p. 229)

Thus, Alhazen proposed that the two eyes acted together in order to achieve single vision, and that the movements of the eyes were coordinated to this end. He supported the proposal, it would seem, by observing the eyes of another person while they were inspecting an object. An empirical method for confirming the coordinated movements of the eyes was described by Robert Smith (1689–1768)—placing a finger over the closed eyelid and feeling the movement when the open eye scanned a scene. He elaborated on the analysis of binocular single vision by recourse to the stimulation of corresponding points in the two eyes, and he related the misalignment of the two eyes to double vision:

The axis of the eye is a line drawn through the middle of the pupil and of the crystalline, and consequently falls on the middle of the retina. And the axes of both eyes produced are called the optick axes. When the optick axes are parallel or meet in a point, the two middle points of the retinas, or any two points which are equally distant from them, and lye on the same sides of them either toward the right hand or left hand, or upwards or downwards, or in any oblique direction, are called corresponding points. Now we find by experience that an object or point of an object appears single when its pictures fall upon corresponding points of the retinas, and double when they do not. For when we view an object steadily, we have acquired a habit of directing the optick axes to the point of view; because its picture falling upon the middle points of the retinas are then distincter than if they fell upon any other places; and since the pictures of the whole object are equal to one another and are both inverted with respect to the optick axes, it follows that the pictures of any collateral point of the object are painted upon corresponding points of the retinas. This habit of directing the optick axes to the point in view is so strong that it is very difficult to do otherwise; insomuch as when one eye is shut and the other is in motion one may feel by ones fingers laid upon the eye-lid, that the eye which is shut, always follows the motions of the eye that is open. But if by squinting or depressing an eye with ones finger, the optick axes are not directed to the same point; in these cases objects appear double: and now it is plain that the pictures are not painted on corresponding places of the retina. (Smith, 1738, pp. 46–47)

Smith was bringing together several strands of interest in binocular vision. Singleness of vision with two eyes was considered to be a consequence of stimulating corresponding points on the two retinas; distinct vision was restricted to the central region of the retina; both eyes moved in unison to retain correspondence; this could be demonstrated by feeling the movements of the closed eye; double vision occurs when one eye is moved out of alignment with the other. Such squinting can be induced artificially (by displacing one open eye with the finger) and it also occurs naturally.

The study of binocular vision has been of continuing concern to students of optics since antiquity. While it has been informed by the studies of Ptolemy, Alhazen, and a host of others, the interest has been largely confined to the phenomenon of binocular single vision—the experience of a single world despite receiving two different projections from it. The situation was transformed by the invention of the stereoscope and the description of stereoscopic depth perception (see Wade, 1983). Charles Wheatstone (1802–1875; Fig. 2.5, left) demonstrated that slightly different images presented to each eye were seen in depth rather than seen double. Such stereoscopic depth could be seen much more easily with the aid of a stereoscope (Fig. 2.5, right), and the factors involved in binocular combination could be examined with an experimental precision that had not been available previously.

From the seventeenth to the early nineteenth century binocular vision had been interpreted in terms of convergence of the eyes

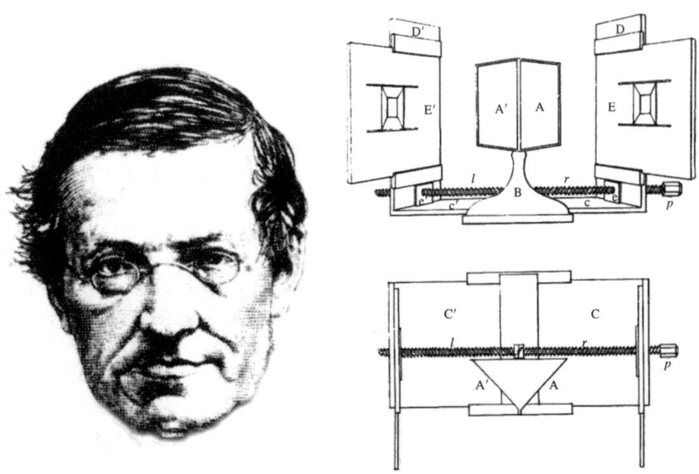

Figure 2.5
Left, Charles Wheatstone (1802–1875) after a portrait in *The Illustrated London News* (1868). Right, his mirror stereoscope as viewed from the front and above (from Wheatstone, 1838). The reflections of the paired pictures (E and E′) were viewed through the mirrors A and A′.

and the stimulation of corresponding points on the two retinas. Descartes (1637) presented the analogy of a blind person holding two sticks in order to feel the singleness of an object at a distance. Berkeley (1709) had championed the influence of convergence in determining visual distance. The two eyes were considered to operate like a range finding device, and it is clearly the case that convergence varies with distance. Vieth (1818) and Müller (1826*a*, 1840) gave a geometrical analysis of binocular single vision, defining a circle passing through the point of fixation and the centres of rotation of each eye: points on the circumference of this binocular circle stimulated corresponding points. Wheatstone interpreted stereoscopic depth perception in terms of psychological processes that enabled combination of the disparate images. The phenomena proved to be damaging to theories of binocular vision that were based on singleness determined by the stimulation of corresponding points (see Wade, 1987). Wheatstone formed afterimages (by prolonged fixation) of differently coloured paired images and observed stereoscopic depth when they were viewed with closed eyes.

Nonetheless, alternatives, in terms of eye movements, were soon proposed. Ernst Brücke (1819–1892; 1841) attacked Wheatstone's theory by arguing that the state of convergence changes very rapidly when viewing either solid objects or stereopairs, thereby changing the binocular visual directions of the disparate parts. Much the same position was maintained by David Brewster (1781–1868), who added changes in accommodation to those of convergence. With regard to the observation of a truncated cone, or stereopairs of one, he stated:

> Each eye, acting alone, sees the cone single, and the various points of its outline are seen more or less distinct, according as they are more or less remote from the point to which the eye is for the instant adjusted. But so rapid is the motion of the eye, and so quickly does it survey the whole of the solid, that it obtains a most distinct perception of its form, its surface, and its solidity. When we view the cone with *both eyes*, we have the same indistinctness of the outline when the optic axes are converged to a single point: but in addition to this, we have the greater indistinctness arising from every point of the figure being seen *double*, except the single point to which the axes are converged. But this imperfection, too, is scarcely visible, from the rapid view which the eyes take of the whole solid, converging their axes upon every point of it, and thus seeing each point in succession single and distinct. (Brewster, 1844, p. 363, original italics)

The arguments of Brücke and Brewster were maintained even though Heinrich Dove (1803–1879; 1841) had reported seeing depth in stereopairs that were briefly illuminated by an electric spark. Moreover, some years later Alfred Volkmann (1800–1877; 1859) invented the tachistoscope to examine precisely this problem. He confirmed Dove's observation of depth in briefly exposed stereoscopic images. Tachistoscopes were generally employed thereafter to present stimuli for periods that were too short to enable eye movements over them.

As was mentioned in Chapter 1, Helmholtz (Fig. 2.6, left) devoted a considerable portion of volume 3 of his *Handbuch der physiologischen Optik* (Helmholtz, 1867*a*, 1925, 2000) to a discussion of eye movements and also stereoscopic vision. His primary concern was with determining the position assumed by the eye following an eye movement (see Chapter 4) and he also considered the motions of two eyes (Helmholtz, 1864). Using after-images projected onto a grid of vertical and horizontal lines he determined that the vertical meridia in each eye differed slightly in orientation (Fig. 2.6, right). Helmholtz wrote: 'Therefore not the *really vertical* meridians of both fields of view correspond, as has been supposed hitherto, but the *apparently* vertical meridians. On the contrary, the horizontal meridians really correspond, at least for normal eyes which are not fatigued' (1864, p. 196, original italics). As was the case with earlier studies of binocular eye movements, Helmholtz's interest was directed to the issue of

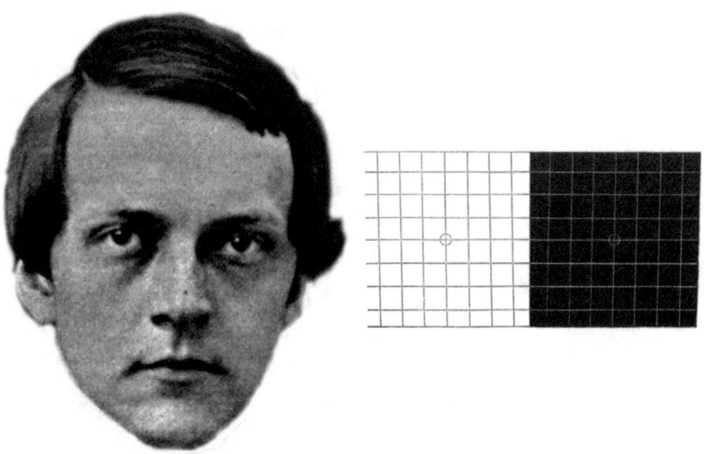

Figure 2.6
Left, Herman Ludwig Ferdinand Helmholtz (1821–1894) after a daguerreotype in Koenigsberger (1902). Right, his diagram of the tilted vertical meridians in the left and right eyes (from Helmholtz, 1864).

retinal correspondence, and he was able to use the stereoscope to assist in his studies.

Prior to Wheatstone's invention of the stereoscope, binocular eye movements were considered in terms of aligning the eyes so that corresponding regions of each retina could be stimulated by the same object. When this did not occur double vision (diplopia) ensued. Strabismus was a naturally occurring (and relatively common) condition involving misalignment of the eyes and unco-ordinated movements of them. It is in cases of strabismus that the breakdown of binocular vision was examined in greater detail, and this resulted in further study of eye movements themselves.

2.2.1 Strabismus

Ophthalmology has a longer recorded history than optics: several surviving papyri dating from the second millenium BC describe disorders of the eye and treatments of them. For example, the Ebers papyrus described dimness of sight and strabismus (see Bryan, 1930). A millenium later, there were specialists in diseases of the eye practicing in Egypt. An illustration of a cataract operation of the type that was probably performed almost two thousand years ago was redrawn by Thorwald (1962), and written records indicate that such operations had been conducted a thousand years earlier (see Magnus, 1901). Greek medicine profited greatly from these earlier endeavours, and added to them. Neither Egyptian nor Greek ophthalmology was free from the mystical and metaphysical, and observation was frequently subservient to philosophical doctrine.

Strabismus, squint, or distortion of the eyes, was recorded in antiquity, but its reported association with problems of binocular vision are more recent (see Duke-Elder and Wybar, 1973; Hirschberg, 1899; Noorden, 1996; Shastid, 1917). The eye specialists in Babylonia, Mesopotamia, and Egypt must have had a working knowledge of ocular anatomy in order to carry out the operations they are known to have performed. However, the records that have survived (such as the Ebers papyrus) relate mainly to the fees they charged and the penalties they suffered for faulty operations rather than the conditions they cured. Their skills and understanding would have been passed on to Greek physicians, who both developed and recorded them. Many Greek texts, through their translations, have been transmitted to us, but

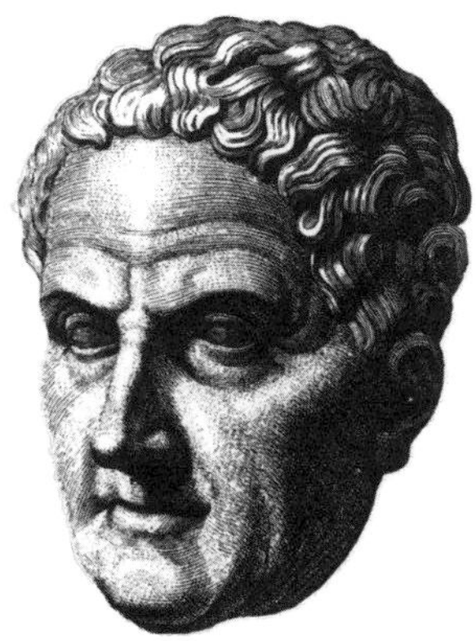

Figure 2.7
Claudius Galen (ca. 130–200) after an engraving in Pettigrew (1840*a*).

any illustrations that they might have included have not survived. Aristotle described many features of perception, including strabismus and the ensuing diplopia: 'Why do objects appear double to those whose eyes are distorted? Is it because the movement does not reach the same point on each of the eyes?' (Ross, 1927, p. 958b). This reflected Aristotle's belief that the eyes operated as a unit rather than independently.

Claudius Galen (ca. 130–200; Fig. 2.7) was renowned as an authority on anatomy, and his works served as the yardstick of truth for over a thousand years, despite the errors they contained. His interests in both normal and abnormal binocular vision might have derived from his contact with Ptolemy, as both were active in Alexandria at around the same time. Galen provided some astute observations on binocular vision, drawing attention to the slight differences in the views of each eye. He also recorded that deviations of the eyes in strabismus were always nasal or temporal. However, he did state that those with strabismus rarely make errors in object recognition:

> Those who squint, either by an acquired anomaly or from the earliest period of foetal life, never commit any errors in the knowledge of objects looked at, for, in such cases, neither of the pupils stands higher than the other, but the fault consists only in this, that the one eye looks too much toward the nose or is directed away from it. (Galen translated in Shastid, 1917, p. 9383)

Corrections for the deviation of an eye were advocated by Paulus Ægineta (ca. 625–690). He recommended the use of a mask for children, which had small apertures so that the eyes would need to align themselves appropriately to see objects. A similar scheme was introduced and illustrated by Ambroise Paré (1510–1590; Fig. 2.8, left) in the sixteenth century (Fig. 2.8, right).

More elaborate masks, shown in Fig. 2.9, right, were prescribed by Georg Bartisch (1535–1606; Fig. 2.9, left). They indicate that he was aware of convergent and divergent squint and he recognized that strabismus was more amenable to correction in children than in adults:

> Therefore in childhood and youth one can prevent and modify the usual state [of squinting] more than in adulthood . . . If one notices a child who sees poorly and with a squint, then as soon as this is recognized, one should make a hood or mask out of thick paper or similar material to cover the head externally . . . If both eyes deviate towards the nose, as is generally seen, then the two holes for the eyes should be arranged more towards

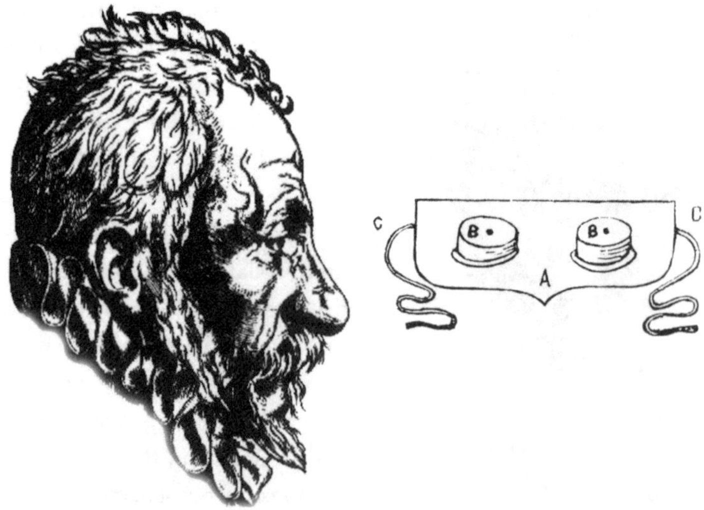

Figure 2.8
Left, Ambroise Paré (1510–1590) after a portrait in Paré (1951). Right, the type of mask he used for the correction of strabismus (from Shastid, 1917).

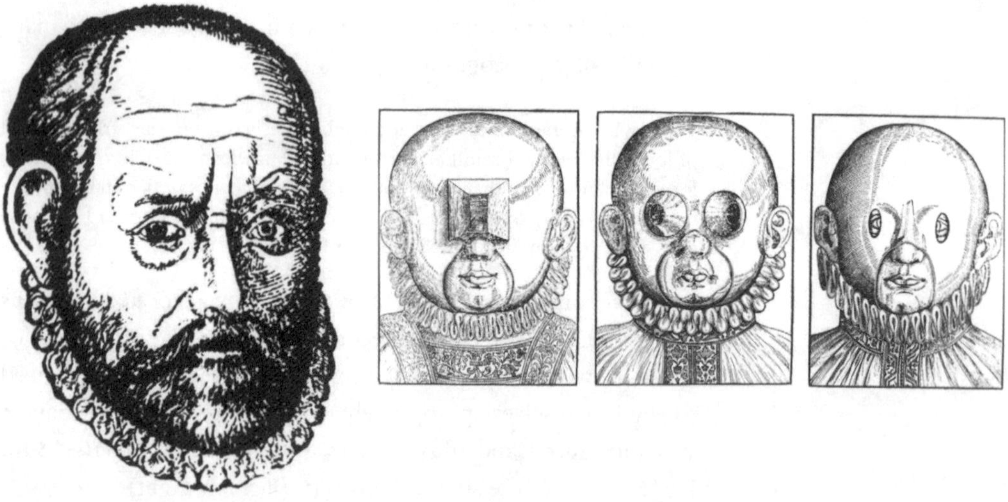

Figure 2.9
Left, Georg Bartisch (1535–1606) after an illustration in Hirschberg (1908). Right, masks for correcting diverging and converging strabismus recommended by Bartisch (1583).

the ears . . . However, if the squint is in one eye alone the hole in the mask should be made straight ahead for the good eye and to the side for the deviating eye . . . When the eyes are directed outwards towards the ears then a special mask must be made for this condition. (Bartisch, 1583, pp. 14–16)

From the eighteenth century attention was directed to the manner in which those with strabismus saw objects singly.

There were many possible causes of squint, most of which were enumerated by Porterfield:

> *First*, This Disease may proceed from Custom and Habit, while in the Eye itself or in its Muscles, nothing is preternatural or defective.... *Secondly*, The *Strabismus* may proceed from a Fault in the first Conformation, by which the most delicate and sensible Part of the *Retina* is removed from its natural Situation, which is directly opposite to the Pupil, and is placed a little to a side of the *Axis* of the Eye, which obliges them to turn the Eye away from the Object they would view, that its Picture may fall on this most sensible Part of the Organ.... *Thirdly*, This Disease may proceed from an oblique Position of the *Crystalline*.... *Fourthly*, This Disease may arise from an oblique Position of the *Cornea*.... *Fifthly*, This Want of uniformity in the Motions of our Eyes may arise from a Defect, or any great Weakness or Imperfection in the Sight of both, or either of the Eyes.... *Sixthly*, Another Cause from which the *Strabismus* may proceed, lyes in the Muscles that move the Eye. When any of those Muscles are too short or too long, too tense or too lax, or are seized with a *Spasm* or *Paralysis*, their Equilibrium will be destroyed, and the Eye will be turned towards, or from that Side where the Muscles are faulty. (Porterfield, 1737, pp. 239–240, 241–242, 243, 245, 247, and 249, original italics)

There were those who adopted one or other of these possibilities. Some believed that the non-deviating eye suppressed the signals from the deviating one. Other commentators considered that there was a refractive difference between the eyes. Yet others considered that the new pattern of stimulation could be learned (by association) to yield singleness of vision. Accordingly, nature and nurture could vie to determine why the eyes were awry. Thomas Reid (1710–1796; 1764) devoted many pages of his *Inquiry* to both theoretical and practical aspects of strabismus. He raised eleven theoretical queries about the condition, and also expressed some success at training squinters to bifixate on objects. In the context of squinting he wrote:

> We see young people in their frolics learn to squint, making their eyes either converge or diverge, when they will, to a very considerable degree. Why should it be more difficult for a squinting person to learn to look straight when he pleases.... one who squints, and originally saw objects double by reason of that squint, may acquire such habits, that when he looks at an object, he shall see it only with one eye: nay, he may acquire such habits, that when he looks at an object with his best eye, he shall have no distinct vision with the other eye at all.... Having examined about twenty persons that squinted, I found in all of them a defect in the sight of one eye. Four only had so much of distinct vision in the weak eye, as to be able to read with it, when the other was covered. (Reid, 1764, pp. 351, 356, and 358)

The overriding historical concern with squinting has been with its medical treatment, rather than its relevance to theories of vision or eye movements. It was in this medical context that Erasmus Darwin (1778) investigated squinting in a young child who had alternating dominance. Darwin reported the outcome of a treatment regime that he had applied to correct it:

> The child was then about five years old, and exceedingly tractable and sensible, which enabled me to make the following observations with great accuracy and frequent repetition. 1. He viewed every object which was presented to him with only one eye at a time. 2. If the object was presented on his right side, he viewed it with his right eye. 3. He turned the pupil of that eye, which was on the same side with the object, in such a direction, that the image might fall on that part of the bottom of the eye where the optic nerve enters it. 4. When an object was held directly before, he turned his head a little to one side, and observed it with but one eye, *viz.* with that most distant from the object, turning away the other in the manner above described; and when he became tired with observing it with that eye, he turned his head the contrary way, and observed it with the other eye alone, with equal facility; but never turned the axes of both eyes on it at the same time. 5. He saw letters, which were written on bits of paper, so as to name them with equal ease, and at equal distances, with one eye as with the other. 6. There was no perceptible difference in the diameters of the irises, nor in the contractibility of them, after having covered his eyes from the light. These observations were carefully made by writing single letters on shreds of paper, and laying wagers with the child that he could not read them when they were presented at certain distances and directions. . . . A paper gnomon was made, and fixed to a cap; and when this artificial nose was placed over his real nose, so as to project an inch between his eyes, the child, rather than turn his head so far to look at oblique objects, immediately began to view them with that eye which was next to them. . . . by wearing the artificial nose, he had greatly corrected the habit of viewing objects with the eye farthest from them; and had more and more acquired the voluntary power of directing both his eyes to the same object, particularly if the object were not more than four or five feet from him; and will, I believe, by resolute perseverance, entirely correct this unsightly deformity. (Darwin, 1778, pp. 86–87, 88, and 96)

Squinting was not only a medical condition that warranted treatment but it provided a naturally occurring example of retinal noncorrespondence to which theories could be addressed. In this way, the study of strabismus not only aided understanding of this condition, but also promoted further research into eye movements themselves and generated new insights into the normal operation of the eyes. Given these early interests in the binocularity of vision and its disruption in strabismus, it is perhaps unsurprising that attention soon turned to the musculature responsible for eye movements.

2.3 Oculomotor anatomy and physiology

The eyes are, of course, moved by muscles, although this aspect of their anatomy did not receive as much attention as the structure of the eye itself. Unfortunately, the anatomical drawings of the eye presumably made by Greek physicians have not survived. Some written accounts, on the other hand, did survive and were translated into many languages. Magnus (1901) has reconstructed the diagrams from the extant texts and few detail the muscles with precision. Magnus' reconstruction of the eye according to Galen is shown in Fig. 2.10. Despite the paucity of graphical detail regarding the ocular musculature, Galen gave a lucid written description of the six extraocular muscles, indicating the three axes around which the eye can rotate:

Well then, since there are four movements of the eyes, one directing them in toward the nose, another out toward the small corner, one raising them up towards the brows, and another drawing them down toward the cheeks,

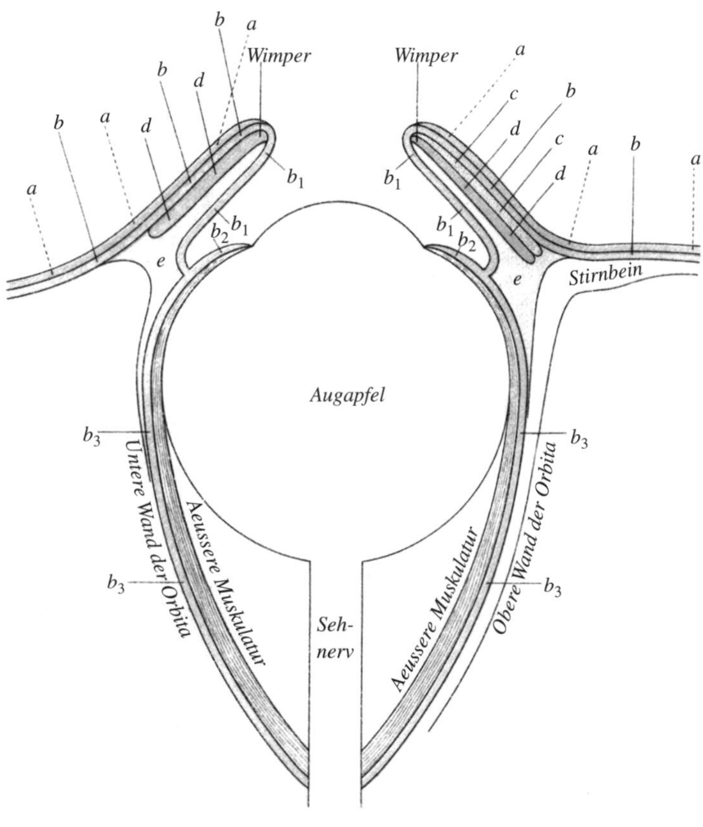

Figure 2.10
The eye and extraocular muscles according to Galen. The illustration is based upon Galen's description and was drawn by Magnus (1901).

> it was reasonable that the same number of muscles should be formed to control these movements. And so two were formed at the sides (one at each corner) [*recti, medialis* and *lateralis*], and one of the other two above [*rectus superior*] and the other below [*rectus inferior*], but they all become tendinous to make one broad, circular tendon that ends in the *iris* [the ciliary region]. Since it was better that the eye should also rotate, Nature made two other muscles [*obliqui, superior* and *inferior*] that are placed obliquely, one at each eyelid, extending from above and below toward the small corner of the eye, so that by means of them we turn and roll our eyes just as readily in every direction. (May, 1968, p. 483, original italics)

Most of Galen's dissections were on rhesus monkey (Singer, 1956), although the results were subsequently adopted as applying to humans. Galen's anatomy informed science and medicine for well over a thousand years, largely due to the restrictions that were subsequently placed on dissections. It resulted in a reliance on his works on anatomy, which were recounted dogmatically until the time of Vesalius (1543). The journey from Galen to Vesalius was tortuous, not least for those who required surgery. The disinterest in science and medicine after the sacking of Rome in the fifth century left Europe in what have been called the 'Dark Ages'. Greek anatomical wisdom was retained by Islamic scholars, who translated many books into Arabic and eventually transmitted them to late mediaeval students (O'Leary, 1949). Galen's medical works were translated into Arabic by Hunain ibn Is-hâq (ca. 807–877). The earliest surviving diagrams of the eye are to be found in Islamic manuscripts (see Meyerhof, 1928; Polyak, 1942, 1957), of which that by Hunain ibn Is-hâq is probably the oldest (Fig. 2.11). It is essentially a functional diagram, since it adopts different viewpoints for different parts of the eye. This could be the reason why the pupil and the lens are shown in circular form, and the lens is situated in the middle of the eye. The extraocular muscles are also shown extended from the eyeball. The illustration was copied several times in the centuries that followed. Thus, Arabic accounts of the eye drew on Galen for inspiration, but their illustrations reflect a greater concern with geometry than anatomy. Throughout this period, the nature of light was not understood, and the gross anatomy of the eye and its attachments were not accurately depicted.

As indicated in Chapter 1, visual science underwent a revolution in the seventeenth century. Two critical features necessary for understanding vision were uncovered in its first two decades by

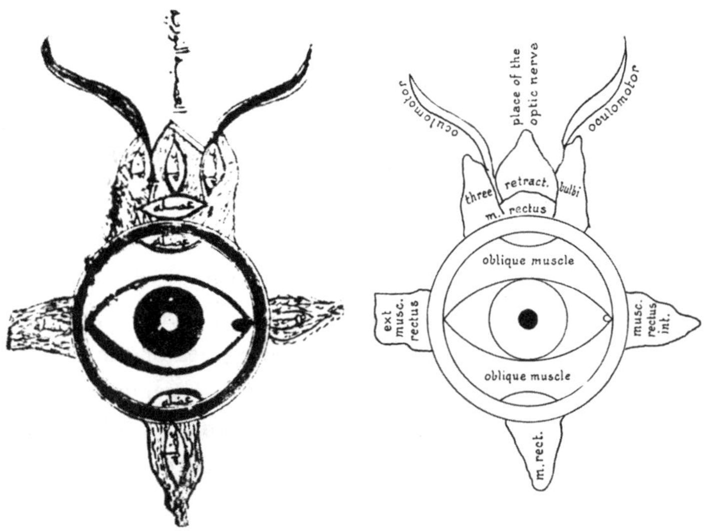

Figure 2.11
Left, the eye and extraocular muscles according to Hunain ibn Is-hâq (ca. 808–873), and right, the diagram with English labels for the various structures (both figures after Meyerhof, 1928).

Kepler (1604, 1611) and thereafter by Scheiner (1619, 1630). Kepler described how the eye operated as an optical instrument, focusing light onto the retina to form an image. His primary concern was to construct better optical instruments, and he analysed how images might be formed in the eye (see Park, 1997; Wade, 1998). His insight led him to the *camera obscura* (or pinhole camera), which in turn stimulated the thought that the eye with its aperture must function in a fairly similar but imperfect way. He tried to understand how the crystalline lens focused rays of light by using water-filled glass flasks. Kepler not only constructed what can be thought of as an early artificial eye, but was probably the first Western scientist to analyse pinhole images correctly (Lindberg, 1968, 1976; Smith, 1998).

In 1619, Scheiner provided a considerably more accurate illustration of the vertebrate eye (see Fig. 1.3). The anterior and posterior curvatures of the lens were now correctly represented and the optic nerve was shown leaving the eye nasally. This diagram has often been described as the first correct representation of the human eye despite the fact that Scheiner stated he had never dissected any human eyes:

> The observation of most animals' eyes tells us all these things; indeed these processes happen in the eyes of cows, sheep, goats, and pigs, on which I have done many experiments in the presence of other people; logical reasoning leads me to suppose a similar process for the human eyes as well, because in

every man's eye there is a hole, through which the optical nerve comes out, placed in the same position as in animals; indeed the cavities of each eye are placed in the skull along the sides of the bone which shapes the nasal projection, although in the case of man we have to rely on reasoning more than on observation, because I have never had the opportunity to test a human eye. (Scheiner, 1619, p. 18)

Some years later, Scheiner (1630) was able to demonstrate the image forming properties of the eye by placing an excised animal's eye in the aperture of a *camera obscura* and noting how an image could be seen on the exposed rear surface of the retina. He also gave detailed diagrams comparing the optics of the eye with that of a camera with a lens. His demonstration of image formation in an excised eye was considered so valuable that it was repeated and illustrated seven years later by Descartes (see Fig 1.4), who refined it by replacing the retina with an eggshell in some experiments (Descartes 1637/1902). He was concerned with the mechanics as well as the optics of the eye. He provided a speculative mechanistic account of how the paired muscles work by means of reciprocal action. Two diagrams depicting the action are shown in Fig. 2.12: the illustration on the left is from *De homine* (Descartes, 1662) and that on the right is from *Traité de l'homme* (Descartes, 1664/1909); they are radically different in detail, but the principle that they depict was remarkably prescient, despite reference to Galen's animal spirits.

The function that eye movements served was also stressed by many writers—namely to direct the eyes to objects of interest, so that they can be seen distinctly (see Section 2.5.1). As early as the thirteenth century, John Pecham (ca. 1230–1292) speculated that the shape of the eyeball facilitated rapid movements over a scene: 'Because of the many things that must be quickly perceived, the eye must be round so that it can easily turn and move' (translated in Lindberg, 1970, p. 111). This became a recurrent theme, and it was related to the known differences in visual acuity in central and peripheral vision. Only those points which were near the optic axis were clearly visible. Scheiner (1619) made this point explicitly: 'The movement of the eye is adapted for every variation of position so that the optical axis is directed to a selected part of an object making it most distinctly perceived' (p. 243). Robert Hooke (1635–1703) was similarly explicit in his *Micrographia*: 'Now, as we accurately distinguish the site or position

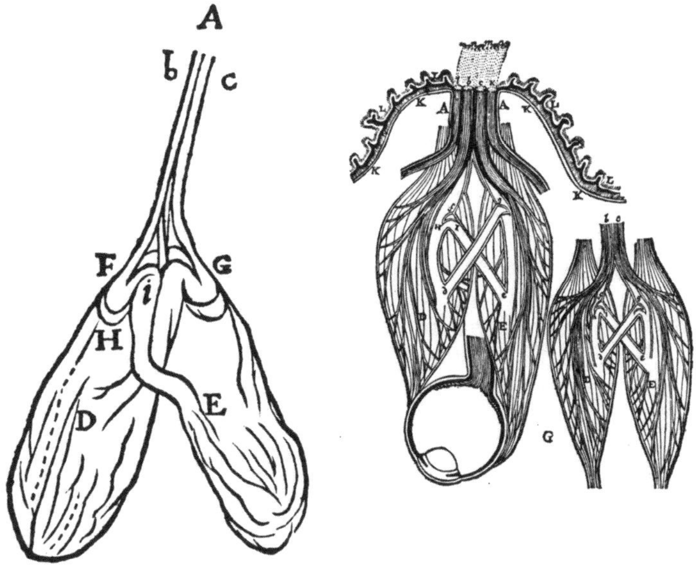

Figure 2.12

Illustrations of reciprocal action of eye muscles taken from Descartes: left from *De homine* and right from *Traité de l'homme*. The description of the figures is taken from *De homine*, as translated in Fulton (1966): 'Let us imagine a tube or small nerve, bf, flowing into the muscle D—which I am supposing is one of those which move the eye, and there dividing into several branches, loose in texture, which stretch or shrink according to the quantity of animal spirits which flow in or out of them, and whose ramifications are so arranged that the animal spirits flowing into them cause the whole body of the muscle to swell and shorten, thus pulling the eye to which it is attached towards it; on the other hand when the animal spirits flow out of the muscle it shrinks and lengthens. Besides bf, there is another tube, ef, through which the animal spirits flow into muscle D, and there is yet another tube, dg, by which they flow out of it. Muscle E, which I assume moves the eye in the opposite direction to muscle D, receives the animal spirits from the brain through the tube cg, while those from muscle D flow through dg to E, which returns them to D by ef. . . . if the animal spirits from the brain tend to flow with more force through bf than cg, they close the valve g and open f—either more or less, in proportion to their strength—through which the spirits in muscle E pass to muscle D by the tube ef, at a speed in proportion to the size of the opening at f, so that the muscle D shortens, because the spirits cannot flow out of it, while E lengthens, and thus the eye is turned towards D. On the other hand if the spirits flow with greater force through cg than through bf they close valvule f and open g, so that the spirits from muscle D go back at once by the tube dg to muscle E, which thus becomes shortened and pulls the eye towards that side.' (Fulton, 1966, pp. 263–264).

of an Object by the motion of the Muscles of the eye requisite to put the optick Line in a direct position' (1665, p. 179). Such concern with eye movements was more in terms of accounting for differences in visibility in different parts of the visual field than in determining the ways the eyes actually moved. However, this understanding of the necessity to move the eyes in order to provide clarity of vision was a crucial development in the

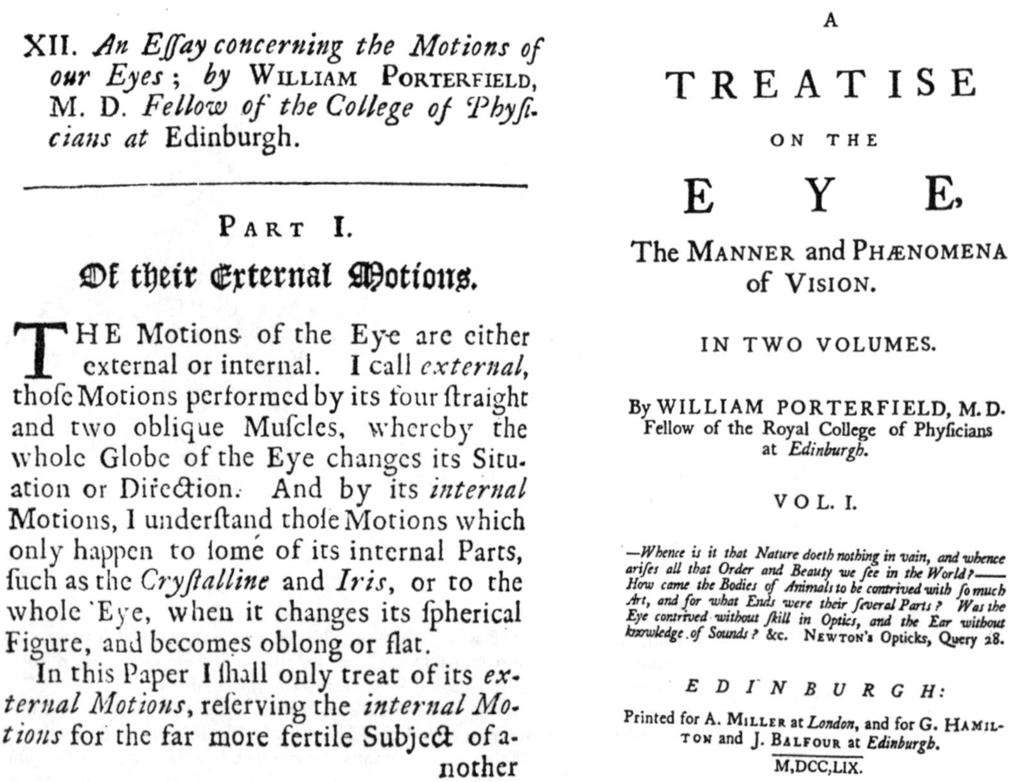

XII. *An Eſſay concerning the Motions of our Eyes*; *by* WILLIAM PORTERFIELD, M. D. *Fellow of the College of Phyſicians at* Edinburgh.

PART I.

Of their External Motions.

THE Motions of the Eye are either external or internal. I call *external*, thoſe Motions performed by its four ſtraight and two oblique Muſcles, whereby the whole Globe of the Eye changes its Situation or Direction. And by its *internal* Motions, I underſtand thoſe Motions which only happen to ſome of its internal Parts, ſuch as the *Cryſtalline* and *Iris*, or to the whole Eye, when it changes its ſpherical Figure, and becomes oblong or flat.

In this Paper I ſhall only treat of its *external Motions*, reſerving the *internal Motions* for the far more fertile Subject of another

A

TREATISE

ON THE

EYE,

The MANNER and PHÆNOMENA of VISION.

IN TWO VOLUMES.

By WILLIAM PORTERFIELD, M.D.
Fellow of the Royal College of Phyſicians at *Edinburgh*.

VOL. I.

—Whence is it that Nature doeth nothing in vain, and whence ariſes all that Order and Beauty we ſee in the World?——How came the Bodies of Animals to be contrived with ſo much Art, and for what Ends were their ſeveral Parts? Was the Eye contrived without ſkill in Optics, and the Ear without knowledge of Sounds? &c. NEWTON's Opticks, Query 28.

EDINBURGH:

Printed for A. MILLER at *London*, and for G. HAMILTON and J. BALFOUR at *Edinburgh*.

M,DCC,LIX.

Figure 2.13

Left, the title of Porterfield's (1737) first article on eye movements, published in *Edinburgh Medical Essays and Observations*. Right, the title page of the first volume of Porterfield's (1759*a*) *Treatise* published 22 years later.

understanding of eye movements and an important precursor for later studies of the details of eye movements themselves.

From the late seventeenth century there was greater concern with the detail of eye movements. This involved both the internal and external movements of the eyes, as well as voluntary and involuntary movements. Porterfield (1737, 1738) distinguished between the external and internal motions of the eye, and treated the external first. The title page of Porterfield's first article is shown in Fig. 2.13, left, together with that of his better-known *Treatise*, published over twenty years later (Fig. 2.13, right). We will examine them in the reverse order, as less attention is now directed to the internal than to the external motions. The mechanism of accommodation is reasonably well understood and it is confined mainly to the level of physiology. It might be said that the greater the understanding of a process that serves functional adaptation, the less the psychological interest in it.

2.4 Internal motions of the eye

Porterfield examined both motions of the iris and of the lens under this heading. It is the latter that attracted the most concerted attention in the period up to the mid-nineteenth century. Indeed the term 'accommodation' was coined by Porterfield to describe the process of focusing: 'our Eyes change their Conformation, and accommodate themselves to the various Distances of Objects' (Porterfield, 1738, p. 126). How this change took place was to prove an enduring problem. Interest in accommodation, like that in external eye movements, derived from an aspect of everyday perception: when we can see objects clearly at one distance those at other distances are indistinct. Moreover, the ability to focus on objects at different distances changes with ageing. These phenomenal distinctions were assigned added significance when the operation of the eye as an optical instrument was accepted (see Smith, 1998; Wade, 1998).

2.4.1 Accommodation

The great anatomist John Hunter (1728–1793) described the situation succinctly at the end of the eighteenth century. He planned to present his theory of accommodation in the Croonian lecture to the Royal Society in 1793, but death intervened. The lecture was delivered by his brother-in-law, Everard Home (1756–1832), who held quite contrary views to those Hunter wished to be expressed. Hunter wrote:

> The laws of optics are so well understood, and the knowledge of the eye, when considered as an optical instrument, has been rendered so perfect, that I do not consider myself capable of making any addition to it; but still there is a power in the eye by which it can adapt itself to different distances far too extensive for the simple mechanism of the parts to effect. (Extract of a letter from John Hunter to Joseph Banks in 1793, published by Home, 1794, p. 24)

The solution to the enigma of accommodation was provided in the middle of the nineteenth century when Antonie Cramer (1822–1855; 1853) and Helmholtz (1855) independently proposed that the lens was elastic and under tension. Helmholtz, in one of his *Popular lectures*, reflected the significance of accommodation in visual science when he noted: 'The mechanism by which this is accomplished... was one of the greatest riddles of the physiology of the eye since the time of Kepler... No problem in optics has given rise to so many contradictory theories as this' (1873, p. 205).

In the early eighteenth century, at the time Porterfield was writing, the major candidate mechanisms for accommodation had been stated. Kepler (1611) proposed that the lens moved forward and backward in the eye itself, as if the lens was of fixed curvature as in a camera. Scheiner (1619) observed pupil constriction when focusing on near objects, and associated this with accommodation. Descartes (1637) speculated that the lens changed in curvature, without any evidence of actual changes in the shape of the lens. Descartes' apologist, Jacques Rohault (1620–1675; 1671), entertained the possibility that the eye could lengthen or shorten. Isaac Newton (1642–1727) examined many aspects of image formation in the eye in his *Opticks* (Newton, 1704). His advocate, Jean Théophile Desaguliers (1683–1744; 1719), suggested that the corneal curvature was increased when viewing near objects thereby increasing refraction. In addition to these theories, Phillipe de La Hire (1640–1718; 1685) argued that there is no active process of accommodation because of pupil constriction when viewing near objects and the ability to ignore blurred images. The greater depth of focus with a constricted pupil was well known at that time from the operation of cameras. Although Scheiner had observed the constriction of the pupil with fixation on near objects, he still inclined toward Kepler's view that the lens moved in the eye. He did, however, entertain the notion that the lens could become more convex when focusing on near objects.

Systematic studies of accommodation are often reported as commencing with Thomas Young (1773–1829; 1793, 1801), but Porterfield (1738) and Wells (1792) carried out sophisticated experiments before Young. Porterfield devised and named an instrument called an optometer for determining the near and far points of vision. The instrument was potentially a boon to practitioners, but it was not widely adopted by them. It was based on an observation made by Scheiner (1619), who had described the consequences of viewing an object through two closely-spaced apertures. This has become called 'Scheiner's experiment' and it has been crucial in the elucidation of accommodation. The experiment was clearly described by Helmholtz:

> Two pinholes are made in a card at a distance apart less than the diameter of the pupil of the eye. With one eye closed, the observer looks through both holes at a small object sharply delineated against a contrasting background, for example, at a needle held in front of a bright window. The needle should be adjusted at right angles to the line joining the two holes. If the eye is focused on the needle itself, it appears single; but if it is focused on something else, nearer or farther away, the needle appears double. (1924*a*/2000, pp. 124–125)

Porterfield improved on Scheiner's experiment by using as a stimulus a small luminous point on a dark background, and on this basis made the first optometer. It consisted of a metal plate with two narrow and close vertical slits in it so that when it was held close to the eye their separation was less than the pupil diameter. The stimulus viewed was a vertical slit illuminated by a candle in a lamp housing. The distance of the vertical light line from the vertical slits could be changed so that the near and far points of vision could be measured; that is, the nearest and farthest positions at which the line could be seen as single; variations in pupil diameter were not controlled.

Young (1801) improved on Porterfield's instrument by incorporating a lens and a graduated scale. Young's new optometer provided measurements across the range over which accommodation could operate, and he provided tables to assist in the prescription of lenses for myopic and presbyopic eyes. Wells (1792) considered that Porterfield's experiments were the most accurate that had been conducted. Nonetheless, he was critical of Porterfield's endeavours with the optometer, in part because they had not been conducted with sufficient thoroughness, and also because only one of Porterfield's eyes had been examined. Wells developed an alternative stimulus for determining the near and far points of vision—the image of a candle flame reflected from the bulb of a small thermometer. With this he determined the different ranges of distinct vision for his own left and right eyes, and the intermediate accommodation that attends binocular viewing of objects within the range of one eye but not the other.

Porterfield (1738) was able to discount hypotheses based on the involvement of structures other than the crystalline lens by recourse to sight following removal of the lens. The operation was performed in order to restore vision by removal of a cataract. Porterfield examined such an individual in one of whose eyes the crystalline lens had been removed. The individual was unable to accommodate at all when using the aphakic eye (the one without a lens) although accommodation was possible with the normal eye. Accommodation with the aphakic eye required the aid of a convex lens, the power of which needed to be modified for objects at different distances:

> A Man having a Cataract in both Eyes, which intirely deprived him of Sight, committed himself to an Oculist, who finding them ripe, performed the Operation, and couched the Cataracts with all the Success could be desired; but after they were couched, he could not see Objects distinctly, even at an ordinary Distance, without the Help of a very convex *Lens*. . . . Seeing that nothing happens in the Eye, in couching the Cataract, but that the Crystalline is depressed, it follows, that the Change made in our Eyes, according to the Distance of Objects, must be attributed to this Humour. (Porterfield, 1738, pp. 182–184 and 186, original italics)

Thus, Porterfield concluded that since elongation of the eye was still possible for such a person, as was variation in corneal curvature, they could not be the basis for accommodation; therefore, the crystalline lens must be involved.

Nonetheless, uncertainty remained concerning the manner in which the lens functioned. Porterfield was led to the conclusion, on anatomical grounds, that the lens moved forward and backward in the eye. Moreover, it was believed that any changes in the shape of the lens would be a consequence of muscular action within it, the evidence for which was wanting: 'If it can be said, that the Crystalline changes its Conformation, and becomes more or less convex, by the Action of certain muscular Fibres that enter its Composition, it is incumbent on those who entertain this Opinion to show us these Fibres' (Porterfield, 1738, pp. 191–192). Eight reasons for supporting his view were stated and Porterfield concluded: 'As to the *efficient Cause* it has been already demonstrated, that this lyes in the *Ligamentum ciliare*, which being muscular, does by its Contraction change the Situation of the *Crystalline*, according as Objects are nearer or further off' (1738, pp. 212–213, original italics).

In 1793 a paper by the nineteen-year-old Thomas Young, regarding some 'Observations on vision', was presented to the Royal Society; in it Young argued that accommodation of the eye was achieved by changes in the curvature of the crystalline lens. Young took Porterfield's evidence to be consistent with variations in lens curvature rather than the alternative, and suggested that the lens was muscular. This might have been an error of youthful arrogance or exuberance but it was repeated when he re-examined the topic some years later (Young, 1801). The surmise reflected Young's preference for elegant speculation over systematic experiment in this and his other scientific enquiries. As he himself remarked in a letter late in his life 'the acute suggestion was then—and indeed always—more in the line of my ambition than experimental illustration' (Jones, 1871, p. 256). His hypothesis was based on a critical survey of earlier theories and from Porterfield's study of accommodation in an aphakic individual. Moreover he examined the crystalline lens taken from an ox with a magnifier and stated that the arrangement of fibres could only be accounted for on the supposition of muscular fibres within it. The idea of changes in lens curvature was not new, but the proposal of a muscular lens was.

Young's 'acute suggestion' that the lens changed its curvature to effect accommodation was rediscovered by the foremost authorities on physiological optics in the second half of the nineteenth century—Frans Cornelis Donders (1818–1889) and Helmholtz. Donders remarked that:

> Previously to the time of Young it [changes in lens curvature] could be considered as little more than a loose assertion, to which no value was attached. The force of Young's experiments was, however, not understood... Perhaps the necessary attention was not paid to Young's demonstration, because physiologists, not being acquainted with any muscular elements in the eye, could scarcely imagine by what mechanism the crystalline lens should change its form, and they were little inclined to believe with Young in the contractility of the fibres of the lens. (1864, p. 11)

Helmholtz, who also had great respect for Young and proceeded to resurrect his trichromatic theory of colour vision, had this to say about Young's (1801) second paper on the optometer and accommodation: 'This is a work of astonishing perspicacity and originality, which was qualified to settle the question as to accommodation even at that time, but, on account of its conciseness, it is often hard to follow, and, moreover, it presupposes the most thorough knowledge of mathematical optics' (Helmholtz, 1924*a*, 2000, p. 167).

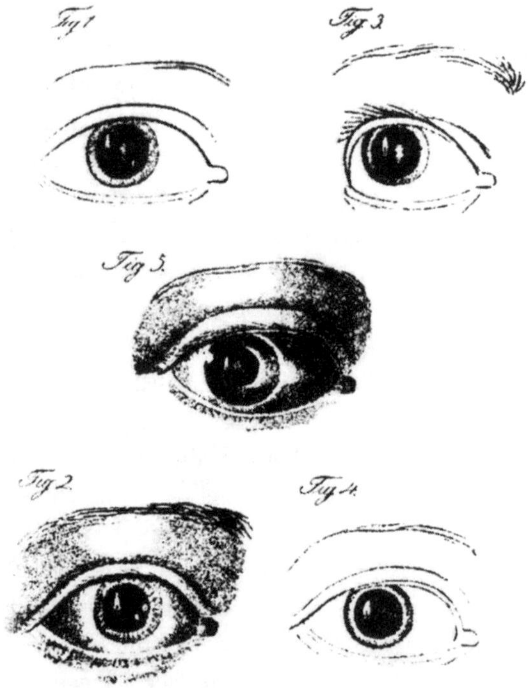

Figure 2.14
Purkinje images. The reflections of a candle flame from the structures of the eye. The images were described by Purkinje in 1823, and reprinted in his *Opera Omnia* (1918).

One of the methods Young used to discount any changes in the curvature of the cornea during accommodation involved examining reflections of light from its surface. He noted that the image of a candle flame reflected from the cornea did not change in size as the eye focused on near or distant objects. Shortly afterwards, Brewster used the changing size of corneal reflections to diagnose the condition of keratoconus or conical cornea (cited in Wardrop, 1808).

Reflected images became of greater significance following Purkinje's (1823*b*) description of less intense ones from the front and back surfaces of the lens (Fig. 2.14). The practical importance of the multiple reflected images was not lost on Purkinje, who wrote:

> These methods for the observation of the surfaces of the lens will not be without use, I think, in therapeutic investigation, especially where one wants to differentiate precisely whether only the capsule of the lens is involved, the lens itself, its posterior surface, or the vitreous humor. From the exact measurements of the flame reflections on the lens of a living human subject one can determine with considerable labor its shape and its relation to the acuity of vision. The distance of the lens from the surface of the iris one can judge from the speed of change which the image of the flame undergoes when the candle is brought closer or moved away. (Translated in John, 1959, p. 61)

Within a few decades, vastly improved methods for studying the reflections were introduced, first by Cramer (1853) and then by Helmholtz (1855). They were based on the observation that a light source held in front and a little to the side of the eye will produce four reflections, although not all equally bright. The brightest reflection comes from the front of the cornea, the transparent outer part of the eye. Two other images, both considerably fainter, come from the front and the back surfaces of the crystalline lens, between the two chambers of the eye. The image from the posterior corneal surface is barely visible because the refractive indices of the cornea and aqueous humour are very similar.

Despite Purkinje's clear indication of the use of reflected images to determine the changes of the surfaces of the lens during accommodation, his account was not cited by Helmholtz either in his *Popular lectures* or in the three editions of his *Handbuch*. In 1849, Max Langenbeck (1818–1877) reached a similar conclusion to Purkinje, and Langenbeck was said by Helmholtz to be the first 'who drew the correct inference that the anterior surface of the lens is, therefore, more convex in near vision' (1924*a*/2000, p. 164). The only mention Helmholtz made of Purkinje was to his book of 1825, and Purkinje was listed with many others as supporting the theory that the lens changed curvature during accommodation.

The crucial experiments on changes in lens curvature during accommodation were performed a few years later by Cramer (1853). He viewed the reflections from the surfaces of the lens through a telescopic tube, mounted on a quadrant, which magnified the images up to twenty times. By measuring both the locations and sizes of the images reflected from the front and back surfaces of the lens under different conditions, he correctly concluded that the lens increases in curvature for accommodation on near objects (see Donders, 1864).

Helmholtz (1855) reached exactly the same conclusion, and he did so independently. Moreover, he devised an even better measuring instrument, which he called an ophthalmometer. He described it in his *Handbuch* in the following way:

> The author has constructed an instrument whereby it is possible to make these and other measurements of the eye accurately and quite independently of small movements of the head, and which is therefore called an ophthalmometer . . . [It] is essentially a telescope, adapted to vision at short distances,

having two glass plates placed close together, in front of its objective. (1924*a*/2000, p. 10)

The conclusions reached by Helmholtz were the same as those of Cramer. Helmholtz wrote the following about the mechanism by which accommodation is achieved:

On contraction, the ciliary muscle could pull the posterior end of the zonule forwards nearer the lens and reduce the tension of the zonule . . . If the pull of the zonule is relaxed in accommodating for near vision, the equatorial diameter of the lens will diminish, and the lens will get thicker in the middle, both surfaces becoming more curved. (1924*a*/2000, p. 151)

The problem that had beset students of vision for three and a half centuries was finally resolved. The general principles of the process of accommodation had been described by Cramer and Helmholtz.

2.5 External motions of the eye

Many early researchers followed the sensory-motor theory of perception as advanced by Berkeley. However, not all students of the senses accepted Berkeley's theory. Prominent among these was Porterfield, who rejected Berkeley's theory that touch teaches vision the dimensions of space on logical grounds: he argued that touch is as arbitrary in its representation of space as is vision, and therefore cannot teach vision external dimensions.

Like Erasmus Darwin, Porterfield was part of the medical tradition of examining eye movements. Unlike Darwin, he had an acute awareness of optics and its integration with vision and its defects. He also appreciated the historical background in which the research was placed. Porterfield's (1737) first article on eye movements considered 'their external motions'; it started with a detailed account of the structure of the eye and its muscles, often drawing on comparative anatomy. However, it is not Porterfield's anatomy that was of primary interest to him, but his integration of eye movements and vision. Eye movements were considered important because of the function they served in vision, and his essay involved many digressions into areas of perception. Following an account of the four straight muscles (recti) he speculated on the torsional function of the oblique muscles, then on to the location of the optic disc, scanning eye movements, convergence and distance perception, binocular single vision,

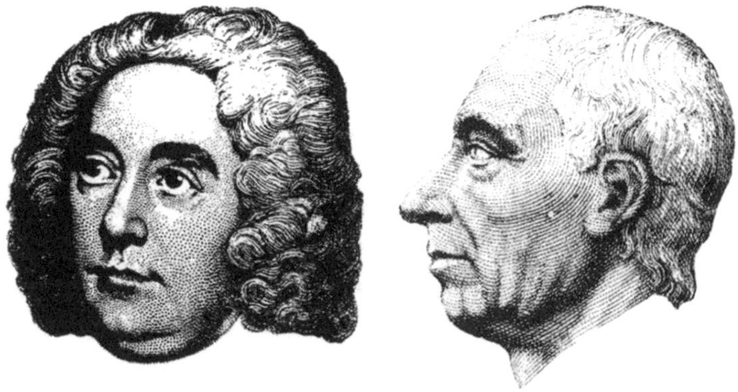

Figure 2.15
Left, George Berkeley (1685–1753) after an engraving in Fraser (1871). Right, Thomas Reid (1710–1796) after a frontispiece engraving in Stewart (1800).

visual direction, colour vision, strabismus, and vision and touch. In short, Porterfield's principal aim was philosophical; he inveighed against the empiricist theory of vision advanced by Berkeley (Fig. 2.15) by proposing that visual location is innate:

> *The Judgment we form of Objects being placed without the Eye in those perpendicular Lines, or, which is nearly the same thing, the Judgment we form of the Situation and Distance of visual Objects, depends not on Custom and Experience, but on an original connate and immutable Law, to which our Minds have been subjected from the Time they were first united to our Bodies.* (Porterfield, 1737, p. 215, original italics)

The law is: '*Every Point on an Object appears and is seen without the Eye nearly in a straight Line, drawn perpendicularly to the* Retina, *from that Point of it where its Image falls*' (Porterfield, 1737, p. 208, original italics). The origins of the law can be traced to Kepler's (1611) analysis of visual direction, and Porterfield applied the principle to account for a range of phenomena from double vision in strabismus to upright perception on the basis of an inverted retinal image. Porterfield's defence of a geometrical theory of space perception based on innate processes of visible direction, in opposition to Berkeley's theory, was followed by Thomas Reid (Fig. 2.15) and others (see Cantor, 1977). For Porterfield both direction and distance were considered to be innate, whereas for Reid (1764) it was the monocular (two-dimensional) visible direction that was inborn (see Pastore, 1971). This principle of visual direction was attacked by Wells (1792) on empirical grounds. First, it could not predict the diplopia experienced by individuals with strabismus after they have aligned an object in each eye separately. Second, it could not account for the apparent direction of afterimages following voluntary movements of the eyes (see Ono, 1981).

Porterfield's principle of visual direction was also brought to bear in reconciling upright perception with an inverted retinal image. Reid (1764) adopted essentially the same sentiments in rejecting both the retina as the site of seeing and Berkeley's theory that all seeing is learned. Porterfield (1737) realized that as acuity declined with retinal eccentricity then it would be difficult to perceive clearly all parts of a large object at once. Accordingly, he considered that vision was dependent upon scanning objects by moving the eyes. A second factor that was implicated in this was the importance of visual persistence in yielding a unified percept during scanning:

> Now, though it is certain that only a very small Part of any Object can at once be clearly and distinctly seen, namely, that whose Image on the *Retina* is in the *Axis* of the Eye; and that the other Parts of the Object, which have their Images painted at some Distance from this same *Axis*, are but faintly and obscurely perceived, and yet we are seldom sensible of this Defect; and, in viewing any large Body, we are ready to imagine that we see at the same Time all its Parts equally distinct and clear: But this is a vulgar Error, and we are led into it from the quick and almost continual Motion of the Eye, whereby it is successively directed towards all the Parts of the Object in an Instant of Time. (Porterfield, 1737, pp. 185–186, original italics)

Most of those who discussed perception and eye movements in the eighteenth and nineteenth centuries continued to commit this 'vulgar Error'. It was not until the pattern of eye movements could be measured with greater precision that substance could be supplied to Porterfield's shrewd surmise, as will be described in Chapter 4.

2.5.1 Distinct vision

Porterfield, in the last quotation, specified the key phenomenon that informed studies of eye movements: the restriction of high visual resolution (distinct vision) to a small part of the retina. If only a small part of the scene can be resolved in detail, how do we form an impression of a well-defined scene? Porterfield provided the answer—by moving the eyes rapidly over the scene. Thus, distinct vision informed studies of eye movements. In modern parlance, visual acuity declines from the region around the fovea towards the periphery. However, Porterfield's answer introduced other questions: how can a unitary experience of the visual world be maintained with 'the quick and almost continual Motion of the Eye'? This is a thorny issue that will be returned to in Chapter 6.

Classical considerations of visual resolution were in terms of distance. When an object recedes from view it eventually ceases to be seen. The Greek mathematician, Euclid (ca. 323–283 BC), stated that: 'Every object seen has a certain limit of distance, and when this is reached it is no longer seen' (translated in Burton, 1945, p. 357). Ptolemy was more precise: 'What is seen by the central rays on the visual axis is seen more clearly than objects at the side' (Lejeune, 1956, p. 20). Alhazen used his board (Fig. 2.4, right), constructed to examine binocular vision, to investigate reading in peripheral vision. Words could be placed at peripheral locations on the board, and Alhazen determined what could be seen clearly:

> The experimenter should then gently move the strip [with a word written on it] along the transverse line in the board, making sure that its orientation remains the same, and, as he does this, direct his gaze at the middle strip while closely contemplating the two strips. He will find that as the moving strip gets farther from the middle, the word that is on it becomes less and less clear . . . as the moving strip gets farther from the middle, the word that is on it decreases in clarity until he ceases to comprehend or ascertain its form. Then if he moves it further, he will find that the form of that word becomes more confused and obscure. (Sabra, 1989, pp. 244–245)

The term *distinct vision* was in general use from at least the seventeenth century. Rohault (1671) related it to the optical dispersion in the eye, which was least on the optical axis. Porterfield and his contemporaries used it to refer to the superior visual acuity for fixated objects. Wells (1792) described it thus: 'bodies to be distinctly or perfectly seen, not only require, that their pictures should be accurately formed upon the retina, but that they should fall upon a particular part of it' (p. 132).

Rohault was a strong supporter of Cartesian philosophy, and some of the early speculations on the limits of visual resolution were made by Descartes (1637, 1965). The problem he addressed related to distinguishing between single and double stars and he assigned the limits of visual resolution to the dimensions of the receptive fibres in the retina. Descartes assumed that the retina consisted of the endings of the fibres of the optic nerve. Since these were of a particular size, he argued that no object smaller than a fibre could be resolved. The possibility of measuring this limit to visual resolution was initially undertaken by Descartes' correspondent, the mathematician, musician, and Minim, Marin Mersenne (1588–1648). Mersenne (1651) acknowledged that it was difficult to determine 'the smallest angle that is visible' because of differences in the acuteness of eyes. Nonetheless, he stated that a grain of sand (with an estimated diameter of 0.225 mm) could be seen from a distance of 10 or 12 feet. Mersenne calculated that a grain at this distance subtended an angle of 15″ at the eye.

Hooke (1705), too, saw the significance of Descartes' speculation to his measures of visual acuity, and he drew attention to them in his lectures on light:

The discerning Power of the Sense is not capable of making Distinction of Parts when they are smaller than such a Bulk, the Terminus of which, I find to my Eye, to be when the Representation is about the Bigness of the smaller Pores of Wood. . . . But the Eye being then at most but capable of seeing or distinguishing those Pores; it follows, that (if the Cause of that Distinction be from the ends of the Filaments of the Optic Nerve, as *Des Cartes* ingeniously supposes) the Filaments cannot be smaller than the Microscopical Pores of Wood, and that the Eye is incapable of distinguishing the Parts of any Picture that are smaller than those: So that any Object being so far removed from the Eye as to make the Picture of it on the Retina less than a Microscopical Pore, that Object becomes invisible. . . . The Power of the Eye is limited to a certain Magnitude of Appearance, under which nothing can be distinctly perceived: Whatsoever Object therefore affects the Eye under a less Angle than that Eye can distinguish, becomes invisible or not seen. Now whereas most Eyes distinguish not a less Angle than a Minute, or the 60th part of a Degree, or the 21600 part of a Circle, therefore whatever is sensated or seen by it, is seen of that Bigness or under that Angle: And so if there be 2 or 3, or 10 or 100 small Stars so near together as that they are all comprised within the Angle of one Minute, the Eye has a Sensation of them all, as if they were one Star, and distinguishes them not one from another. . . . And the *Retina* being like a piece of Plush, with the ends of the Threads turn'd towards the *Crystalline*, all the other ends of them being terminated in the *Brain*, there can be no more distinct Sensations than there are distinct Threads to convey the Impression on them: So that if the whole Picture of the Object be smaller than one single Thread of this Plush, it cannot affect or move a less part than one of those small Threads or Filaments of the *Retina*, and therefore the Sensation is the same as if the Object did take up or cover the whole end of the Thread or Filament, though it affect but a tenth part of it provided it be strong. (Hooke, 1705, pp. 12, and 97–98, original italics)

Porterfield (1738) assumed that the limits of visual acuity were based on the size of the retinal elements themselves, and 'this Experiment of Dr. *Hook*'s, serving to determine the *minimum visibile*, affords us a pretty certain Proof of the Magnitude of our nervous Fibres' (p. 250, original italics). The existence of retinal receptors was not known at that time, and the retina was thought to be composed of the terminations of the optic nerve fibres. The value

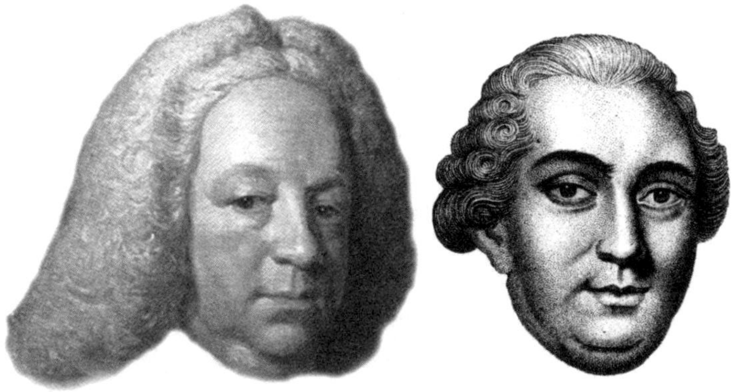

Figure 2.16
Left, James Jurin (1684–1750) after an illustration in Robinson (1980). Right, Comte de Buffon (George Louis Leclerc; 1707–1788) after a frontispiece engraving in Le Clerc (1866).

he derived for a minimum visible of one minute was one 7,200th part of an inch 'which is a surprizing and almost inconceivable Smallness' (p. 252). He also noted that birds of prey are likely to have both more acute vision and even smaller retinal fibres. Smith (1738) determined the limit of visual acuity to be about two-thirds of a minute, a value that was confirmed by James Jurin (1684–1750; Fig. 2.16, left) in his *Essay on distinct and indistinct vision*, appended to Smith's *Opticks*. However, Jurin (1738) noted that different values were obtained for detecting a separation between two pins and detecting a single pin.

Porterfield assumed that the most distinct vision was found on the optic axis. The optic axis is the line passing through the centres of all the optical elements of the eye. It does not coincide with the visual axis, which is the line passing from the point of fixation to the fovea. The two lines intersect at the nodal point of the eye (see Howard and Rogers, 1995). Wells (1792) described a simple procedure for distinguishing between them: when a candle flame is aligned with its reflection in a mirror, the reflected corneal image is not in the centre of the cornea. The observation was astute because the angular difference is only about 5°.

Nonetheless, the distinction between the optic and visual axes was rarely made even by those who are known for advancing visual science. For example, Purkinje (1823*a*) stated:

> Firstly, it is to be noted that every movement by means of which the centre of the visual field, where vision is clearest, is directed appropriately back and forth to those contours and lines of external objects. With small objects, e.g., letters, it is only with the greatest difficulty that these movements can be sensed in your own eyes, but it is much easier with larger objects. (pp. 158–159)

Purkinje included a section on eye movements in his book on subjective vision (see Wade and Brožek, 2001), and described the differences between scanning shapes like circles and lines. He suggested that it was easier to follow the contours of a circle than those of a line. This topic was to be returned to in the following century, as will be described in Chapter 4. Purkinje's speculations on eye movements were cursory and so it remains a paradox that one of the main modern methods employed to measure eye movements utilizes Purkinje images. The use to which he put them himself was in determining the movements of the lens in accommodation (see Section 2.4.1).

A similar sentiment regarding eye movements and distinct vision was expressed by Ernst Heinrich Weber (1795–1878; 1834):

> Eyes have the most acute vision in a particular structure: an object that falls on the axis of the retina is distinguished very clearly, but objects located beside it lose clarity the further from the retinal axis their image falls. If we observe very carefully, we notice that the part of the retina where the images are clearly distinguished is very small. So if we wish to perceive any line accurately and take in its length with the eye, we move the eye so that individual parts of the line fall on the retinal axis in turn. We get to know the length of the line by the movement of the eye, of which we are conscious, in the same manner as we discover the length of an object by movement of the finger. (Translated in Ross and Murray, 1978, p. 101)

Weber (1846) was able to draw on further information, particularly that gathered by Hueck (1840), who determined visual acuity at a range of eccentricities, noting that the value at 5° was three times worse than that at the centre. Weber also made a statement about the lack of awareness of eye movements over a scene that was almost the same as that given by Porterfield (1737) a century earlier. Volkmann examined not only visual resolution in distinct vision but he also charted its change with eccentricity. The stimuli he used were threads from a spider's web and he determined the minimum visible as 8″ (Volkmann, 1836). In later studies he assessed visual resolution in the peripheral retina for both point and thread stimuli (Volkmann, 1846). Using a black dot two observers were in reasonably close agreement for the measures taken from 0° to 60°. Acuity dropped off gradually in the first 5°, and then more rapidly; at 15° it was ten times worse than when fixating.

While studies of distinct vision and oculomotor anatomy provided key insights into the functions of eye movements and the necessity for making them, they did not address the details of the eye movements themselves. For this, methods for objectively measuring the eye movements were required (see Chapter 4). As we discussed in Chapter 1, one of the earliest such methods was to use an afterimage of a bright source of illumination. The displacement of the afterimage during eye movements could then be used to provide insights into the nature of these movements.

2.6 Afterimages

Afterimages can be seen following either brief, intense illumination of the eye or prolonged fixation on an illuminated stimulus. Thus, looking briefly at a bright light can result in its continued visibility when the eyes are closed, or directed away from the light to a uniform surface. The term 'afterimage' (Nachbild) itself was used by Purkinje (1823*a*) in the final section of his book on subjective vision, and it was taken up by Fechner (1838) in his more detailed study of them; it has since superceded the other names given to them. They are phenomena that have thrown light on the understanding of vision and eye movements. A survey of afterimages is beyond the purview of this book but their importance in unravelling the nature of eye movements cannot be overemphasized. Aristotle provided a description of the phenomenon:

> When we have looked steadily for a long while at one colour, e.g., at white or green, that to which we next transfer our gaze appears to be of the same colour. Again if, after having looked at the sun or some other brilliant object, we close the eyes, then, if we watch carefully, it appears in a right line with the direction of vision (whatever this may be), at first in its own colour; then it changes to crimson, next to purple, until it becomes black and disappears. (Ross, 1931, p. 459b)

Aristotle said that the colour of the afterimage was the same as that of the stimulus previously fixated; in modern parlance this would be called a positive afterimage. These are less often seen following fixation on coloured than on black and white stimuli. The consequences of looking at an intense light were also described: the afterimage was visible with closed eyes, and it appeared in whatever direction the eyes were pointing. Moreover, there is a suggestion that the sequence of colours is rapid, and this has been corroborated by many others (see Berry, 1922; Plateau, 1878). Indeed, it was called the flight of colours by Helmholtz (1867*a*).

A technique that was rapidly adopted, once it had been described by Franciscus Aguilonius (1567–1617; 1613), was to form a patterned afterimage following fixation on a paned window: a negative afterimage resulted from such observation. That is, the parts of the afterimage that corresponded to the glass panes looked dark, whereas the bars appeared brighter. In 1639 Benedetto Castelli (1557–1643; see Ariotti, 1973) pursued this in a more systematic manner in his remarkable study of afterimages which also set out a number of their critical features. He used a stimulus (a lead framed window) which afforded good fixation: with the eyes closed, the afterimage retained the shape of the window and it passed through a sequence of colours. The visibility of the afterimage was itself cyclical: it faded from view only to reappear and fade again. With the eyes open, the apparent size of the afterimage varied with the distance of the surface onto which it was projected. This last observation was made with greater precision in the late nineteenth century (Emmert, 1881), and it is commonly referred to as Emmert's law.

The dangers of looking at the sun are evident from the description given by an acquaintance of Robert Boyle (1627–1691; 1663) who was foolish enough to observe the sun through a telescope. The fact that he was able to see the effects of this unwise procedure a decade later suggests strongly that he destroyed the retinal cells in the observing eye; what he noted subsequently was the scotoma so formed. Nonetheless, both Newton (1691) and Nicolas Malebranche (1638–1715; 1699) followed a similar procedure. Newton viewed the sun's image reflected in a mirror, as he described in a letter to John Locke. His interest in the phenomenon was a consequence of reading Boyle's account, which he repeated 'with the hazard of my eyes'. He might well have damaged his eyesight since the 'phantasm' remained visible long after the initial observation of the sun. Having formed the afterimage, Newton noted that it could be retained for longer by winking, and that it seemed to be influenced by attention. He was so disturbed by the phenomenon that he shut himself in a dark room for three days 'to recover the use of my eyes'. He wrote that:

> I looked a very little while upon the sun in the looking-glass with my right eye, and then turned my eyes into a dark corner of my chamber, and

winked, to observe the impression made, and the circles of colours which encompassed it, and how they decayed by degrees, and at last vanished. This I repeated a second and a third time. At the third time, when the phantasm of light and colours about it were almost vanished, intending my fancy upon them to see their last appearance, I found to my amazement, that they began to return, and by little and little to become as lively and vivid as when I had newly looked upon the sun. But when I ceased to intende my fancy upon them, they vanished again. After this, I found that as often as I went into the dark, and intended my mind upon them, as when a man looks earnestly to see any thing which is difficult to be seen, I could make the phantasm return without looking any more upon the sun; and the oftener I made it return, the more easily I could make it return again. And at length, by repeating this without looking any more upon the sun, I made such an impression on my eye, that if I looked upon the clouds, or a book, or any bright object, I saw upon it a round bright spot of light like the sun; and, which is still stranger, though I looked upon the sun with my right eye only, and not with my left, yet my fancy began to make the impression upon my left eye, as well as upon my right. For if I shut my right eye, or looked upon a book or the clouds with my left eye, I could see the spectrum of the sun almost as plain as with my right eye, if I did but intende my fancy a little while upon it; for at first, if I shut my right eye, and looked with my left, the spectrum of the sun did not appear till I intended my fancy upon it; but by repeating, this appeared every time more easily. (1691/1829, pp. 217–218)

Newton not only described the phenomenal characteristics of afterimages with accuracy but he also gave an indication of the central involvement in their visibility; generating an afterimage in one eye resulted in its visibility when the other eye was used. In the eighteenth century the general features of afterimages were adumbrated by both Jurin and Comte de Buffon (1707–1788; Fig. 2.16, right). Jurin's contribution was to propose the principle of reciprocal action for afterimages:

These, and many more *phænomena* of like kind, seem to depend upon the principle, that when we have been for some time affected with one sensation, as soon as we cease to be so affected, a contrary sensation is apt to arise in us, sometimes of itself, and sometimes from such causes, as at another time would not produce the sensation at all, or at least not to the same degree. (Jurin, 1738, p. 169, original italics)

The afterimage of the window was in the opposite contrast to that seen under normal viewing, and so the processes in the retina that produced the afterimage were the reverse of those generated by the primary stimulus. Buffon (1743) stated a similar relation with respect to coloured afterimages: objects of one colour produce afterimages that are complementary. Buffon introduced the term accidental colours to describe them, and to distinguish them from natural colours.

With the establishment of the basic features of afterimages, they began to be used as a tool to investigate other aspects of vision—particularly those involving eye movements. The apparent motion of afterimages with voluntary eye movements was seen by some, like Wells, to offer the opportunity of maintaining a stable retinal image despite eye movements. A distinction could then be made between effects due to eye movements and those that were a consequence of motion over the retina. Wells (1792) provided a clear example of this by applying afterimages to examine aspects of binocular visual direction. He also distinguished between the effects of active and passive eye movements on the visual direction of afterimages.

The two nineteenth century researches who conducted the most extensive investigations into afterimages were Joseph Plateau (1801–1883; Fig. 2.17, left) and Gustav Fechner (1801–1887; Fig. 2.17, right), both of whom suffered sorely for their science, as did Newton before them. Fechner was a professor of physics at Leipzig University when he conducted his afterimage experiments. However, the frequency with which he had observed the sun damaged his eyesight, and might have played a part in inducing a crisis that resulted in resignation from his chair, and in his shunning of company and comforts for some years. When he did emerge from this crisis his concerns shifted first towards philosophy and then to psychophysics (Fechner, 1860), which transformed the study of the senses.

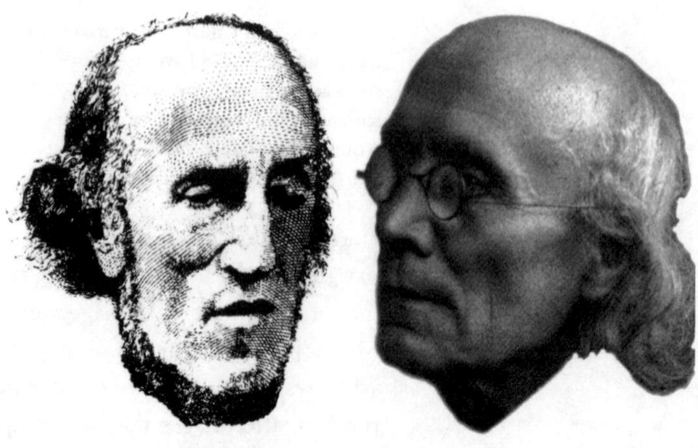

Figure 2.17

Left, Joseph Antoine Ferdinand Plateau (1801–1883) after an engraving in Nuttin (1961). Right, Gustav Theodor Fechner (1801–1887) after a frontispiece photogravure in Kuntze (1892).

The most complete historical survey of afterimages was presented by Plateau (1878); he gave a brief summary of accounts before 1800, and an annotated bibliography is provided for those between 1800 and 1876. It is a sad irony that Plateau himself was blind when he compiled his history. Although he considered that his blindness was a consequence of forming afterimages by observing the sun, this is unlikely to have been the case. In the course of conducting his doctoral research on visual persistence (Plateau, 1829) he often looked at the sun for as long as half a minute, following which he suffered from retinitis. However, his blindness, which became total in 1843, would seem to have been due to uveitis (Verriest, 1990).

2.7 William Charles Wells

Throughout this book we will champion the case for Wells as being one of the founders of research on eye movements. Alas, as with William Porterfield, it appears that no portrait of him was either made or exists. An approximation of his likeness might be found in Fig. 2.18, left, which is of his sister, and the title page of his book on binocular vision is shown there too (Fig. 2.18, right). Wells was born to Scottish parents (from south-west Scotland) in Charlestown, South Carolina. He spent his early years in Charlestown but was educated in Scotland. He was sent to school at Dumfries and then to Edinburgh University where he graduated in medicine in 1780. He next spent four years in his native America before returning to Britain to practise medicine in London. He was elected a Fellow of the Royal Society in 1793 (on the basis of his *Essay upon single vision with two eyes*) and of the Royal Society of Edinburgh in 1814 (following publication of his *Essay on dew*). His medical practise was not successful, which gave him time to prosecute experiments and observations on a wide range of natural phenomena. His *Essay upon single vision* is relatively rare, and the text has been reprinted in Wade (2003*a*). Wells distinguished between the optical and visual axes of the eye, clarified the action of belladonna on accommodation, related eye movements to binocular visual direction, and examined eye movements during visual vertigo.

Wells (1792) understood that afterimages could be used as a tool to investigate various aspects of vision—particularly those

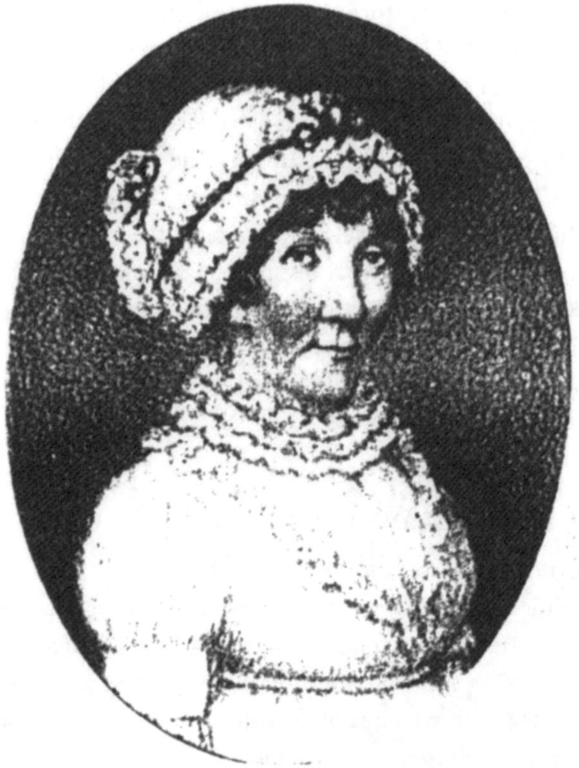

AN

ESSAY

UPON

SINGLE VISION WITH TWO EYES:

TOGETHER WITH

EXPERIMENTS

AND

OBSERVATIONS

ON

SEVERAL OTHER SUBJECTS IN OPTICS.

By WILLIAM CHARLES WELLS, M. D.

LONDON:

PRINTED FOR T. CADELL, IN THE STRAND.

1792.

Figure 2.18

Left, Louisa Susannah Wells (1755–1831), the sister of William Charles Wells, in 1815 (after a frontispiece illustration in Wells, 1906). Right, the title page of Wells' *Essay upon single vision with two eyes*.

involving eye movements. The source generally used by Wells was a candle flame, which was viewed for many seconds to generate an afterimage. For example, he generated afterimages in each eye and noted that the single impression moved with voluntary movements of the eyes, and remained single even with passive movements of one eye. When the afterimage was projected onto a white surface and one eye was displaced, the singleness of the afterimage remained even though the paper onto which it was projected appeared double. This was one of the many subtle demonstrations Wells made with afterimages, and he pursued their implications with penetrating logic.

Wells conducted a series of elegant experiments on eye movements and vertigo, published in 1792 and 1794, which paved the way for much subsequent research, although his publications have been woefully neglected. Wells demonstrated how the eyes moved following rotation of the body around a vertical axis. This was achieved by comparing afterimages (formed before body rotation) with real images (viewed following rotation). He described fast and slow phases of nystagmus, and provided the first account of discontinuous eye movements in vertigo. He related the direction of visual vertigo to head position during rotation. He found that nystagmus could be suppressed by attending to targets. He demonstrated torsional nystagmus by noting the rotation of a horizontal afterimage following rotation with his head tilted backwards. He described the suppression of vision during the fast phase of nystagmus—what we would now call saccadic suppression. These aspects of his research will be described in more detail in Chapter 3.

2.8 Erasmus Darwin's *Zoonomia*

Robert Waring Darwin (1766–1848) presented a paper on ocular spectra (afterimages) to the Royal Society in 1786; its title page is shown in Fig. 2.19, left. The paper was reprinted in its entirety in the first volume of Erasmus Darwin's *Zoonomia*, published in 1794. Erasmus Darwin's portrait was shown in Fig. 1.12. He was born at Elston, near Newark, Nottinghamshire on 12 December 1731. At the age of nine he went to Chesterfield School, proceeding to St John's College, Cambridge in 1750. He studied medicine at Edinburgh University for two years from 1754, and practised as a physician at Lichfield from 1756–1781. His house, close by Lichfield Cathedral, has been restored and is now a museum that reflects many aspects of his rich and rewarding life. Darwin built a successful medical practise at Lichfield, but his interests were not confined to medicine. He formed friendships with major engines of the industrial revolution, like James Brindley (1716–1772), Matthew Boulton (1701–1759), James Watt (1736–1819), Josiah Wedgwood (1730–1795), and Joseph Priestley (1733–1804). From around 1765 onwards they met on the nearest Monday to the full moon; the group later became the Lunar Society of Birmingham (see Uglow, 2002). The final twenty-one years of his life were spent practising medicine at Derby. It was during this period that his fame as a poet and his authority as a physician were firmly established. Darwin's epic poem on vegetable life, *The botanic garden*, was published in two

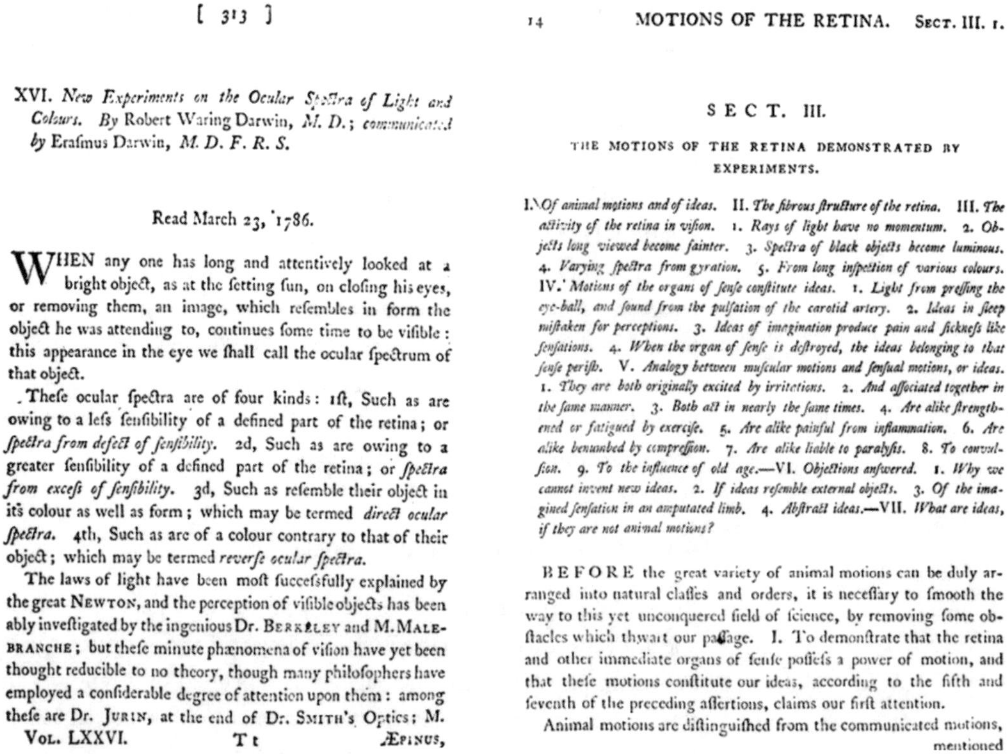

[313]

XVI. *New Experiments on the Ocular Spectra of Light and Colours. By* Robert Waring Darwin, *M. D.; communicated by* Eraſmus Darwin, *M. D. F. R. S.*

Read March 23, 1786.

WHEN any one has long and attentively looked at a bright object, as at the ſetting ſun, on cloſing his eyes, or removing them, an image, which reſembles in form the object he was attending to, continues ſome time to be viſible: this appearance in the eye we ſhall call the ocular ſpectrum of that object.

Theſe ocular ſpectra are of four kinds: 1ſt, Such as are owing to a leſs ſenſibility of a defined part of the retina; or *ſpectra from defect of ſenſibility.* 2d, Such as are owing to a greater ſenſibility of a defined part of the retina; or *ſpectra from exceſs of ſenſibility.* 3d, Such as reſemble their object in its colour as well as form; which may be termed *direct ocular ſpectra.* 4th, Such as are of a colour contrary to that of their object; which may be termed *reverſe ocular ſpectra.*

The laws of light have been moſt ſucceſsfully explained by the great NEWTON, and the perception of viſible objects has been ably inveſtigated by the ingenious Dr. BERKELEY and M. MALEBRANCHE; but theſe minute phænomena of viſion have yet been thought reducible to no theory, though many philoſophers have employed a conſiderable degree of attention upon them: among theſe are Dr. JURIN, at the end of Dr. SMITH's Optics; M.

VOL. LXXVI. Tt ÆPINUS,

14 MOTIONS OF THE RETINA. SECT. III. 1.

SECT. III.

THE MOTIONS OF THE RETINA DEMONSTRATED BY EXPERIMENTS.

I. *Of animal motions and of ideas.* II. *The fibrous ſtructure of the retina.* III. *The activity of the retina in viſion.* 1. *Rays of light have no momentum.* 2. *Objects long viewed become fainter.* 3. *Spectra of black objects become luminous.* 4. *Varying ſpectra from gyration.* 5. *From long inſpection of various colours.* IV. *Motions of the organs of ſenſe conſtitute ideas.* 1. *Light from preſſing the eye-ball, and found from the pulſation of the carotid artery.* 2. *Ideas in ſleep miſtaken for perceptions.* 3. *Ideas of imagination produce pain and ſickneſs like ſenſations.* 4. *When the organ of ſenſe is deſtroyed, the ideas belonging to that ſenſe periſh.* V. *Analogy between muſcular motions and ſenſual motions, or ideas.* 1. *They are both originally excited by irritations.* 2. *And aſſociated together in the ſame manner.* 3. *Both act in nearly the ſame times.* 4. *Are alike ſtrengthened or fatigued by exerciſe.* 5. *Are alike painful from inflammation.* 6. *Are alike benumbed by compreſſion.* 7. *Are alike liable to paralyſis.* 8. *To convulſion.* 9. *To the influence of old age.*—VI. *Objections anſwered.* 1. *Why we cannot invent new ideas.* 2. *If ideas reſemble external objects.* 3. *Of the imagined ſenſation in an amputated limb.* 4. *Abſtract ideas.*—VII. *What are ideas, if they are not animal motions?*

BEFORE the great variety of animal motions can be duly arranged into natural claſſes and orders, it is neceſſary to ſmooth the way to this yet unconquered field of ſcience, by removing ſome obſtacles which thwart our paſſage. I. To demonſtrate that the retina and other immediate organs of ſenſe poſſeſs a power of motion, and that theſe motions conſtitute our ideas, according to the fifth and ſeventh of the preceding aſſertions, claims our firſt attention.

Animal motions are diſtinguiſhed from the communicated motions, mentioned

Figure 2.19

Title pages of (left) Robert Darwin's article on afterimages, published in the *Philosophical Transactions of the Royal Society* in 1786, and (right) the opening page of Erasmus Darwin's chapter on eye movements in *Zoonomia* (1794).

parts in 1789 and 1791, and the two volumes of *Zoonomia*, dealing with animal life, appeared in 1794 and 1796. Robert Darwin was the third son of his first marriage. His wife, Mary, died in 1770 and Erasmus married Elizabeth Pole in 1781. Details of Darwin's life can be found in King-Hele (1999, 2002).

Erasmus Darwin's work conflates two traditions regarding the study of eye movements—the philosophical and the medical. Empiricist philosophers have used muscular movements as an explanatory tool for educating vision about three-dimensional space. Paradoxically, the concerns of physicians have been more empirical, that is, more practical. They have observed movements of the eyes, particularly when they have been abnormal. This usually applied to squint, or strabismus, which was one of the first topics Darwin addressed. He was an empiricist in the mould of Bishop Berkeley (1709). He believed that our perception of space was a consequence of motions within it. Darwin incorporated motion as a fundamental part of perception: 'The word *perception* includes both the action of the organ of sense in consequence of the impact of external objects, and our attention to that action; that is, it expresses both the motion of the organ of sense, or idea, and the pain or pleasure that succeeds or accompanies it'. (E. Darwin, 1794, p. 12, original italics)

The sections of *Zoonomia* concerned with vision embraced the dimension of motion in general and eye movements in particular. One was entitled 'The motions of the retina demonstrated by experiment' (Fig. 2.19, right) and the other was on 'Vertigo'. *Zoonomia* itself has an interesting history. The first volume was published in 1794, with the second edition of it in 1796; the first edition of the second volume appeared in that year too. Volume 1 contained Darwin's survey of organic life, and volume 2 presented his classification of diseases. The third edition was published in four volumes in 1801. Some significant changes in the sections on vision were made over the three editions. Erasmus Darwin commenced the section on motions of the retina:

> BEFORE the great variety of animal motions can be duly arranged into natural classes and orders, it is necessary to smooth the way to this yet unconquered field of science, by removing some obstacles which thwart our passage. I. To demonstrate that the retina and other immediate organs of sense possess a power of motion, and that these motions constitute our ideas. (1794, p. 14)

Thus, Darwin embraced the long philosophical tradition that held eye movements close to its theoretical heart. Eye movements were of value to the empiricists, but prior to Darwin they were rarely examined empirically. That is, the ways in which the eyes moved were not investigated. Rather, eye movements provided a useful theoretical weapon with which empiricists could attack nativist ideas about the perception of space, and it provided a vehicle for explaining perceptual learning. Muscular sensations could be associated with visual stimulation, and the third dimension of space could slowly be learnt.

Prior to the publication of *Zoonomia*, Darwin (1778) had written an article on squinting, and he had established an enduring interest in afterimages. In a letter to Benjamin Franklin (1706–1790), in January 1774, he noted that:

> I have another very curious Paper containing Experiments on the Colours seen in the closed Eye after having gazed some Time on luminous Objects, which is not quite transcribed, but which I will send you, if you think it is

likely to be acceptable to the [Royal] Society at this Time, but will otherwise let it lie by me another year. (Willcox, 1978, p. 25).

This paper was not published under his name but was, perhaps, expressed indirectly through the article by his son (R. Darwin, 1786). This article was reprinted in its entirety as Section XL of *Zoonomia*, and large parts of the section on 'Motions of the retina' were derived from it. Robert's son, Charles, suggested that rather more than a little help was provided by Erasmus to Robert in both the article, and the dissertation on which it was based. In his *Life of Erasmus Darwin* Charles wrote of the article that 'I believe he was largely aided in writing it by his father' (C. Darwin, 1887, p. 84). In the footnote to the reprint of Franklin's letter (which is published in Franklin, 1765/1970), Willcox (1978) suggests that they collaborated on it. The language of the article bears a close similarity to that in which Erasmus cloaks diseases in *Zoonomia*. We cannot determine the extent to which it corresponds to Robert's later publications, because there were none. The article described positive and negative afterimages in both their achromatic and chromatic aspects, the fragmentation of patterned afterimages, and the variation in the apparent size of the afterimage with the distance of the surface on which it is projected. A simple 'tadpole' demonstration was described in which a black shape was fixated for some time and then projected on to white paper; a negative afterimage could be seen, and it appeared whiter than the paper itself. The interpretation of this effect was essentially in terms of differential retinal adaptation. The visibility of afterimages could be revived by intermittent stimulation (moving the hand in front of the eyes), and it was noted that there can be a latency before the afterimage is initially visible.

Erasmus Darwin also devoted considerable space to the topic of vertigo in *Zoonomia*. Like afterimages, this phenomenon had a long observational history but relatively little advance had been made in determining its cause. This was largely because little was known about the functions of the vestibular system (Wade, 2000*b*, 2003*b*). Vertigo assumed a role of enormous importance in understanding the dynamics of eye movements, and it will be treated in detail in Chapter 3. Again, afterimages proved to be the essential tool for distinguishing between the fast and slow phases of nystagmus, and they were demonstrated by Wells, who became an opponent of Erasmus Darwin.

Neither Darwin (1794) nor Wells (1792) set out to study eye movements. Like many writers before them, their initial perceptual interests were in binocular vision and its breakdown as a consequence of strabismus. Wells' monograph was on binocular single vision, a topic that had a long history at that time. However, he was concerned with examining the relative positions of the eyes during single vision, and it is in this context, as well as the interest that Darwin and Wells shared in vertigo, that key early insights into the details of eye movements were revealed. Prior to Darwin and Wells the field lacked a means of determining how the eyes moved with any degree of objective precision. However, Darwin and Wells were able to provide the crucial first steps towards objective measurements of eye movements in their use of afterimages to study visual vertigo.

3

Nystagmus

3.1 Introduction

The first phenomenon to lend support to Porterfield's suggestion that the eyes engaged in a 'quick and almost continual motion' was nystagmus, although Porterfield did little to hasten its experimental support. Nystagmus refers to the slow movements of the eyes in one direction followed by their rapid return. The term derives from the nodding movements of the head when in a drowsy state—the head drops slowly and then is jerked back. The similar smooth and jerky movements of the eyes can be elicited in a number of ways and are associated with a variety of maladies. The visual and postural disturbances that accompany nystagmus are referred to as vertigo. A simple way of inducing nystagmus is to rotate the upright head and body around a vertical axis with the eyes open. This results first in the eyes remaining fixed on an external object and therefore rotating slowly in the direction opposite to the body and then they jerk rapidly in the direction of body rotation, only for this cycle to be repeated. If the body rotation continues for very long then nausea is produced. However, when the body stops rotating suddenly the eyes do not: they engage in similar phases of fast and slow rotations but in the directions opposite to those that were induced during rotation. This has been called after-nystagmus (Duke-Elder, 1932) and its slow phase is in the direction of prior body rotation. It is accompanied by an apparent rotation of the surroundings (visual vertigo) and its investigation by Wells led to the first systematic accounts of discontinuous eye movements.

The attraction of Wells' (1792) experiments on eye movements was that he distinguished between subjective impressions of how the eyes moved, derived from some feeling of movement within the orbit, and a more objective method of assessing them. Porterfield (1759*b*) had relied upon the former: following body rotation the eyes did not feel as though they were moving, but the rotation of the visual world was compelling. Wells was able to confirm this, but it was due to a 'happy accident' that he was led to doubt the value of such subjective impressions. Wells was conducting an experiment on binocular afterimages, formed by fixating a candle flame for some time. While the afterimage was still visible he had a bout of dizziness, or giddiness as he called it, during which the afterimage was observed to move, but he did not have any feeling that his eyes were moving. As a consequence, he placed little trust in his subjective impressions of eye rotations, and sought to use the afterimage as a technique for examining the ways in which the eyes did move: 'During a slight fit of giddiness I was accidentally seized with, a coloured spot [afterimage], occasioned by looking steadily at a luminous body, and upon which I happened at that moment to be making an experiment, was moved in a manner altogether independent of the positions I conceived my eyes to possess' (Wells, 1792, p. 95).

There was yet another obvious method for examining eye movements: to observe the eyes of another person. Although this is obvious to us, it was rarely employed in studies of vertigo. Wells did use this to confirm his own afterimage observations of post-rotational eye movements. He asked another person to rotate until they felt giddy, when they stopped Wells observed their eyes: 'To have the same thing proved in another way, I desired a person to turn quickly round, till he became very giddy; then to stop himself and look stedfastly at me. He did so, and I could plainly see, that, although he thought his eyes were fixed, they were in reality moving in their sockets, first toward one side, and then toward the other' (Wells, 1792, p. 97).

The experiments conducted by Wells should have heralded a new chapter in eye movement research but they did not. His observations and experiments were not used as a springboard for more detailed investigations. They were ignored in a manner that seems with hindsight to be inexplicable. The method he adopted was to compare the movement and position of an afterimage with that of a real image. The method was to be rediscovered in the nineteenth century, first in the context of eye position following an eye movement (see Chapter 4), and later for noting the pattern of eye movements themselves.

3.2 Visual vertigo

Vertigo involves not only apparent visual motion but apparent body motion too. When extreme it can induce nausea, vomiting, and disturbances of balance. It has been a source of interest since antiquity and it is a phenomenon that is associated with the first measurements of eye movements. Because it is a condition that accompanies many diseases, vertigo has been a source of constant interest and speculation, particularly in medical circles. Vertigo can be induced in healthy individuals in a variety of ways. For example, Aristotle (Fig. 3.1, left) described the vertiginous effects of alcohol: 'Why is it that to those who are very drunk everything seems to revolve in a circle, and as soon as the wine takes a hold of them they cannot see objects at a distance?... objects near at hand are not seen in their proper places, but appear to revolve in a circle' (Ross, 1927, p. 892*a*).

According to the fourth century Roman commentator, Diogenes Laertius, Aristotle's pupil Theophrastus (ca. 370–286 BC; Fig. 3.1, right) had written a book on vertigo but it had been lost by that date. This is a great loss, as Theophrastus was an astute and critical observer, as is evident from his book *On the senses* that has survived (Stratton, 1917).

In addition to vertigo caused by alcohol, an even simpler way of inducing it has long been known to children—whirling the body around quickly and then stopping suddenly. The Roman

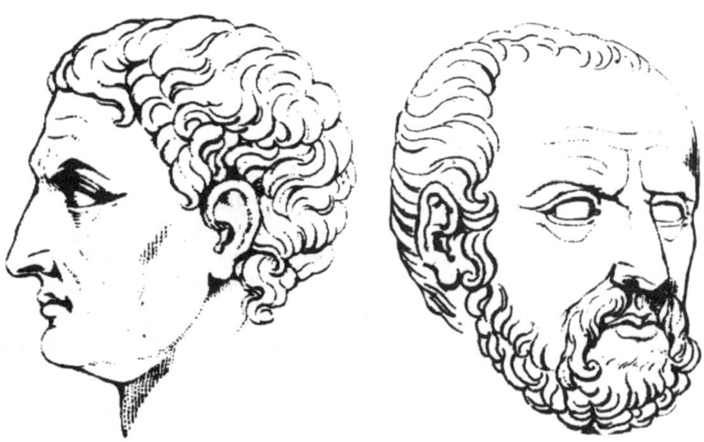

Figure 3.1
Left, Aristotle (ca. 384–322 BC) after an engraving in *The historic gallery of portraits and paintings*. Vol. 5. (1810) London: Vernor, Hood, and Sharpe. Right, Theophrastus (ca. 370–286 BC) after an engraving in *The historic gallery of portraits and paintings*. Vol. 4. (1809) London: Vernor, Hood, and Sharpe.

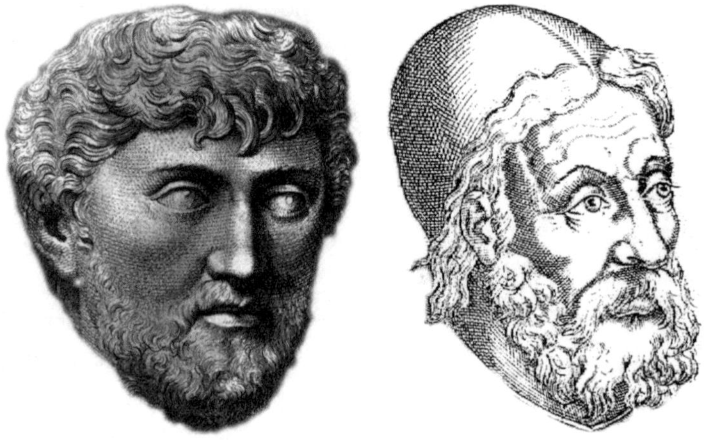

Figure 3.2
Left, Titus Carus Lucretius (ca. 98–55 BC) after an illustration in Wood (1880). Right, Claudius Ptolemy (ca. 100–170) after an engraving kindly provided by the Bibliothèque nationale de France.

poet, Titus Carus Lucretius (ca. 98–55 BC; Fig. 3.2, left), commented on the consequences of such body rotation: 'The room seems to children to be turning round and the columns revolving when they themselves have ceased to turn, so much so that they can hardly believe all the building is not threatening to fall in upon them' (1975, pp. 307–309). Somewhat later, Ptolemy (Fig. 3.2, right) indicated that vertigo could be caused by visual stimulation: 'A particular type of continuous sweep of the visual ray gives the impression that the visible object is moving. This sort of sweep sometimes occurs at the very source of the visual flux, as happens, for instance, in the case of vertigo and fainting, whose effect reaches the eye itself'. (Smith, 1996, p. 119)

Galen also made reference to vertigo caused by observing whirling patterns as well as body rotation. These were described in the context of diseases which lead to dizziness:

> All these affections start obviously in the head and especially the affection which is called *skotoma* (vertigo), the name of which indicates its nature. People who are subject to this ailment are affected by *skotoma* of their vision on account of the smallest causes, so that they often fall, especially when they turn round. Then, what happens to other people only after having turned round a great many times, that will overcome these people after one single turn. They can even be affected by vertigo, when they see another person or a wheel turning or anything else which whirls, even when their head had been overheated for any other reason . . . There is general agreement upon the fact that such frequent turning movements provoke an unequal, tumultuous and disorderly flow of humors and pneuma. Therefore it is only natural that people subject to skotoma are on guard against any motion of this kind. (Siegel, 1970, p. 138, original italics)

3.2.1 Early history of vertigo

All these effects have been reported repeatedly since antiquity, and occasionally novel sources of inducing vertigo have been described. For instance, Paulus Ægineta (ca. 680) noted that:

> Vertigo is occasioned by a cold and viscid humour seizing upon the brain, whence the patients are ready to fall down from a very slight cause, such as sometimes from looking at any external object which turns round, as a wheel or top, or when they themselves are whirled round, or when their head has been heated, by which means the humours or spirit in it are set in motion. (1844, p. 374)

Felix Platter (Fig. 3.3, left) and Thomas Willis (1621–1675; Fig. 3.3, right) heralded the early modern era by suggesting mechanistic interpretations for vertigo in terms of motion of the animal spirit in the brain. Platter observed that: 'An intense, uniform, and extended movement of the head transfers itself in a similar way to the spiritus. Despite holding the head still afterwards, it appears to continue moving for a while, before it eventually feels still. This is the basis for dizziness, if one rotates the head and body in a circle for a long time'. (Koelbing, 1967, p. 89)

Willis defined vertigo as 'an affection in which visible objects appear to rotate' (1672, p. 353), and devoted a chapter to describing its pathology and the conditions that can induce it in healthy individuals, including body rotation. Platter and Willis interpreted vertigo in Galenic terms: motion of the animal spirit in the head produced the apparent motion during rotation, rather

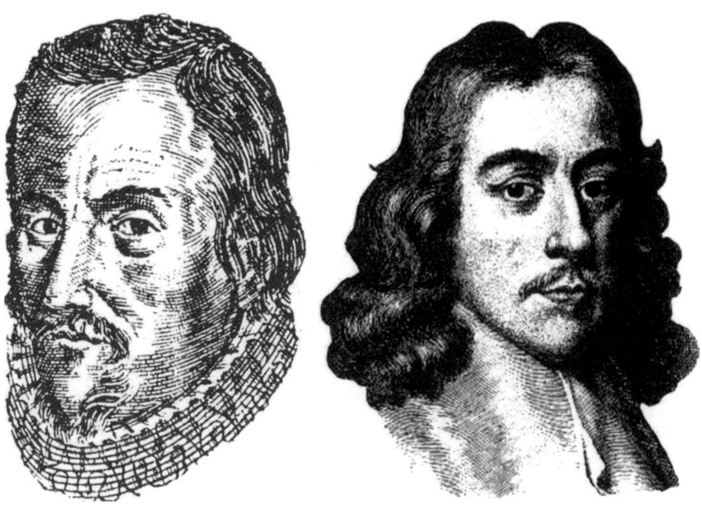

Figure 3.3
Left, Felix Platter (1536–1614) after an engraving in Freher (1688). Right, Thomas Willis (1621–1675) after an engraving in Birch (1743).

like smoke in a flask lagging behind that of the rotating vessel. Willis described the visual motion that continues after body rotation ceases, and this was attributed to the continued motions of the animal spirit relative to the stationary head. He accounted for it graphically in his Oxford lectures:

> Vertigo arises from the circular motion of the spirits, and, as it were, their rotations in the brain and its medullary part. It takes place just as smoke and vapour contained in a glass or phial are sent into similar motion if you spin the vessel round. This motion lasts longer in the smoke or vapour than in the vessel. Thus we find people whose spirits are very thin, and therefore flexible and weak, pass into vertigo as soon as the body or head is rotated and this sensation persists after the body has ceased its turning motion. (Dewhurst, 1980, pp. 113–114)

So little was then known about the functions of the brain that this interpretation was held for a long time. Even when the attraction of the animal spirit was waning the logic of the explanation was retained. In his medical text on vertigo Herz (1786) modified the interpretation slightly by referring to movement of nervous humours in the brain rather than animal spirits, but how these humours moved remained mysterious.

Towards the end of the eighteenth century, Boissier de Sauvages (1772*a*,*b*) discussed vertigo in his classification of diseases, and described it as: 'An hallucination which takes place when stationary objects appear to move and rotate around us... The cause of vertigo is nothing other than an impression on the retina which is equivalent to that excited by objects that paint their images successively on different parts of that membrane' (Boissier de Sauvages, 1772*b*, p. 50). He drew parallels with visual persistence with rapidly moving lights, and suggested that the sensitivity of the retina was changed by the retrograde movements of blood in the vessels supplying it. He did discuss the effects of body rotation, and the possibility of unconscious eye movements during and after rotation were entertained. An alternative to speculating on processes in the retina or brain was to study the phenomenon of vertigo itself. Interest in vertigo was principally medical, and most observations upon it were made in that context. For example, Robert Whytt (1714–1766; Fig. 3.4) included giddiness amongst the symptoms for nervous diseases:

> Many people of a delicate, nervous, and vascular system, after stooping and suddenly raising their head, are apt to be seized with a *vertigo*, which is

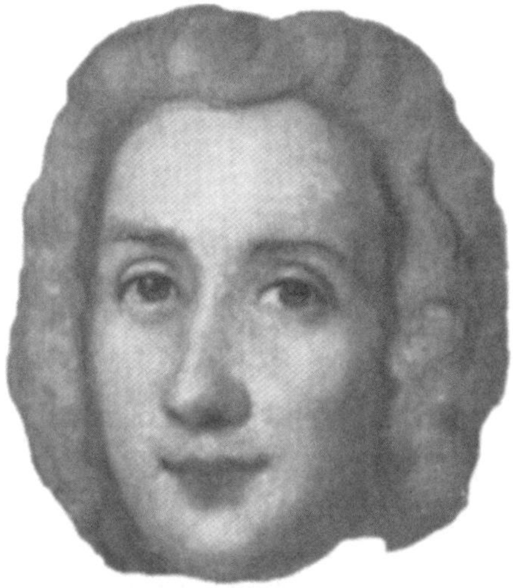

Figure 3.4
Robert Whytt (1714–1766) after an illustration in Comrie (1932).

sometimes accompanied by faintness. In this case, the vessels of the brain being too weak, seem to yield more than usual to the weight of the blood, when the head is inclined; and afterwards, when it is suddenly raised, and the blood at once descends towards the heart, those vessels do not contract fast enough, so as to accommodate themselves to the quantity of blood remaining in them: At the same time the brain, on account of its too great sensibility, is more affected than usual, by any sudden change in the motion of the fluids through its vessels. (1765, p. 309, original italics)

At least these were mechanistic interpretations relating vertigo to processes, like blood flow, that were open to experimental enquiry. However, it was Porterfield's (1759*b*) observations and speculations regarding the link between eye movements and post-rotational visual motion that stimulated renewed interest in the visual dimension of vertigo. Motion was the last of the phenomena of vision described in the second volume of Porterfield's *Treatise*, and his analysis of it was subtle: 'Our eyes do never inform us of what Magnitude or Celerity of Motion is, considered absolutely and in itself, but only what it is relatively, when compared to some other Motion' (1759*b*, p. 417). He went on to list a range of motion phenomena, including a lucid definition of visually induced motion. Vertigo was the final phenomenon discussed:

But, before I dismiss this Subject, I shall endeavour to explain another *Phænomenon* of Motion, which, tho' very common, and well known, yet, so far as I know, has not as yet had any Solution given to it. If a Person turns swiftly round, without changing his Place, all Objects about will seem to move in a Circle to the contrary Way, and the Deception continues, not only when the Person himself moves round, but, which is more surprising, it also continues for some time after he stops moving, when the Eye, as well as the Objects, are at absolute Rest. (Porterfield, 1759*b*, pp. 424–425, original italics)

Porterfield sought to accommodate visual vertigo within his broad analysis of visual motion. He appreciated that visual motion was not restricted to motion over the retina, and that vertigo was a consequence of an error in the assignment of motion:

By the Sight alone, we can never determine how far this Motion belongs to the Object, how far to the Eye, or how far to both. If we imagine the Eye at rest we ascribe the whole Motion to the Object, tho' it be truly at rest; if we imagine the Object at rest, we ascribe the whole Motion to the Eye, tho' it belongs entirely to the Object; and when the Eye is in Motion, tho' we are not sensible of its Motion, yet if we do not imagine that it moves so swiftly as it really does, we ascribe only Part of the Motion to the Eye, and the rest to the Object, tho' it be truly at rest. And this last is what happens in the present Case when the Eye turns round; for tho' we are sensible of the Motion of the Eye, yet we do not apprehend that it moves so fast as it truly does; and therefore the Bodies about appear to move in the contrary Way, as is agreeable to Experience. But the great Difficulty still remains, *viz.* Why, after the Eye ceases to move, Objects should for some Time still appear to continue in Motion, tho' the Pictures on the *Retina* be truly at rest, and do not at all change their Place. This, I imagine, proceeds from a Mistake we are in, with respect to the Eye; which, tho' it be absolutely at rest, we nevertheless conceive it as moving the contrary way to that in which it moved before: From which Mistake with respect to the Motion of the Eye, the Objects at rest will appear to move in the same way, which the Eye is imagined to move in, and consequently will seem to continue their Motion for some Time after the Eye is at rest. (Porterfield, 1759*b*, pp. 425–426, original italics)

In modern terminology Porterfield was suggesting that it was the signals for eye movements, rather than the eye movements themselves, that generated the post-rotational visual motion, and he supported his analysis with an illustration (see Fig. 5.8). The relationship between eye movements and visual motion illusions will be examined in greater detail in Chapter 5.

3.3 Wells on vertigo

There is little in the title of Wells' *Essay* to indicate that it is concerned with vertigo and eye movements. Indeed, even the full title (*An essay upon single vision with two eyes: together with experiments and observations on several other subjects in optics*) provides scant indication of the import his experiments and observations bore on subsequent eye movement research. The 'several other subjects in optics' were four in number and addressed visual position and motion, visual persistence, convergence and accommodation, and finally distinct vision. Vertigo, or giddiness as he calls it, was discussed under the first of these. His experiments and observations were so concisely described that they bear repeating in full, despite the fact that small sections have been given earlier.

It being my intention to treat, in the present article, of several facts relative to visible position and motion, which seem to me to need explanation, without regarding whether or not they depend upon any common cause; I pass to the consideration of the apparent rotation of objects, when we have become giddy, by turning ourselves quickly and frequently round. Some of the older writers upon optics imagined the visive spirits to be contained in the head, as water is in a vessel, which therefore, when once put in motion by the rotation of our bodies, must continue in it for some time after this has ceased; and to this real circular movement of the visive spirits, while the body is at rest, they attributed the apparent motions of objects in giddiness. Dechales saw the weakness of this hypothesis, and conjectured, that the phenomenon might be owing to a real movement of the eyes, but produced no fact in proof of his opinion. Dr. Porterfield, on the contrary, supposed the difficulty of explaining it to consist in showing, why objects at rest appear in motion to an eye which is also at rest. The solution he offered of this representation of the phenomenon, is not only extremely ingenious, but is, I believe, the only probable one which can be given. It does not apply, however, to the fact which truly exists; for I shall immediately show, that the eye is not at rest, as he imagined. The last author, I know of, who has touched upon this subject, is Dr. Darwin. His words are, 'When any one turns round rapidly on one foot till he becomes dizzy, and falls upon the ground, the spectra of the ambient objects continue to present themselves in rotation, or appear to librate, and he seems to behold them for some time in motion.' I do not indeed pretend to understand his opinion fully; but this much seems clear, that, if such an apparent motion of the surrounding objects depends, in any way, upon their spectra, or the illusive representations of those objects, occasioned by their former impressions upon the retinas, no similar motion would be observed, were we to turn ourselves round with our eyes shut, and not to open them till we became giddy; for in this case, as the surrounding objects could not send their pictures to the retinas, there would, consequently, be no spectra to present themselves afterward in rotation. But whoever will make the experiment, will find, that objects about him appear to be equally in motion, when he has become giddy by turning himself round, whether this has been done with his eyes open or shut. I shall now venture to propose my own opinion upon this subject. If the eye be at rest, we judge an object to be in motion when its picture falls in succeeding times upon different parts of the retina; and if the eye be in motion, we judge an object to be at rest, as long as the change in the place of its picture upon the retina, holds a certain correspondence with the change of the eye's position. Let us now suppose the eye to be in motion, while, from some disorder in the system of sensation, we are either without those feelings, which indicate the various positions of the eye, or are not able to attend to them. It is evident, that, in such a state of things, an object at rest must appear to be in motion, since it sends in succeeding times its picture to different parts of the retina. And this seems to be what happens in giddiness. I was first led to think so from observing, that, during a slight fit of giddiness I was accidentally seized with, a coloured spot, occasioned by looking steadily at a luminous body, and upon which I happened at that moment to be making an experiment, was moved in a manner altogether independent of the positions I conceived my eyes to possess. To determine this point, I again produced the spot, by looking some time at the flame of a candle; then turning myself round till I became giddy, I suddenly discontinued this motion, and directed my eyes to the middle of a sheet of paper, fixed upon the wall of my chamber. The spot now appeared upon the paper, but only for a moment; for it immediately after seemed to move to one side, and the paper to the other, notwithstanding I conceived the position of my eyes to be in the mean while unchanged. To go on with the experiment, when the paper and spot had proceeded to a certain distance from each other, they suddenly came together again; and this separation and conjunction were alternately repeated a number of times; the limits of the separation gradually becoming less, till, at length, the paper and spot both appeared to be at rest, and the latter to be projected upon the middle of the former. I found also, upon repeating and varying the experiment a little, that when I had turned myself from left to right, the paper moved from right to left, and the spot consequently the contrary way; but that when I had turned from right to left, the paper would then move from left to right. These were the appearances observed while I stood erect. When I inclined, however, my head in such a manner, as to bring the side of my face parallel to the horizon, the spot and paper would then move from each other, one upward and the other downward. But all these phenomena demonstrate, that there was a real motion in my eyes at the time I imagined them to be at rest; for the apparent situation of the spot, with respect to the paper, could not possibly have been altered, without a real change of the position of those organs. To have the same thing proved in another way, I desired a person to turn quickly round, till he became very giddy; then to stop himself and look stedfastly at me. He did so, and I could plainly see, that, although he thought his eyes were fixed, they were in reality moving in their sockets, first toward one side, and then toward the other. (Wells, 1792, pp. 92–97)

In the course of a few pages Wells provided the basis for subsequent research on vertigo as well as eye movements. He is clearly critical of the theories presented by Porterfield (1759b) and Darwin (1786) and provided strong evidence to refute them. Nonetheless, it was not Robert Darwin who responded to Wells' criticism but Erasmus Darwin.

3.4 Darwin on vertigo

Eye movements interact with afterimages, and it was this aspect that attracted Robert Darwin (1786) to Porterfield's account of post-rotational visual motion. As we have seen in Section 2.8,

Darwin presented a detailed account of afterimages (which he referred to as ocular spectra), distinguishing between their positive and negative phases, relating their visibility to differential retinal adaptation, and describing how their apparent size was related to the distance of the surface onto which they were projected. In addition, he offered an alternative interpretation of post-rotational apparent motion. He suggested that the sequence of light entering the eyes during body rotation was visible as a moving afterimage when the body came to rest: 'When any one turns round rapidly on one foot, till he becomes dizzy and falls upon the ground, the spectra of the ambient objects continue to present themselves in rotation, or appear to librate, and he seems to behold them for some time still in motion' (Darwin, 1786, p. 315).

Robert Darwin's (1786) article was reprinted in full as the final chapter in the first volume of his father's book *Zoonomia*, which was published in 1794, two years after Wells' *Essay upon single vision*. *Zoonomia* was the culmination of many years of thought and writing, and so the chapter entitled 'Vertigo' reflected ideas that had been nurtured prior to the appearance of Wells' *Essay* in 1792. Darwin commenced by noting that 'the disease called vertigo or dizziness has been little understood' (1794, p. 231). In the chapter Darwin listed the conditions which can induce vertigo and the symptoms accompanying it. The inducing conditions are visual, as in looking down from a tall tower or viewing a whirling wheel, or postural, as in seasickness or rotating the body. These were all related to the importance of vision in maintaining postural equilibrium. He also described the vertigo and double vision that accompanies drunkenness. The example of post-rotational vertigo is described thus:

> When a child moves round quick upon one foot, the circumjacent objects become quite indistinct, as their distance increases their apparent motions; and this great velocity confounds both their forms, and their colours, as is seen in whirling round a many coloured wheel; he then loses his usual method of balancing himself by vision, and begins to stagger, and attempts to recover himself by his muscular feelings. This staggering adds to the instability of the visible objects by giving a vibratory motion besides their rotatory one. The child then drops to the ground, and the neighbouring objects seem to continue for some seconds of time to circulate around him, and the earth under him appears to librate like a balance. In some seconds of time these sensations of a continuation of the motion of objects vanish; but if he continues turning somewhat longer, before he

falls, sickness and vomiting are very liable to succeed. (Darwin, 1794, p. 235)

The emphasis throughout Darwin's chapter is on the visual and muscular aspects of maintaining balance, and in learning to associate them with one another. However, it was in the '*Additional observations on* VERTIGO, *which ought to have been inserted in Sect*. XX.6. [Of vertigo]', which were appended to the reprint of Robert Darwin's article that Erasmus supported his (son's) theory against the attack of Wells. Erasmus gave some of the results of Wells' experiments and addressed his observation that post-rotational visual motion still occurred after rotating with the eyes closed.

After revolving with your eyes open till you become vertiginous, as soon as you cease to revolve, not only the circum-ambient objects appear to circulate around you in a direction contrary to that, in which you have been turning, but you are liable to roll your eyes forwards and backwards; as is well observed, and ingeniously demonstrated by Dr. Wells in a late publication on vision. The same occurs, if you revolve your head with your eyes closed, and open them immediately at the time of your ceasing to turn; and even during the whole time of revolving, as may be felt by your hand pressed lightly on your closed eyelids. To these movements of the eyes, of which he supposes the observer to be unconscious, Dr. Wells ascribes the apparent circumgyration of objects on ceasing to revolve. The cause of thus turning our eyes forwards, and then back again, after our body is at rest, depends, I imagine, on the same circumstance, which induces us to follow the indistinct spectra, which are formed on one side of the center of the retina, when we observe them apparently on clouds . . . and then not being able to gain more distinct vision of them, we turn our eyes back, and again and again pursue the flying shade . . . Doctor Wells imagines, that no spectra can be gained in the eye, if a person revolves with his eyelids closed, and thinks this is a sufficient argument against the opinion, that the apparent progression of the spectra of light or colours in the eye can cause the apparent retrogression of objects in the vertigo above described; but it is certain, when any person revolves in a light room with his eyes closed, that he nevertheless perceives differences of light both in quantity and colour through his eyelids, as he turns round; and readily gains spectra of those differences. And these spectra are not very different except in vivacity from those, which he acquires, when he revolves with unclosed eyes, since if he then revolves very rapidly the colours and forms of surrounding objects are as it were mixed in his eye; as when the prismatic colours are painted on a wheel, they appear white as they revolve. (Darwin, 1794, pp. 571 and 573).

That is, afterimages could still be formed with the eyes closed and they would be in the peripheral parts of the retina. Then there is a tendency to pursue but never to locate a peripheral afterimage even when it is very weak. Darwin was unjust in considering that

Wells proposed that eye movements were the cause of vertigo, rather than a correlate of it.

Darwin listed several other reasons challenging the involvement of eye movements in post-rotational visual motion. First, he contended that visual motion continued for longer than eye movements. Second, he considered that the eyes rotated with equal velocity in both directions, and he did not distinguish between the slow and fast phases of nystagmus. Third, giddiness could be experienced by a blind person. Finally, he provided what he considered to be crucial evidence that eye and visual motions were not related. Darwin denied the occurrence of ocular torsion or rolling of the eyes and so he conducted an ingenious experiment

> in which the rolling of the eyes does not take place at all after revolving, and yet the vertigo is more distressing than in the situations above mentioned. If any one looks steadily at a spot in the ceiling over his head, or indeed at his own finger held up high over his head, and in that situation turns round till he becomes giddy; and then stops, and looks horizontally; he now finds, that the apparent rotation of objects is from above downwards, or from below upwards; that is, the apparent circulation of objects is now vertical instead of horizontal, making part of a circle round the axis of the eye; and this without any rolling of his eyeballs. The reason of there being no rolling of the eyeballs perceived after this experiment, is, because the images of objects are formed in rotation round the axis of the eye, and not from one side to the other of the axis of it; so that, as the eyeball has not the power to turn in its socket round its own axis, it cannot follow the apparent motions of these evanescent spectra, either before or after the body is at rest. (Darwin, 1794, p. 572)

Thus, Darwin considered that if ocular torsion was not possible then rotary motion could not be associated with it. Accordingly, Darwin dismissed the correlation between eye movements and visual motion for all forms of post-rotational vertigo.

3.5 Wells and Darwin

The first volume of *Zoonomia*, containing Darwin's deliberation on vertigo, appeared in May or June of 1794. Wells must have read it with mounting indignation, as he wrote two rejoinders as letters to the September and October issues of *The Gentleman's Magazine* for the same year. Wells dismissed Darwin's arguments that eye movements were not correlated with visual vertigo, both on logical and experimental grounds. In the first letter, Wells (1794*a*) demonstrated that visual vertigo occurs with rotation in darkness, contrary to Erasmus Darwin's speculation. The letter was concerned principally with the logic of Darwin's theory, although it did mention some experimental observations too. In the second letter (Wells 1794*b*) he described experiments indicating not only that the eyes moved following body rotation (discounting Porterfield's position) but also gave more details about how they moved. Darwin had argued that even weak stimuli can induce afterimages. Wells refuted this experimentally by rotating his body in darkness and then moving into a lighted room and experiencing visual vertigo.

Wells examined Darwin's theory with far greater scrutiny than Darwin himself had entertained. Moreover, Wells addressed some deep perceptual issues in the course of the rebuttal. One concerned the extent to which one perceptual phenomenon can be considered to cause another. A second was on induced motion, and the interaction between real and apparent motions. A third touched on the issue of motion afterimages, which were to become a popular explanatory device in the nineteenth century. Wells examined the last concept of motion afterimages with a degree of rigour that was rarely evident in nineteenth century works (see Chapter 5).

Wells' second letter addressed the specific arguments that Darwin had raised against Wells' theory. Not only was each of the criticisms countered, but Wells also added several additional facts about eye movements and vertigo. First, post-rotational eye movements involve slow rotation in one direction and rapid rotations in the reverse direction; vision is suppressed during the rapid return. Second, the eyes can undergo torsional nystagmus. Third, nystagmus (and the apparent rotation that accompanies it) can be suppressed by directed attention. Fourth, the extent of torsional nystagmus is less than that of horizontal nystagmus.

Wells provided a succinct summary of his own theory at the beginning of the second letter:

> When we stop ourselves while giddy from turning, our eyes do not return to a state of rest along with our bodies, but continue to move for some time after. Of this, however, we are not conscious; and hence we imagine the relative motion between ourselves and objects at rest to be possessed by the latter; in like manner as a person gliding down the stream of a smooth and swift river fancies its banks are passing by him. (Wells, 1794*b*, p. 905)

He then went through each of Darwin's objections, and paid particular regard to the experiment which induced vertigo by rotating the body with the head tilted backwards. Wells' description warrants repetition:

As Dr. Darwin gives no proof, from experiment, that the eye does not roll upon its axis during the giddiness which has been produced in the above-mentioned situation, I presume he rests his belief of the fact altogether upon the inability of the eye to perform such a motion. But surely the parts which connect the eye-ball to the socket are sufficiently flexible to allow it to move in some degree round its axis; and, whoever bestows the least consideration upon the origin, progress, and termination, of the oblique muscles of the eye must perceive that they have the power of giving it such a motion. That the eye actually does roll upon its axis, is shewn by the following experiment: I placed a long thin rule parallel to the horizon, its edge being towards me, and gave it such a position, in other respects, that it was the only object intervening between my eyes and a bright sky. I afterwards fixed my eyes upon a mark in the middle of its edge, and having obtained in this way a long narrow luminous spectrum, I turned myself, having my eyes pointed to a spot over my head, till I became giddy. I then stopped and directed my eyes to the middle of a perpendicular line drawn upon the wall of my chamber. A luminous line, the spectrum of the rule, now appeared upon the wall, crossing the real and perpendicular line at right angles, or nearly so. The two lines, however, did not for a moment preserve the same position with regard to each other, but continually moved round their common point of intersection, in such a manner that the extremities of the one alternately approached and receded from the extremities of the other; the motion of those of the spectral line having therefore a direction contrary to that of the apparent motion of the extremities of the real line, and of the apparent motion of every other body within my view. When the spectrum of the line ceased to move, the apparent rotation of objects likewise ceased. Now it is evident from this experiment that, during the time the surrounding objects seemed to move in a vertical circle, the centre of which was in the axis of the eye, there was a real motion of the eye in the contrary direction round its axis; and consequently, that Dr. Darwin's chief argument against my opinion tends only to confirm it. (Wells, 1794*b*, pp. 906–907)

We should be grateful to Darwin for so singling out Wells' theory for criticism. Without that spur, Wells would not have penned his defence to *The Gentleman's Magazine*, and we would not have available the elaboration of his theory and the elegant experiment demonstrating torsional nystagmus. It was following the second retort that Wells and Darwin were referred to as 'the vertiginous philosophers' by the correspondent T. J. in a letter to *The Gentleman's Magazine*. In addition to naming them thus, T. J. raised another important issue concerning adaptation to rapid rotation:

I would ask one or both of the vertiginous philosophers, who have lately so much opposed each other in your Magazine on the subject of vision, how the intoxicated man sees double? and, when he has tumbled on the floor, and

> scrambles lest he should fall lower, what could have occasioned those *moving spectra* to a body at rest? And yet we have seen at Sadler's Wells, and such places, a tumbler spin like a top for a quarter of an hour together, at the same time balancing naked swords and drinking-glasses over his head, and not be affected in the least. (T. J., 1794, p. 1093, original italics)

Darwin had not, in fact, communicated with *The Gentleman's Magazine* on this issue, but Wells had printed the two letters above attacking Darwin's theory of vertigo. Darwin had mentioned, in *Zoonomia*, that the effects of rotation could be reduced by experience. In citing the child's game of rotating on one foot and then stopping, he noted that:

> In some seconds of time these sensations of a continuation of the motion of objects vanish; but if he continues turning round somewhat longer, before he falls, sickness and vomiting are very liable to succeed. But none of these circumstances affect those who have habituated themselves to this kind of motion, as the dervises in Turkey, amongst whom these swift gyrations are a ceremony of religion. (Darwin, 1794, p. 235)

Darwin (1796) made some minor additions to his chapter on vertigo in the second edition of *Zoonomia*, and in the third edition (1801*a*) he returned to the issue of post-rotational perception and briefly addressed Wells' objections to his theory. Darwin's views were modified slightly, but he remained convinced that visual vertigo was not associated with eye movements: 'Whence I conclude, that vertigo may have for its cause either the ocular spectra of the sense of vision, when a person revolves with his eyes open; or the auricular murmurs of the sense of hearing, if he is revolved near a cascade; or the evanescent titillations of the sense of touch, if he revolves blindfold' (1801*a*, p. 346). In suggesting that bodily sensations generated visual vertigo in the last condition, Darwin failed to recognize the significance of Wells' afterimage experiments.

Wells (1794*b*) summarized his conclusions in his second letter to *The Gentleman's Magazine*. He had established that the eyes undergo involuntary motion following rotation, with resulting apparent motion of the environment; the eye movements involve slow rotation in one direction, with rapid return (nystagmus); the direction of apparent motion is dependent upon the orientation of the head during rotation; involuntary eye movements can be vertical, horizontal, or torsional; and, the eye movements can be suppressed by concentrated fixation.

Wells' experimental variations on this theme should be considered as laying the foundations for vestibular research, which are usually attributed to Purkinje. It seems likely that Purkinje did not read English in the early part of his career, and so would not have had access to Wells' book and articles. Purkinje (1820) did cite the translation into German of the first volume of Darwin's *Zoonomia* (1795), but there was little in it to suggest the subtlety of Wells' initial experiments in 1792.

Erasmus Darwin's aims were on a grand scale, and he did not wish to be diverted by detail. His *Zoonomia* commenced: 'The purpose of the following pages is an endeavour to reduce the facts belonging to ANIMAL LIFE into classes, orders, genera, and species; and by comparing them with each other, to unravel the theory of diseases' (1794, p. 1, original capitals). The four classes of diseases he proposed were those of irritation, sensation, volition, and association. In the third edition Darwin listed the various forms of vertigo, and concluded that 'The links of association, which are effected in the vertigo occasioned by unusual motion, are the irritative motions of the sense of vision, those of the stomach, and those of the heart and arteries' (1801*b*, p. 255).

Darwin (Fig. 3.5, upper) did make a material contribution to studying the link between vestibular stimulation and eye movements with his design of the first human centrifuge. This was described and illustrated in volume four of the third edition of *Zoonomia* (Darwin, 1801*b*). He called the device a rotative couch; he did not, however, construct one or perform experiments with it. The proposed function of the rotative couch was to increase pressure on the brain. He described it thus:

> Another experiment I have frequently wished to try, which cannot be done in private practice, and which I therefore recommend to some hospital physician; and that is, to endeavour to still the violent actions of the heart and arteries, after due evacuations by venesection and cathartics, by gently compressing the brain. This might be done by suspending a bed, so as to whirl the patient round with his head most distant from the centre of rotation, as if he lay on a mill-stone... For this purpose a perpendicular shaft armed with iron gudgeons might have one end pass into the floor, and the other into a beam in the ceiling, with a horizontal arm, to which a small bed may be readily suspended. By thus whirling the patient with increasing velocity sleep might be produced, and probably the violence of the actions of the heart and arteries might be diminished in inflammatory fevers. (1801*b*, pp. 436–437)

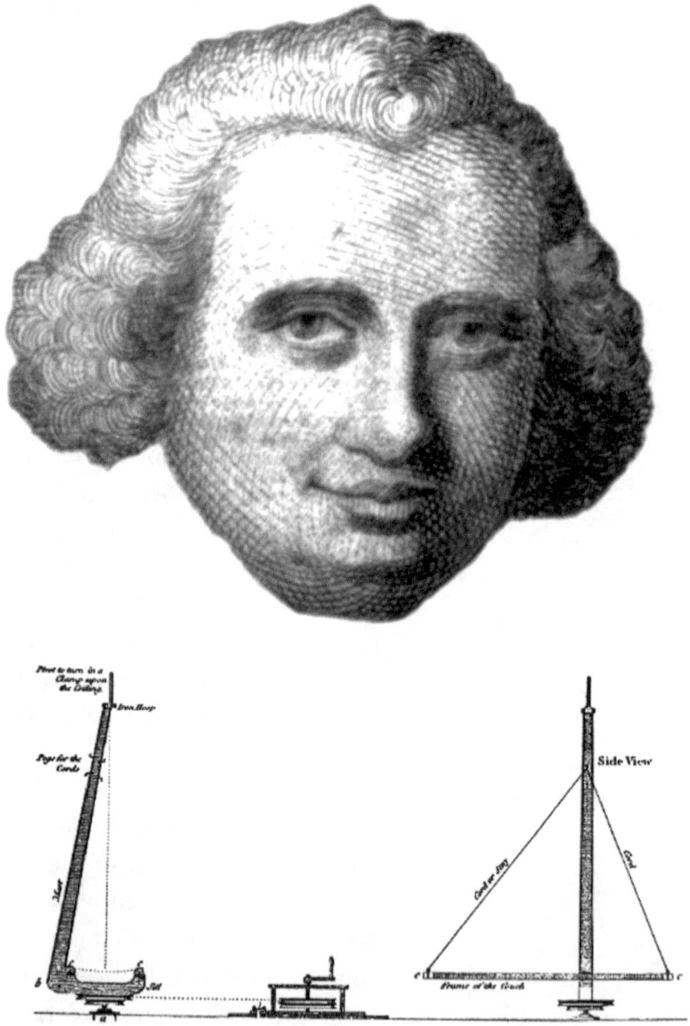

Figure 3.5

Upper, Erasmus Darwin after an engraving in *The European Magazine and London Review*, **27**, 75. Lower, Darwin's design for a human centrifuge or 'rotative couch' from Darwin (1801*b*).

Detailed engineering drawings were made by Darwin's friend, James Watt, and are shown in the lower part of Fig. 3.5. It is clear that Darwin's device was not stimulated by his concern with vertigo, rather it was driven by his theory of disease, in which any means of inducing sleep was considered efficacious. Indeed, it was a conversation with his engineer friend—James Brindley—that led to the invention of the rotative couch:

Another way of procuring sleep mechanically was related to me by Mr. Brindley, the famous canal engineer, who was brought up to the business of a mill-wright; he told me that he had more than once seen the experiment of a man extending himself across the large stone of a corn-mill, and that by

> gradually letting the stone whirl, the man fell asleep, before the stone had gained its full velocity, and he supposed would have died without pain by the continuance or increase of the motion. In this case the centrifugal motion of the head and feet must accumulate the blood in both those extremities of the body, and thus compress the brain. (1801*b*, p. 314)

The basis for Darwin's invention of the rotating chair or bed might have been idiosyncratic but its subsequent application has been widespread, and it has provided the foundation on which much vestibular research has progressed (see Section 3.8).

It is instructive to note that those who sought to make links between post-rotational eye movements and visual motion (Porterfield, Wells, and Purkinje), although trained in medicine, were principally concerned with vision. All three had written about specifically visual phenomena before they considered visual vertigo, and all had some acquaintance with the study of eye movements. In the cases of Porterfield and Wells, eye movements, both internal and external to use Porterfield's (1737, 1738) terms, had been examined in considerable detail. Those whose interests were in disease, like Erasmus Darwin, either ignored or rejected the involvement of eye movements in visual vertigo.

The extent to which Wells' investigations on the eye movements consequent on vestibular stimulation has been neglected is remarkable. It is as if he had not written anything on the subject. He had, in fact, recorded nystagmus for the first time, but it was not given that name. Boissier de Sauvages (1772*a*) did describe a disease he called nystagmus, which 'consists of a spasmodic and alternate movement of the eye' (p. 6), but he did little more than provide a brief description of abnormal rapid eye movements. The term did not come into common currency until the nineteenth century. Wells restricted his description to the involuntary, slow drift of the eyes in one direction and their ballistic return. In addition, the eyes can drift with equal speed in opposite directions, which is referred to as pendular nystagmus. The jerky nystagmus can be elicited by visual or vestibular stimulation, and accompanies some neurological disorders. The term itself is an old one, but it referred to the nodding of the head in a drowsy state.

The person who has been accorded credit for describing optokinetic nystagmus, post-rotational eye movements, and the dependence of their direction on prior head position, is Purkinje (see Wade and Brožek, 2001). This has been repeated so many times and by so many historians that it generally accepted without question. Perhaps this is because two of the most notable figures in subsequent vestibular research (Mach and Bárány) have added their authority to this belief.

3.6 Purkinje and Flourens

The phenomenal effects of vestibular stimulation, during and after body rotation, were studied long before the system that signalled angular accelerations of the head had been identified. Experiments on vertigo were conducted by Purkinje (Fig. 3.6, left) and he is linked with Pierre Flourens (1794–1867; Fig. 3.7, left) as a founder of vestibular research. In 1820 Purkinje wrote an extensive article on his observations of vertigo, and it was followed by several other shorter reports. Like Darwin (1794) before him, he distinguished between different inducing conditions for vertigo: those caused by body rotation, by galvanic (electrical) stimulation of the ears, by cerebral ischemia, by looking down from great heights, and from alcohol and other narcotics. Most of his experiments were on the first of these. He produced vertigo by rotating the body voluntarily, on a roundabout, and in a rotating contraption (Fig. 3.6, right). As has been noted, such devices, which were human centrifuges, were invented by Darwin (1801*b*) and used by Joseph Mason Cox (1763–1818; 1804) and others as a treatment for insanity (see Wade et al., 2005). It was

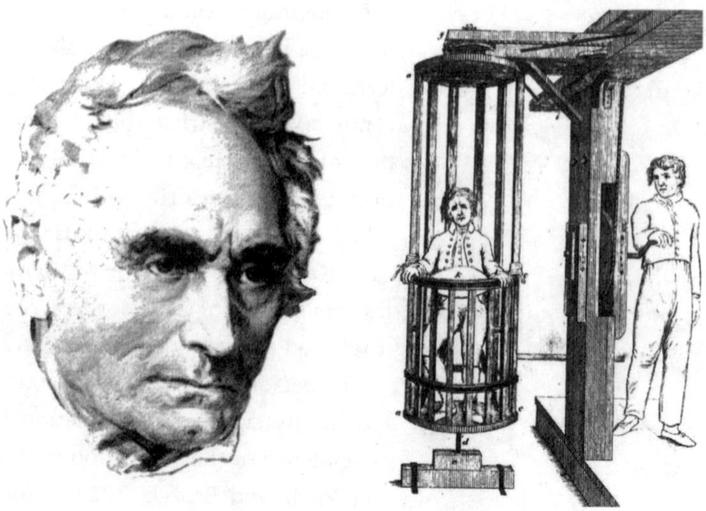

Figure 3.6
Left, Jan Evangelista Purkinje or Purkyně (1787–1869) after an illustration in Psotníčková (1955). Right, a rotating device of the type used in his experiments on vertigo, after an illustration in Kruta (1969).

considered that stimulating the blood supply to the brain provided relief to those suffering from a wide range of mental disturbances.

Purkinje was not primarily interested in the medical applications of rotation, but in the use of the chair to investigate the subjective aspects of visual motion following body rotation. Initially, he examined the introspective reports of post-rotational vertigo and made many experimental manipulations of it, as well as inducing vertigo by rotating the body in the specially designed device. Purkinje described eye movements during and after rotation and suggested that 'visual vertigo is a consequence of the conflict between unconscious involuntary muscular actions and voluntary conscious ones in the opposite direction' (1820, p. 95). In his article, Purkinje cited very few sources of earlier research, but he did make reference to a translation into German of Erasmus Darwin's *Zoonomia* (1795) and Herz's (1786) medical text on dizziness and its treatment.

Purkinje performed many of the experimental manipulations described by Wells, and provided a general principle: 'that the midpoint of the head (considered as a sphere), around which the first movement was performed, invariably determined the direction of apparent motion regardless of the subsequent position of the head' (1820, p. 86). Kruta (1964) referred to this as 'Purkinje's law of vertigo'. There was no clear indication of how such motions in the head could be detected, and Purkinje's interpretation was conceptually little different from Willis' (1672) appeal to movements of the animal spirit in the head: rather than the animal spirit showing inertia relative to the head, Purkinje suggested that motion of the brain itself lagged behind that of the head, with particular influence exerted by the cerebellum. Purkinje concluded his first article with a statement that was soon to be realized: 'It remains for a future work to establish the possible movements in the brain which measure its structure and organization' (1820, p. 125).

Flourens (1824, 1830, 1842) conducted lesion studies, initially on the cerebellum and later on the labyrinth of the inner ear, which established the significance of the semicircular canals for the maintenance of posture and balance. Flourens' most productive period was in the 1820s with his experiments on reptiles, birds, and mammals, and he rarely made distinctions between the

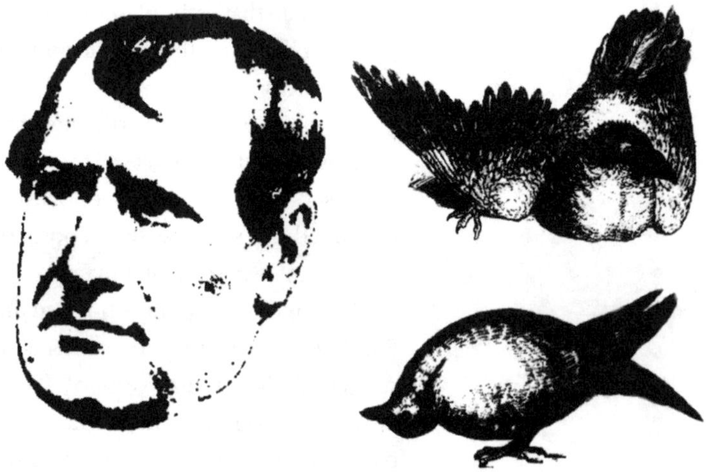

Figure 3.7
Left, Marie Jean Pierre Flourens (1794–1867), after an illustration in Haymaker and Schiller (1970). Right, postures adopted by pigeons following section of the semicircular canals, after an illustration in Kruta (1969).

brains of these animals. Thus, he viewed the brain as having some degree of localized function, but that it acted as a unit. These ideas were to inhibit his association of the functions of the vestibular receptors with the control of equilibrium. In his experiments in the late 1820s he sectioned the semicircular canals of pigeons, and he was able to demonstrate that destruction of a particular semicircular canal elicited eye movements in the same plane as well as disturbances of posture and equilibrium: the body of the experimental animals always turned in the direction of the severed canal (Fig. 3.7, right). Despite such strong experimental indications, the belief that the vestibular receptors were involved in hearing remained. It was even suggested that the orientations of the semicircular canals served the function of locating the direction of sound.

Purkinje (1826, 1827) saw the relevance of Flourens' experiments to his own studies of vertigo, and he was impressed by the selective disturbances of motor coordination produced by lesions of the cerebellum. These led to a change in his interpretation of vertigo: rather than considering that the brain as a whole moved, rather like Willis' fluid in a flask, he attributed the effects to movements associated with the cerebellum. He stated that 'the cerebellum is the seat of the spatial sense' (1826, p. 120), but the manner in which it operated remained a mystery.

Purkinje's experiments on vertigo have been taken as heralding a new era. A new sense, the vestibular system, was exposed by Flourens' scalpel, and Purkinje's investigations of vertigo would eventually be interpreted in the light of semicircular canal function. However, this was not achieved by Purkinje himself, despite his knowledge of Flourens' experiments. In 1826 Purkinje published a detailed review of a German translation of Flourens' (1824) book, in which Purkinje described his experiments (with his student Krauss) confirming the effects of cerebellar lesions on postural control. In the review he outlined the essential features of his earlier (1820) experiments on vertigo, and sought to relate them to Flourens' experiments. At first Purkinje considered that the brain was a light substance, which moved in one direction or another as a consequence of the mechanical forces acting on it. This view was changed to one in which the brain itself either had some internal disturbance or contracted, but he could find no evidence from lesions to indicate how such action took place. Lesions in the cerebellum, on the other hand, had specific effects on vertigo:

> With the first repetition of Flourens' experiments on the cerebellum I was left in no doubt that the subsequent appearance of uncoordinated movements in animals was nothing other than the expression of a powerful vertigo, and that the experience of space was disturbed. The following experiments with lesions in different parts of the cerebellum similarly indicated that the direction of vertigo was so determined. (Purkinje, 1826, p. 122)

In the following year, Purkinje published a longer article on the physiological significance of vertigo in which these ideas were elaborated. His conclusion was that 'The cerebellum has two organic functions, one works through the musculature and stimulates conscious movements, the other acts on the cerebrum and results in the combined sensation and perception of spatial experience' (1827, p. 309). He also related these localized effects to the uncoordinated eye, head, and body movements that occur during epileptic seizures.

3.7 Mach, Breuer, and Crum Brown

Purkinje's experiments with a rotating chair fuelled the interests of others to study visual motion using similar devices. Ernst Mach (1838–1916; Fig 3.8, left) developed his own model for examining the perception of motion (Fig. 3.8, right). The wooden chair could rotate around a horizontal axis; it was mounted in a frame, rr, which could rotate around a vertical axis; this could be adjusted to different positions relative to another frame, RR, that could be

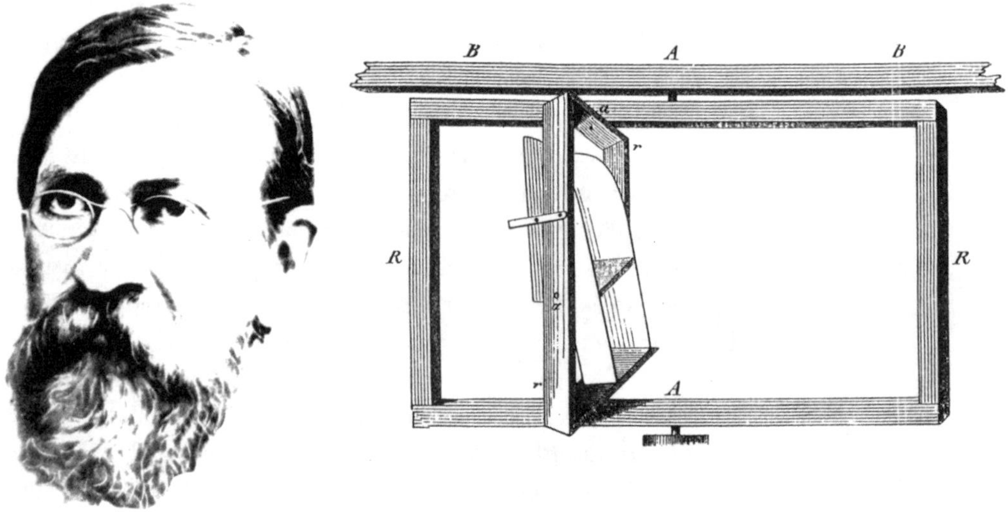

Figure 3.8
Left, Ernst Mach (1838–1916) after a photograph in Schmitz (1983). Right, his device for rotating the body around different axes (from Mach, 1875).

rotated around a vertical axis. With this device he was able to investigate both visual orientation during tilt and the effects of rotation. He demonstrated that vertigo can be induced by visual stimulation alone. Mach made the explicit connection between Purkinje's experiments on vertigo and the function of the semicircular canals.

On the basis of his spinning experiments, Mach (1873, 1874, 1875) advanced a hydrodynamic theory of vestibular function as did Joseph Breuer (1842–1925; Fig. 3.9, left) and Alexander Crum Brown (1838–1922; Fig. 3.9, right) at about the same time and independently. Both examined body rotation, but with less sophisticated machinery than Mach's. Breuer rotated the body actively, and Crum Brown used a revolving stool. Unlike many other independent discoveries these were not a source of dispute. This remarkable trio of scientists all employed eye movements to support their theories (see Henn, 1984; Howard and Templeton, 1966; Young et al., 2001). During head rotation the endolymph in the canals displaces receptors in the ampulla, signalling angular accelerations and exerting control over posture and eye movements. At last there was a theory that was free from the influence of the animal spirit, although the proposed motion of endolymph in the canals was remarkably similar to the fluid analogies made by Willis (1672).

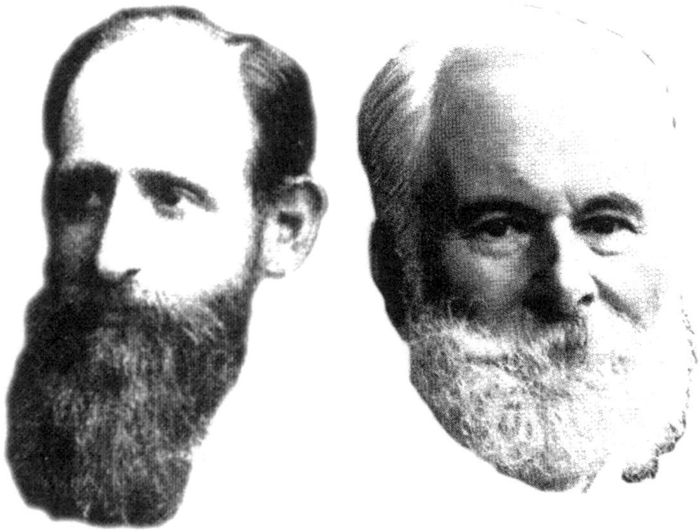

Figure 3.9
Left, Josef Breuer (1842–1925) after a portrait in Lesky (1965); right, Alexander Crum Brown (1838–1922) after a portrait in Comrie (1932).

The involvement of the semicircular canals in the control of eye movements and equilibrium had been growing in the years since Flourens' studies. Prosper Ménière (1799–1862; 1861) had linked experiments involving lesions to the semicircular canals with clinical cases of disorientation and dizziness, now referred to as Ménière's disease. Friedrich Goltz (1834–1902; 1870) had come even closer to providing a hydrodynamic theory. The semicircular canals were clearly implicated in the maintenance of balance, but there was a lingering doubt about whether they had any auditory function. Goltz suggested that the movements of fluids in the canals could stimulate receptors in the ampullae. They could provide a means of detecting motion of the head and its orientation with respect to gravity. In the following year, Eduard Hitzig (1838–1907; 1871) provided a detailed account of galvanic stimulation of the ear, and its effects upon muscle tone, elaborating on the earlier work of Johann Ritter (1776–1810; 1801) and Purkinje (1820). Hitzig also observed the manner and direction of eye movements, giving a poetic analogy of their kinematics. He described the nystagmus induced, and he called it by that name. The eye movements were likened to a fisherman's float drifting slowly with the current and then being snatched back, only to repeat this sequence. The fast phase of nystagmus was always in the direction of the anode during galvanic stimulation.

Thus the scene was set for an integration of the physical, physiological, and psychological aspects of vestibular stimulation achieved by Mach, Breuer, and Crum Brown. All three acknowledged that the experiments of Goltz were the spur to their own work, and all of them examined the effects of body rotation on the maintenance of balance and on the movements of the eyes.

Ernst Mach was a physicist at the University of Prague, where Purkinje was trained and the university to which he returned in 1850. Purkinje was still active there when Mach arrived in 1867. Mach outlined a positivist approach to science, following in the paths of Berkeley and Hume, by arguing that all sciences reduce to sensations. In the context of vision research he defined a new area of form perception, by correlating the appearance of contours with physical variables. Josef Breuer practiced medicine in Vienna, and one of his patients was Sigmund Freud (1856–1939). Breuer is best known for his collaboration with Freud, by interesting him in hysteria. However, before his limited excursion into the study of mental illness, Breuer had earned an independent reputation in physiology and medicine. His work with Hering, on the reflex regulation of respiration, is marked by the Hering-Breuer reflex (see Baumann, 2002). Receptors in the lungs respond to the extent of stretching and signal this to the brain via the vagus nerve setting in train a feedback control of respiration. For his vestibular research, Breuer (1874, 1875) followed in the tradition of Flourens by making systematic lesions of the semicircular canals of pigeons. He also examined the effects of body rotation on eye movements. Breuer distinguished between the canal receptors and the otolith organs of the vestibular system, which detected orientation with respect to gravity. Most of his experimental work was conducted at his practice—even his experiments on vestibular function in pigeons.

Alexander Crum Brown was a chemist at the University of Edinburgh. He is best known for introducing the modern method of symbols connecting atoms in organic chemistry. Crum Brown (1874, 1875) based his analysis on thresholds for detecting body rotation on a revolving stool; the thresholds were lowest when the head was positioned so that one of the semicircular canals was in the plane of rotation. He also proposed that the contralateral canals operated as a pair rather than independently. In his Robert Boyle Lecture at Oxford University, Crum Brown remarked:

This hydrokinetic theory of the function of the semicircular canals was propounded at very nearly the same time by Professor Mach of Prague, Dr. Breuer of Vienna, and myself. I give the names in the order of publication. The views expressed by us were not exactly the same . . . The theory as I have just described it might perhaps have been developed, as I have here developed it, from a consideration of the structure and position of the canals. But as a matter of fact this was not the historical order. It was the experiments of Flourens that first directed attention to these organs as having something to do with equilibrium of the body. (1895*b*, pp. 20–21)

Each of the three founders of hydrodynamic theory was scrupulous in acknowledging the contributions of the others. However, of the three, Mach conducted the most thorough and detailed investigations of human responses to rotation. His book on *Foundations of the theory of movement sensations* was published in 1875, and in it he integrated the psychological and physiological evidence for the function of the semicircular canals; it has now been translated by Young et al. (2001), with a valuable commentary. Mach's device for rotating the body in different axes enabled him to investigate both visual orientation during tilt and the effects of rotation. When Wells was writing, he was not aware of the function of the semicircular canals, nor did he have any specific apparatus for facilitating the study of its functions. Nonetheless, he did describe the consequences of both body tilt and body rotation on perception and on eye movements.

Mach entered into his investigations concerning vertigo without a knowledge of the earlier literature on it. He developed his theory independently of Breuer and Crum Brown, but readily acknowledged their significance. In his assessments of Breuer's description of nystagmus during and following body rotation, Mach (1875) unknowingly rediscovered Wells' method of generating an afterimage prior to rotation and observing its displacement from real images when rotation ceased:

I observed nystagmic movements described by Breuer in the following manner. I produced a strong and lasting afterimage with a piece of flaming magnesium wire. If I now rotate actively about the body axis in a clockwise direction (as seen from above), I notice how the afterimage sticks on an object and then suddenly catches up. The eyes rotate slowly counterclockwise and jerk back clockwise. This movement gradually weakens until finally the afterimage rotates with the observer. After stopping, the afterimage moves slowly across the objects clockwise, interrupted by jerklike movements in the opposite direction. The objects then move counterclockwise. (Young et al., 2001, p. 84)

This is very similar to the description given by Wells (1792) in his *Essay upon single vision with two eyes*. Mach regretted being unaware of Purkinje's experiments when he commenced with his own, and could have avoided unknowingly repeating some of them. The subtlety of Wells' experiments was superior to those of Purkinje, and so Mach's savings would have been all the greater if he had known about them. Nonetheless, Mach did add that he might not have discovered other aspects of motion sensation had he have known about the earlier research on it.

3.8 James and Bárány

Mach, Breuer, and Crum Brown continued to investigate the consequences of the hydrodynamic theory of semicircular canal function, but Crum Brown, in 1878, made a particularly astute prediction: if deaf–mutes have defects in all the parts of the inner ear, then they will not be able to experience vertigo nor have the eye movements characteristically associated with it:

A great deal of valuable information might be obtained by carefully testing the delicacy and accuracy of the sense of rotation in deaf-mutes. Many deaf-mutes have not only the cochlea, but the whole internal ear, destroyed; if, then, the inmates of deaf and dumb establishments were systematically tested by means of such experiments as Mach and Brown made upon themselves, experiments which would, no doubt, greatly interest and amuse them, and if the condition of the internal ear were, in each case of *post-mortem* examination of a deaf-mute, accurately noted, we should soon obtain a mass of information which would do more to clear up the relation between the sense of rotation and the semicircular canals than any number of experiments on animals unable to describe to us their sensations. (Crum Brown, 1878, p. 658, original italics)

A few years later, William James (Fig. 3.10, left) put this to the test with a specially constructed device for rotating the body. Almost all normal observers experienced vertigo. However, of over 500 deaf–mutes tested, almost 200 experienced no dizziness (James, 1882). The results were confirmed by Kreidl (1891), who found that over 80% of congenitally deaf individuals experienced no vertigo following rotation. Moreover, there were no nystagmic eye movements in those who did not experience vertigo. James (1890) provided a general account of eye movements in vertigo

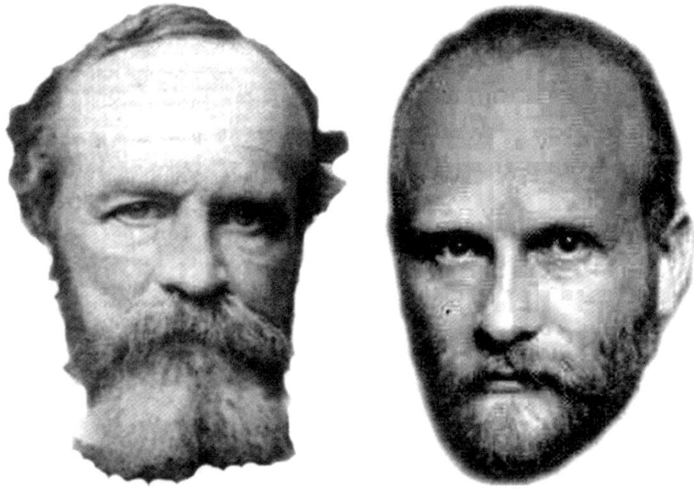

Figure 3.10
Left, William James (1842–1910). Right, Robert Bárány (1876–1936).

in his *Principles of psychology*. He related eye movements following body rotation to those involved in optokinetic nystagmus:

If we look at a waterfall, river, railroad train, or any body which continuously passes in front of us in the same direction, it carries our eyes with it. This movement can be noticed in our eyes by a bystander. If the object keep passing towards our left, our eyes keep following whatever moving bit of it may have caught their attention at first, until that bit disappears from view. Then they jerk back to the right again, and catch a new bit, which again they follow to the left, and so on indefinitely. This gives them an oscillating demeanour, slow involuntary rotations leftward alternating with rapid voluntary jerks rightward. But the *oscillations continue* for a while after the object has come to a standstill, or the eyes are carried to a new object, and this produces the illusion that things now move in the opposite direction. For we are unaware of the slow leftward automatic movements of our eyeballs, and think that the retinal movement-sensations thereby aroused must be due to a rightward motion of the object seen; whilst the rapid voluntary rightward movements of our eyeballs we interpret as attempts to pursue and catch again those parts of the object which have been slipping away to the left. Exactly similar oscillations of the eyeballs are produced in *giddiness*, with exactly similar results. Giddiness is easiest produced by whirling on ones heels. It is a feeling of the movement of our own head and body through space, and is now pretty well understood to be due to irritation of the semi-circular canals of the inner ear. When after whirling, we stop, we seem to be spinning in the reverse direction for a few seconds, and then objects appear to continue whirling in the same direction in which, a moment previous, our body actually whirled. The reason is that our *eyes normally tend to maintain* their field of view. If we suddenly turn our head leftwards it is hard to make the eyes follow. They roll in their orbits rightwards, by a sort of compensating inertia. Even though we *falsely think* our head to be moving leftwards, this consequence occurs, and our eyes move rightwards—as may be observed in anyone with vertigo after whirling. As these movements are unconscious, the retinal movement-feelings which they occasion are naturally referred to the objects seen. And the intermittent voluntary twitches of the eyes towards the left, by which we ever and anon recover them from the extreme rightward positions to which the reflex movement brings them, simply confirm and intensify our impression of a leftward-whirling field of view: we seem to ourselves to be periodically pursuing and overtaking the objects in their leftward flight. (James, 1890, pp. 89–90, original italics)

James believed that the rapid return movements of the eyes were voluntary because 'it often ceases if we voluntarily fix our eyes upon a given point' (p. 90). Wells (1794*b*) had made the same observation but did not reach the same conclusion. James related the eye movements in vertigo to a range of other motion illusions. His analysis of motion perception was essentially similar to that proposed by Porterfield (1759*b*): objects are seen as moving when they move over the retina and the eyes are considered to be still or when they remain stationary on the retina but the eyes are thought to move. James was integrating visual vertigo with his analysis of space perception generally.

An alternative approach was taken by Robert Bárány (1876–1936; Fig. 3.10, right) who examined the medical aspects of vertigo and eye movements. Bárány used nystagmic eye movements as a clinical index of vestibular function and he was awarded the Nobel Prize in 1914 for his research on vestibular function. Indeed, the rotating chair is now called the Bárány chair. In 1906 he refined a caloric method of stimulating the semicircular canals so that the eye movements they induce could be easily observed. Bárány (1913*a*,*b*) wrote two articles on the relationship of vertigo to the semicircular canals, and these also surveyed the history of research on the topics. His history fell short of the standard set by Mach (1875), even though Mach was cited! After remarking that he had come across over one hundred dissertations on vertigo from the sixteenth to the eighteenth centuries, these were dismissed as adding little to what had been known to the ancients:

The reality is that they all say much the same thing. In the Middle Ages one had become fully accustomed to the complete description. Whoever wrote a book studied the texts of his predecessors and wrote more or less the same thing with small variations. For example, regarding the interesting question of vertigo from rotation, many authors have speculated whether it is accompanied by unconscious eye movements. It did not occur to any of them to rotate themselves a few times and to feel if their eyes were moving, or to ask

> his good friend to rotate and observe his eyes. The often shrewd considerations would only be carried out on the writing table. The first to make the observations that will be discussed here was *Purkinje* in 1825. (Bárány, 1913*a*, pp. 396–397, original italics)

Needless to say, it did occur to Wells (1792), who described the involuntary eye movements with greater precision than did Purkinje. It is also a little odd that Bárány has cited the relatively cursory account of vertigo given in Purkinje's (1825) *New contributions to the study of vision in its subjective aspect*, rather than the extensive article of 1820. Nonetheless, in addition to the descriptions of the experiments by Purkinje and Flourens, as well as outlining the hydrodynamic theory of Mach, Breuer, and Crum Brown, Bárány integrated the clinical studies of Ménière (1861). He summarized their endeavours with a musical allusion:

> *Purkinje* and *Flourens* (1825–1828) have devised an ingenious prelude, *Ménière* (1861) has introduced the first phrase, *Goltz* (1870) addressed a new theme, and the theory of *Mach, Breuer*, and *Crum Brown* concluded the movement, with a powerful, full-bodied accord. The second movement is like a fugue, where many voices whirl around one another, at one time with harmonic combination, and a moment later they are in conflict. (1913*a*, p. 399, original italics)

Bárány standardized a form of stimulating the vestibular system that did not involve rotation—irrigation of the ear with warm and cold water. The procedure was known about and had been applied for many years; Goltz (1870) referred to it as common knowledge. This is now called caloric stimulation and it is a standard clinical test for vestibular function. Bárány's experiments using the chair and caloric stimulation were carried out while he was a physician in Vienna, where Hering, Breuer, and Mach had been active experimenters. The award of the Nobel Prize in 1914 was announced while Bárány was a prisoner of war, although his release was expedited thereafter. On his return to Vienna, Bárány was dismayed by the reaction of his colleagues to the Nobel award; they did not consider that he had given adequate acknowledgements to the researches of those who preceded him (see Diamant, 1984). Bárány moved to Uppsala and spent the rest of his academic life in Sweden.

Vertigo was considered to provide insights into motion illusions generally by those with a psychological interest (see Chapter 5). For physicians it was seen as a useful tool for determining the integrity of vestibular function. These two activities became more closely integrated with the perceptual demands of first aircraft and then space flight in the twentieth century. That is, there were practical applications of the knowledge derived from both experimental and medical research on vertigo.

3.9 Griffith and Dodge

Aircraft flight placed demands on the vestibular receptors that were beyond the normal range. Only the human centrifuge had subjected the human frame to similar forces. It had been devised as a treatment for insanity, it was adopted as an instrument for generating vertigo, and now it was applied to simulating the pressures of aircraft flight. It was, therefore, timely for a grand review of what was known about vestibular function. Such a review was compiled and published by Coleman Griffith (1893–1966; Fig. 3.11, left). In 1922 he published *An historical survey of vestibular equilibration*. As he noted in the Foreword: 'The historical task undertaken in this volume was incited by the problem of bodily equilibration in flight, a problem which aroused widespread interest during the World War'.

Griffith's survey listed 1701 publications on, or related to, the vestibular system. The early work is not sampled systematically—for instance Wells (1792) is not cited—but that from the time of Flourens in the 1820s is thorough. The survey essentially commences with the work of Purkinje (1820) and Flourens

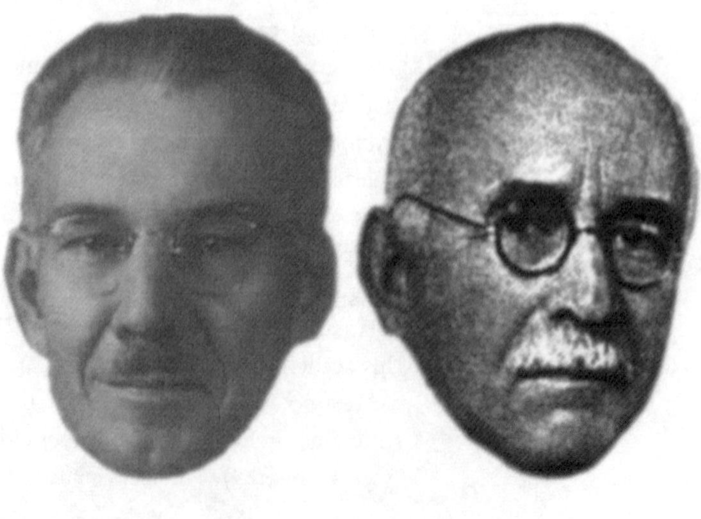

Figure 3.11
Left, Coleman Roberts Griffith (1893–1966). Right, Raymond Dodge (1871–1942) after a portrait in Taylor (1937).

(1824). For example, he stated that 'The method of rotation had its beginning, apparently, in the hands of Purkinje and almost every investigator since his time has used it in one form or another' (p. 9). Many subsequent writers (e.g. Boring, 1942; Howard and Templeton, 1966; Wendt, 1951) have deferred to Griffith's authority on the history of vestibular research. Boring in his *Sensation and perception in the history of experimental psychology* typified this:

The history of what has been called vestibular equilibration, the static sense, ampullar sensation, giddiness, vertigo, the sense of rotation, and the sensibility of the semicircular canals is voluminous and simple. It is voluminous because there has been so much written about it: in 1922 Griffith cited 1685 titles from 1820 on. It is simple because it can all be organized about Purkinje's description of dizziness (1820–1825), Flourens' discovery that lesions of the semicircular canals produce muscular incoordination in the plane of the affected canals (1824–1830), the Mach–Breuer–Brown experiments and their theory of the function of the canals (1873–1875), and the discovery of vertiginous habituation by the psychologists of the U.S. Army (1918), Griffith (1920), and Dodge (1923). (Boring, 1942, p. 535)

That this is the received wisdom is indicated in a major text on the vestibular system (Kornhuber, 1974), which commenced in similar vein:

The history of vestibular research begins early in the nineteenth century. Against a background of the known anatomical structure of the labyrinth in different animals, the work of Purkinje (1820), Flourens (1824)... led to the conclusion that the vestibular end-organs have a different function from hearing, and that they regulate body and eye positions and if disturbed, give rise to vertigo. (p. 3)

Griffith's particular research interest was in vestibular habituation and he had examined this with aircraft pilots. Initially aviators were selected on the basis of their vestibular sensitivity, as determined by tests on a Bárány chair. However, seasoned pilots were not so susceptible to vertigo, and he argued that they had habituated to the repeated rotations to which they had been exposed. In order to examine habituation more rigorously, Griffith (1920) tested students on repetitive rotations in a modified Bárány chair. They were exposed to ten rotations of 20s, alternating in direction, per session and they were tested over many days. Measures of the duration of apparent motion and the number and duration of nystagmic eye movements were recorded after the body was stopped:

We have found that, as turning is repeated from day to day, the duration of after-nystagmus, the number of ocular movements made, and the duration of the apparent movement rapidly decrease. The major part of this decrease occurs within the first few days. The decrease takes place not only from day to day but also within a period of trials on any single day. (Griffith, 1920, p. 46)

In his later work, Griffith continued studying human performance, but his interests shifted towards sports, and he is now remembered as the father of sports psychology.

The topic of vestibular habituation attracted Raymond Dodge (1871–1942; Fig. 3.11, right) and he sought to determine how the eyes moved during and after rotation (Dodge, 1923). The problem of adaptation to rotation is a general one, and relates to the issue raised earlier in this chapter regarding the absence of vertigo in whirling dervishes; it is also relevant to the relative immunity to motion sickness of those, like seafarers, who are regularly exposed to the conditions which can induce it. As he remarked: 'The very existence of habituation to rotation was vigorously denied during the war by those who were responsible for the revolving chair tests for prospective aviators' (Dodge, 1923, p. 15).

Dodge will feature prominently in Chapter 4, as he had previously measured eye movements during reading and was noted for the ingenuity of the recording instruments he made. Recording eye movements during rotation provided a particular challenge:

Just before the War I became particularly interested in recording the *reflex compensatory* eye-movements that occur when the semi-circular canals are stimulated by rotation of the subject. The instrumental problem was peculiarly difficult and intriguing. Since a moving field is more or less in evidence if the eyes are open during rotation of the subject, reflex compensatory movements tend to be complicated by pursuit movements during direct observation, even when a strong convex lens is used to prevent clear vision. To study the reflex in pure form, the first requirement was to record the movements of the closed eyes. (Dodge, 1930, pp. 111–112, original italics)

In examining the possibilities he had noticed that the convexity of the cornea was visible as a moving bulge beneath the lid. Dodge (1921) mounted a mirror over the closed eye lid and was able to record eye movements by the reflections from it. The device he devised is shown in Fig. 3.12. With it he was able to confirm the results of Griffith: without the possibility of visual fixation, after-nystagmus declines with repeated rotations.

In the next chapter it will become evident that Dodge was a pioneer of recording eye movements generally, and during reading

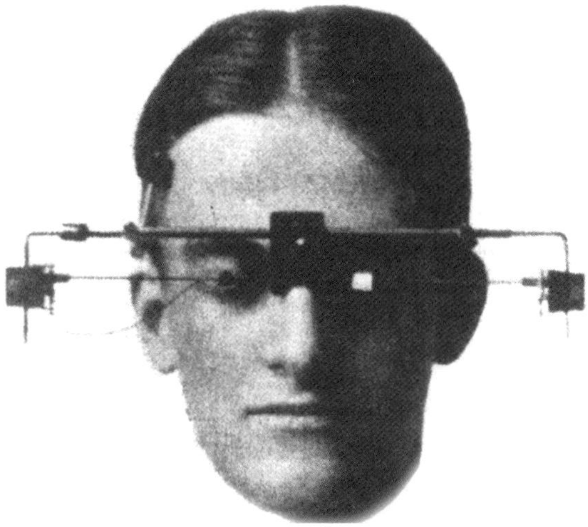

Figure 3.12
Dodge's device for measuring eye movements with closed eyes (after Dodge, 1921).

in particular. It is of interest to note that following his developments in these novel areas he engaged in examining eye movements following body rotation—the problem tackled by previous pioneers over a century earlier. Indeed, Dodge shared with Purkinje a willingness to engage in heroic experiments. When Purkinje gained access to a rotating chair he noted the effects of being rotated for one hour in it. Dodge similarly subjected himself to a gruelling regime: 'The experiment consisted of a six-day training period during which the subject (myself) was rotated in the same direction one hundred and fourteen times each day at as nearly uniform speed as possible' (Dodge, 1923, p. 16). The amplitude of post-rotational nystagmus decreased from day to day throughout the experiment. Any feelings of dizziness also disappeared with prolonged practice, and the experience was said to be soothing.

4

Saccades and fixations

4.1 Introduction

Writers on vision in the eighteenth century drew attention to the rapid motions of the eyes over a scene, but they were not given a name. They are now called saccades. They were not open to the precise measurement that can now be brought bear on them, but they were related to an issue of modern concern—reading. For example, Porterfield (1737) made the following astute observation:

> Thus in viewing any Word, such as MEDICINE, if the Eye be directed to the first Letter M, and keep itself fixed thereon for observing it accurately, the other Letters will not appear clear or distinct . . . Hence it is that to view any Object, and thence to receive the strongest and most lively Impressions, it is always necessary we turn our Eyes directly towards it, that its Picture may fall precisely upon this most delicate and sensible Part of the Organ, which is naturally in the *Axis* of the Eye. (pp. 184–185, original italics and capitals)

In this chapter we present an historical examination of the methods that have been adopted to measure the quick motions of the eyes, and the theoretical consequences that have resulted from appreciating the import of Porterfield's observations. Prior to that, however, we will examine the ways in which eye position has been determined. This is essentially the issue of fixation. In addition, we explore the vital research responsible for revealing the saccade-and-fixate strategy of the oculomotor system, with which we are now familiar; the strategy that evolved as an adaptation to the demands of highly mobile eyes. The development of this knowledge of oculomotor behaviour involved two key breakthroughs allied to Porterfield's insights. The first is that eye movements are discontinuous, involving brief rapid movements and longer static or slow moving periods. The second is the importance of the periods that lie between saccades—fixations or slow pursuit—and their perceptual consequences.

Visual vertigo provided a way of determining that eye movements were not all of the same type. The fast and slow phases of nystagmus could readily be discerned, and it was evident that little was visible during the fast phase. The discontinuous movements were always associated with a change of direction. The examination of eye movements during inspections of objects and text was to show that discontinuities also occurred in the same direction, punctuated by brief periods of fixation.

Afterimages were to prove the key to determining the stability of the eye during fixation, the torsion of the eye in oblique gaze, and the initial attempts to assess the velocity of eye movements. Crum Brown (1895*a*,*b*) extended his studies of eye movements from vertigo to scanning and was able to determine the jerk-like motions of the eyes. There was a sequence of rapid jerks interspersed by brief fixations. Again, this was demonstrated by the use of afterimages. Eventually, the jerks became known as saccades, and it is the emergence of understanding this aspect of eye movements that will be reviewed in the second part of the chapter. While there exist numerous earlier nineteenth century studies of eye movements outside the context of nystagmus, an appreciation of the distinction of saccades as a specialized family of movements, or of their importance in vision is absent from most of these works.

4.2 Fixations

Much of the eye movement research in the nineteenth century was concerned with the position of the eye during fixation, particularly following a rotation of the eye. That is, eye position rather than eye movement was the topic of enquiry. Helmholtz (Fig. 4.6, left) devoted a large section of his *Handbuch der physiologischen Optik* to eye movements both because of their inherent interest and because of the importance they held for his empiricist theory of perception. This was clearly voiced in his opening statement: 'The movements of the eyes play an essential roll in the formation of the perception of space through the sense of sight, so we must become more closely acquainted with them' (Helmholtz, 1867*a*, p. 457). Helmholtz did much to integrate the then extant knowledge of eye movements, and he specified what he considered to be certain laws associated with them. The technique that he adopted with great skill was the use of afterimages as stabilized retinal images.

The seeds for afterimage studies can again be found in Wells' experiments using them to determine the position of the eye. More specifically, when Wells (1794*b*) examined torsional nystagmus he formed an afterimage of a horizontal edge and then noted how it rotated relative to a vertical line drawn on the wall; torsion was evidenced by a change in the relative angles of the two lines. Much the same technique formed the bedrock of eye movement research in the nineteenth century. The experimental situation was simpler too. Typically, an afterimage of a horizontal or vertical line was formed with the eye looking straight ahead and then the eyes rotated to another position where a line was adjusted to the same orientation as the afterimage. This enabled the torsion of the eye to be determined. Although this is not what is usually meant by fixation, it is the aspect of eye position that will be surveyed in Section 4.2.2.

There was another application of afterimages that was described before their use in defining eye position, and this was in the context of the stability of the eyes when fixation is attempted. It is with such instability that we will commence.

4.2.1 The stability of fixation

The general function of eye movements is to retain the stability of the image of salient objects on the region of the retina for which spatial resolution is finest. This needs to be achieved during movements of the head, while pursuing slowly moving objects, and when shifting gaze to novel objects. That is, the restriction of distinct vision to a small region of the eye, around the fovea, has concentrated attention on fixations of the eye. It is, then, a paradox that one of the first aspects of such fixations studied was the instability of the eye. That is, attempts to maintain fixation on an object are not completely successful because of minor movements of the eyes. However, it is not always evident whether some of the early writers were referring to instability during fixation or general movements of the eyes. For example, Du Laurens noted that 'the eye standeth not still but moveth incessantly' (1599, pp. 28–29). It is perhaps more likely that the small involuntary eye movements were described by Edmé Mariotte (1620–1684); he is better known for his account of the blind spot than for his observations on eye movements. He made brief reference to such instabilities, suggesting that they were involuntary: 'The *Eyes* are always in motion, and very hard to be fixt in one place, though it be desired' (Mariotte, 1683, p. 266, original italics). This conclusion was probably reached by careful observation of the eyes of another person.

Afterimages provided a means by which an observer could experience the instabilities in eye position themselves, rather like the effects that can be seen with Fig. 1.8. Robert Darwin used a method much like this to describe the instability of his eyes during fixation:

> When we look long and attentively at any object, the eye cannot always be kept intirely motionless; hence, on inspecting a circular area of red silk placed on white paper, a lucid crescent or edge is seen to librate on one side or the other of the red circle: for the exterior parts of the retina sometimes falling on the edge of the central silk, and sometimes on the white paper, are less fatigued with red light than the central part of the retina, which is constantly exposed to it; and therefore, when they fall on the edge of the red silk, they perceive it more vividly. Afterwards, when the eye becomes fatigued, a green spectrum in the form of a crescent is seen to librate on one side or other of the central circle, as by the unsteadiness of the eye a part of the fatigued retina falls on the white paper. (Darwin, 1786, p. 341)

The illustration he published is shown in Fig. 4.1; it was not coloured, but when Erasmus Darwin (1794) repeated the observation in his *Zoonomia*, a hand-coloured figure was included.

This aspect of eye movement instability received much less attention than other features of afterimages, such as their changes with voluntary eye movements, and the patterns of their disappearances and reappearances (see Wade, 1978, 1998). Nonetheless, it was the problem of fixation instability that led to the experiments on stabilized retinal images in the 1950s. These will be discussed in Chapter 6.

4.2.2 Torsion

Galen had described the oblique muscles that could produce eye rolling or ocular torsion (Section 2.3), but evidence of its occurrence was to wait many centuries. The problem related to reconciling the anatomy of the eye muscles with the difficulty of observing small rotations of the eye around the optic axis.

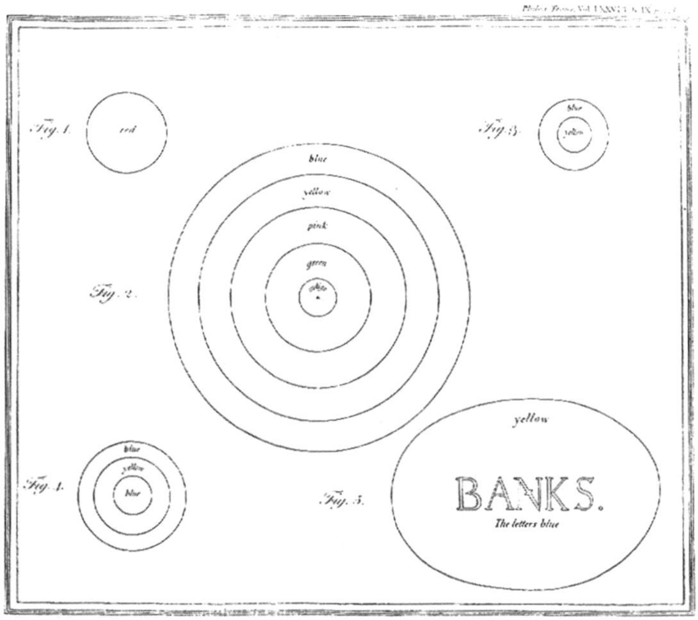

Figure 4.1
The plate published with Robert Darwin's (1786) article on afterimages. That for demonstrating the instability of fixation was *Fig.* 1. The others were for complementary coloured afterimages (*Figs.* 2–4) and for demonstrating the variation in the apparent size of afterimages with the distance of the surface onto which they were projected (*Fig.* 5).

Porterfield (1737) restated the anatomical position in the eighteenth century:

The oblique Muscles of the Eye are two in Number... When it [superior oblique] acts, it rolls the Eye about its *Axis* towards the Nose, and at the same time draws it forwards, and turns its Pupil downwards... The action of this [second oblique] Muscle is to roll the Eye about its *Axis* from the Nose, and at the same time to draw it forwards, and direct its Pupil upwards... Though the Action of these two oblique Muscles seems pretty evident, yet there is scarce any Part of the human Body about which Anatomists have differed more, than in assigning them their proper Offices. (pp. 167–168, and 172, original italics)

Torsion was easier to observe as a consequence of inclining the head, and it is in this context that Scheiner (1619) hinted at its occurrence: 'in an eye movement in which the middle part of the eye remains stationary, it is because it moves by a corresponding head rotation' (p. 245). A more precise description was provided by Hunter (1786) who outlined the function that the oblique muscles could serve: when the head was tilted to one side, they could rotate the eyes in their sockets in the opposite direction to remain more closely aligned to gravity.

Thus when we look at an object, and at the same time move our heads to either shoulder, it is moving in the arch of a circle whose centre is the neck, and of course the eyes would have the same quantity of motion on this axis, if the oblique muscles did not fix them upon the object. When the head is moved towards the right-shoulder, the superior oblique muscle of the right-side acts and keeps the right-eye fixed on the object, and a similar effect is produced upon the left-eye by the action of the inferior oblique muscle; when the head moves in the contrary direction, the other oblique muscles produce the same effect. (Hunter, 1786, p. 212)

It is clear from the dispute between Wells and Darwin (Section 3.5) that Darwin did not accept that torsion occurred at all, and he was by no means alone in this view. It was Wells' (1794*b*) demonstration of torsional nystagmus that should have resolved the dispute. The method he used—forming an afterimage of a horizontal line and then comparing it with a real line—should have opened the way to detailed measurements of eye position. Instead, it was forgotten, only to be rediscovered by Ruete (1845), and applied extensively thereafter.

Bell (1823) argued on the grounds of anatomy and experiment 'that the oblique muscles are antagonists to each other, and that they roll the eye in opposite directions, the superior oblique directing the pupil downwards and outwards, and the inferior oblique directing it upwards and inwards' (p. 174). The experiments he conducted on rabbits and monkeys consisted of either noting changes in tension of the oblique muscles during eye movements or sectioning an oblique muscle in one eye and noting the consequences. Three years later, Johannes Müller (1826*a*) tried to measure torsion by marking the conjunctiva and noting any rotations of the marks. He was unable to see any and concluded that the eyes did not undergo torsion. Much of the remaining part of his book on eye movements was concerned with convergence and binocular single vision.

In contrast to Müller's conclusion, observational studies by Alexander Friedrich Hueck (1802–1842) lent support to the occurrence of torsion. Hueck (1838) examined in more detail rotation of the eyes in the opposite direction to head tilt and tried to measure its magnitude. He stated that the eyes remain in the same relation to gravity for head tilts up to 28°; that is, there was perfect compensation for head inclination:

The observation of actual eye torsion shows that vertical diameter of the eyeball remains vertical if the head is inclined sideways by up to 28°, and therefore during this movement the image maintains its location unchanged. If we incline the head to the side by more than 38°, the eyeball

> can no longer retain its position with respect to the head rotation. (Hueck, 1838, p. 31)

Subsequent experiments have not supported Hueck's claim: while rotation of the eyes does occur, its magnitude is only a fraction of the head tilt. This would now be called ocular countertorsion, and it has a gain of around 0.1 (Howard, 1982). Thus, when the head is tilted laterally by 30° the eyes rotate in the opposite direction by about 3°. It was because the magnitude of countertorsion is small that it was difficult to measure with any degree of precision and there was much debate concerning its occurrence at all. A review of the nineteenth century debates concerning countertorsion was provided by Nagel (1896), who was able to resolve the dispute regarding its occurrence in animals but not in humans. Howard and Templeton (1966) and Howard (1982, 2002) described the techniques that have been applied to measure countertorsion in the twentieth century.

Earlier in the nineteenth century, ocular torsion assumed a greater theoretical importance. Concern with the geometry of eye rotations and with the specification of their constraints led to the formulations of laws that could only be verified by means of measuring its magnitude. Although many were involved in this endeavour, the work was summarized and integrated by Helmholtz (Fig. 4.6, left).

4.2.3 Donders' law and Listing's law

Even though the eyes do not retain precise fixation, due to involuntary movements, the deviations are relatively small. They were essentially ignored in the grand analyses of eye movements undertaken in the nineteenth century by the likes of Donders, Helmholtz, and Hering. A number of preliminary issues required resolving before the geometry of eye movements could be described with accuracy. The first concerned the centre of rotation of the eye. Despite the fact that small translations of the eye occurred, the centre of rotation was determined to be 13.6 mm behind the vertex of the cornea (Helmholtz, 1867*a*). The orbit of the eye can assume a variety of locations as the head moves, and so a further question related to the position the head should adopt for experiments on eye movements. Helmholtz defined the axes of the head with regard to the symmetry between the two sides and the line joining the two eyes. The former was called the median plane and the latter the transverse plane. The head was said to be upright when the median plane was vertical and the transverse plane horizontal.

With the head in this erect position some reference position for the eyes was required as was some system of coordinates for rotations. The primary position was defined as the position of the eyes when they are horizontal and perpendicular to the axis between their centres of rotation (the interocular axis). The adoption of fixed axes around which the eye can rotate is arbitrary. Helmholtz described two systems: the Fick axis system in which the vertical axis is assumed to be fixed to the skull (Fick, 1854) and the Helmholtz system in which the horizontal axis is so fixed. When the eye moves from the primary position along a horizontal or a vertical axis it assumes a secondary position; movements to any other (oblique) location involve the eye in a tertiary position.

Donders (1847; Fig. 4.2, left) measured the eye position in secondary and tertiary locations and provided a general relationship that Helmholtz (1867*a*) elevated to the status of a law:

> The law, given first by Donders and confirmed by all subsequent investigations, is that *when the position of the line of fixation is given with respect to the head, the angle of torsion will invariably have a perfectly definite value for that particular adjustment*; which is independent not only of the volition of the observer but of the way in which the line of fixation arrived in the position in question. (Helmholtz, 1925/2000, p. 44, original italics)

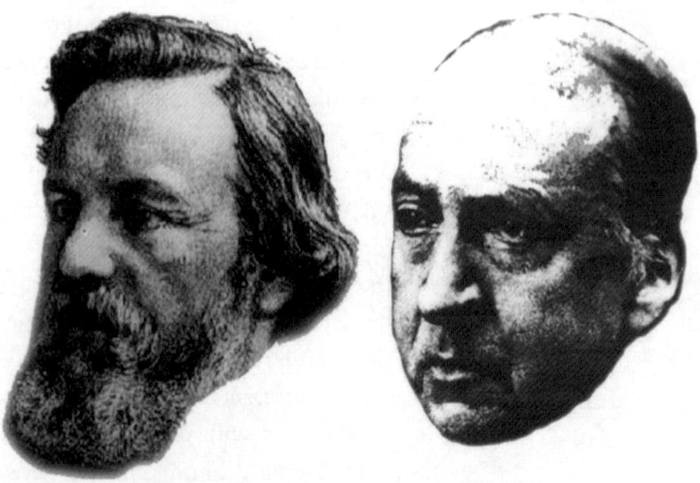

Figure 4.2
Left, Frans Cornelis Donders (1818–1889), right, Johann Benedict Listing (1808–1882), both after a portraits in Schmitz (1983).

Thus, no matter what path the eye pursues to reach a given position, the degree of torsion will be the same. As Helmholtz remarked:

The best way of verifying these facts is by using after-images, as was originally suggested by Ruete. The way to do it is to stand opposite a wall covered with paper on which horizontal and vertical lines can be distinguished, the pattern, however, not being so sharply outlined as to make it difficult to see after-images on it. The best background is one of a smooth pale grey colour. Directly opposite the observer's eye, and on the same level with it, a black or coloured ribbon is stretched horizontally, two or three feet long; standing out in sharp contrast to the colour of the wall-paper . . . Now let the observer look intently for a little while at the middle of the band, and then, without moving his head, turn his eyes suddenly to another place on the wall. An after-image of the band will appear there, and by comparing it with the horizontal lines of the wall-paper, the observer can see whether the after-image is horizontal or not. The after-image itself is developed on those points of the retina belonging to the retinal horizon; and during the motions of the eyes it indicates those parts of the visual field on which the retinal horizon is projected. (Helmholtz, 1925/2000, p. 45)

This is essentially the technique Wells (1794*b*) had used in order to determine the existence of torsional nystagmus. In Helmholtz's case the degree of deviation of the afterimage from

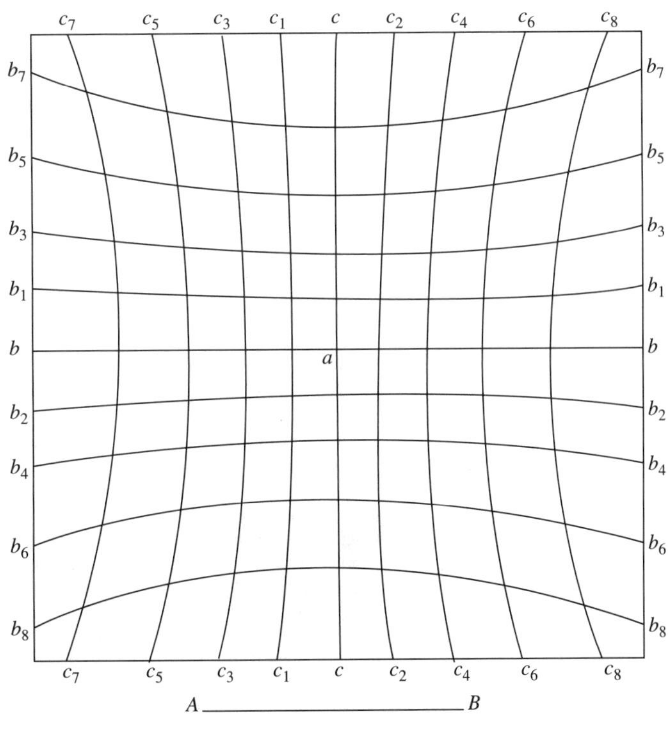

Figure 4.3
Helmholtz's (1867*a*) diagram of eye position in tertiary gaze directions: 'The eye is supposed to be situated on the perpendicular to the plane of the paper at a distance equal to *AB* from the point *a*. In this case the after-images of a horizontal line passing through *a*, when projected on another part of the field, will coincide with the directions of the curves b_1b_1, b_2b_2, etc.; and the after-images of a vertical line passing through *a* will coincide, on the other hand, with the direction of the curves *cc*, c_1c_1, c_2c_2, etc. For normal ocular measurements these curves are hyperbolas' (1925/2000, p. 47).

the rectangular grid could be determined and the diagram he provided to show the degrees of torsion in secondary and tertiary positions is shown in Fig. 4.3. The afterimages remain vertical or horizontal in secondary but not in tertiary positions.

Donders' law was formulated for movements of the eye from the primary position. Another lawful relationship was formulated by Johann Benedict Listing (1808–1882; Fig. 4.2, right). Whereas Donders' law stated that the eye always assumed the same orientation at a particular location, no matter how it had been reached, Listing's law specified the orientation that was adopted in a particular position. Listing (1845) wrote on physiological optics but he did not publish an account of it himself; it was initially described in Ruete's (1853) book on ophthalmology. Again it was Helmholtz who named it Listing's law; it was concerned with describing the axis about which the eye rotates from the primary position (see Fig. 4.4). Helmholtz described it in the following way:

> Accordingly, for the case of a pair of emmetropic eyes with parallel lines of fixation, the law of their motion may be stated as follows: *When the line of fixation is brought from its primary position into any other position, the torsional rotation of the*

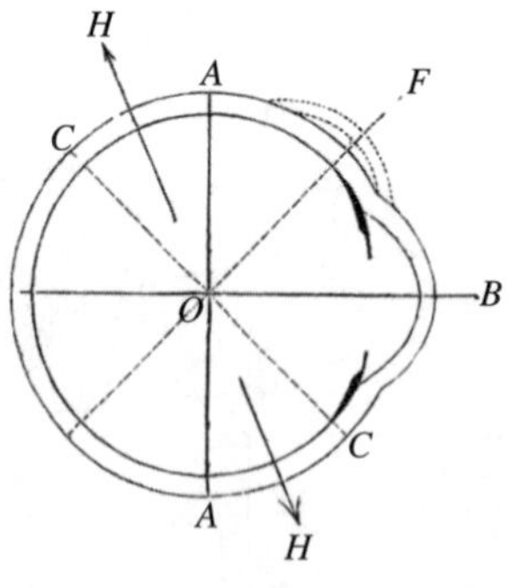

Figure 4.4
The diagram of the eye from Helmholtz (1867*a*) illustrating Listing's law: 'Thus when the eyes turn from the primary position to look in any other direction, according to Listing's law, the axis of rotation will always lie in a plane perpendicular to the line of fixation. Suppose this plane containing the axes of rotation passes through the line *AA* which is perpendicular to the line of fixation OB. Consider a second plane P passing through the eyeball and rigidly connected with it, which coincides with the plane *AA* when the eye is in the primary position. Now if the line of fixation OB is turned into another position OF, the plane P will assume the position represented by CC. In order to pass from this first secondary position to some other position, the eye may turn again around fixed axes all lying in one and the same plane, that is, *in the plane which bisects the angle between the planes AA and* CC, and which therefore intersects the plane of the diagram at right angles in the plane *HH*. This is the plane of the axes of rotation for the given secondary position of the line of fixation OF'. (Helmholtz, 1925/2000, pp. 49–50, original italics)

eyeball in this second position will be the same as if the eye had been turned around a fixed axis perpendicular to the initial and final directions of the line of fixation. This is known as Listing's law of ocular movements, because it was first stated by him in this form. (Helmholtz, 1925/2000, p. 48, original italics)

Both Donders' and Listing's laws apply for eye movements from the primary position; that is, with the eyes parallel and directed to the horizon. Empirical studies generally supported the laws, and Helmholtz reported that eye rotations could be measured to within half a degree using the afterimage method. However, most eye movements are directed to objects that are nearer than optical infinity and so will involve some degree of convergence. Volkmann (1846; Fig. 4.5, left) demonstrated that departures from the laws occur with convergence, as illustrated in Fig. 4.5 (right), taken from Helmholtz (1867*a*).

One of the great advantages that Helmholtz bestowed on eye movement research was the introduction of the bite bar for controlling head position. His model is illustrated in Fig. 4.6 (right) and he described as follows:

In order to fix the direction of the primary position of the line of fixation with reference to the head, I use a little board, with a mark of fixation on it. This planchette is taken between the teeth . . . The length of the board *AB* is 13 cm, and its width is 4 cm. At *A* a portion of the board is cut out in the form of an arc to fit the row of teeth; and at B there is a square wooden post on which a horizontal strip of stiff paper is fastened with wax, so that it can easily be shifted. Both sides of the board at *A* are covered with a layer of warm shellac; and when it begins to harden, the planchette is seized between the teeth so as to get an impression in the shellac. Thereafter, when the mould has hardened, the exact position of the planchette between the teeth can be regained just as it was at first, thus enabling us to resume an experiment where it had been interrupted. (Helmholtz, 1925/2000, pp. 108–109)

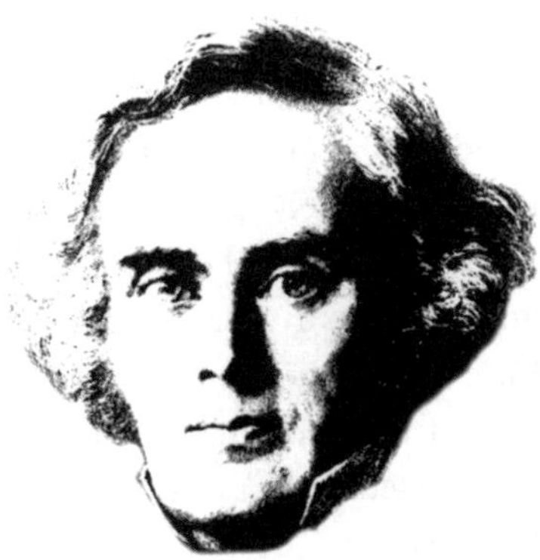

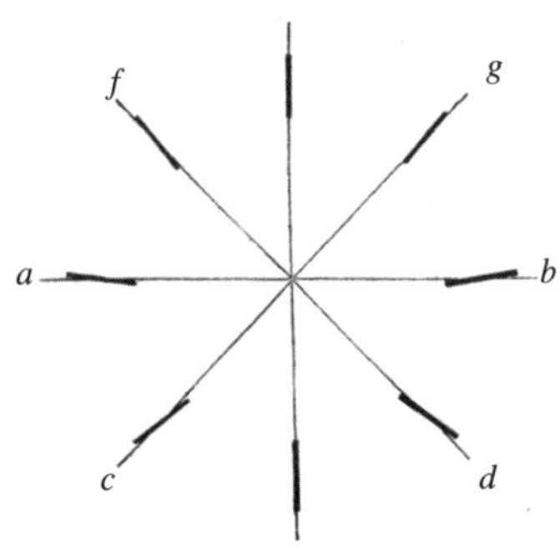

Figure 4.5
Left, Alfred Wilhelm Volkmann (1800–1877) after an illustration kindly supplied by Juri Allik. Right, the diagram from Helmholtz (1867*a*) showing deviations from Listing's law with convergence: 'The short thick lines represent the positions of after-images when the eyes are converged' (Helmholtz, 1925/2000, p. 51).

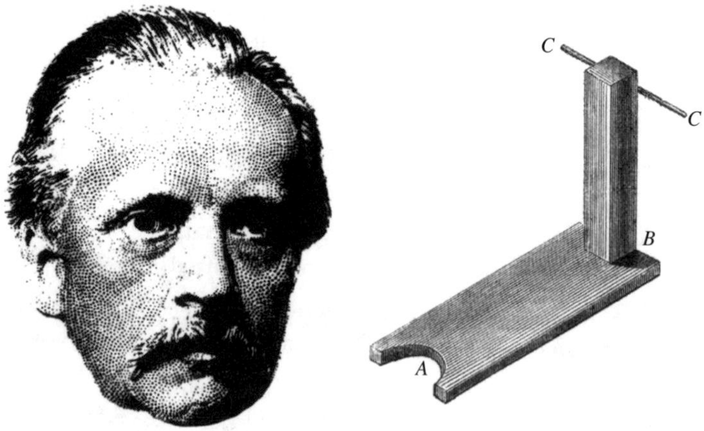

Figure 4.6
Left, Hermann Helmholtz (1821–1894) after an engraving in Koenigsberger (1902). Right, a diagram of the bite board as shown in Helmholtz (1867*a*).

4.2.4 Helmholtz and Hering

One of the remarkable features of this experimental work in the nineteenth century was the reliance on data from a single observer. Helmholtz himself epitomized this tendency. In common with his contemporaries, the processes of perception were considered to be universal so that general principles could be derived from particular observations. Much of the polemic surrounding the heated debates in nineteenth century visual science was based on the conviction that personal perception was pervasive; individual differences were only taken seriously in areas like colour blindness. Novel observations were accepted as fact when they were in turn seen by another investigator. Helmholtz was at his most vulnerable when his observational skills were impugned (see Howard, 1999). He placed great store by his control of fixation and by his ability to assess his eye position with accuracy. This will be evident in the discussion on motion illusions in Chapter 5. He used his inability to see certain depth effects described by Hering (1864*a*) as decisive evidence against nativist theory.

Ewald Hering (1834–1918; Fig. 4.7, left) also wrote and experimented extensively on eye movements, and his views clashed fundamentally with those of Helmholtz (see Turner, 1994). In addition to his five *Beiträge zur Physiologie* (Hering, 1861, 1862, 1863, 1864*a*,*b*) he wrote a very extensive review of the spatial sense and eye movements for Hermann's *Handbuch der Physiologie* (1879*a*). Helmholtz's *Handbuch* was translated into English in 1924/5; Hering's review of eye movements was translated into

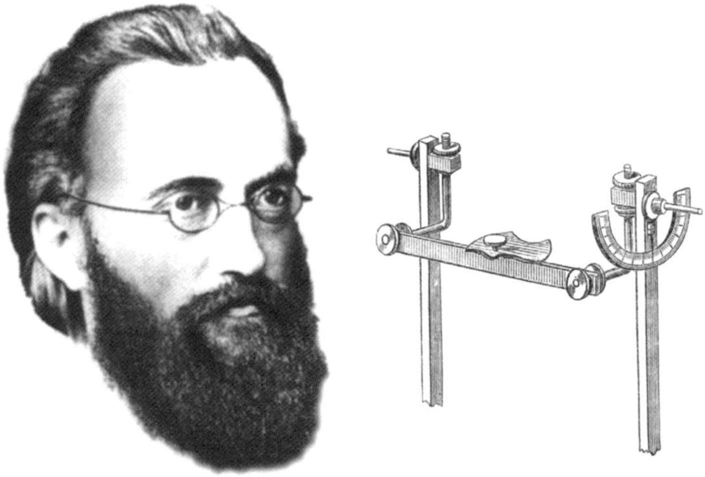

Figure 4.7
Left, Karl Ewald Konstantin Hering (1834–1918) after an illustration in Lesky (1965). Right, an improved bite bar with adjustments for head inclination (from Hering, 1879*a*).

English in 1942. Helmholtz and Hering represented two different philosophical traditions. Helmholtz espoused the empiricist and the associationist views of John Locke and George Berkeley; he believed that each eye was controlled independently and that their binocular coordination was learnt by association; that is, each monocular view was available to consciousness and fusion was a psychical act. Hering, on the other hand, was in the nativist and phenomenological tradition of Immanuel Kant (1724–1804) and Johann Wolfgang Goethe (1749–1832); he contended that each retinal point has local signs for the space values of height, breadth, and depth, and that binocular fusion was physiological. Hering investigated binocular eye movements and argued that the two eyes move as a single unit: his law of equal innervation states that when one eye moves the other moves with equal amplitude and velocity, either in the same or the opposite direction. Eye movements were also implicated in visual direction: the centre of binocular visual direction was called the cyclopean eye.

Hermann Helmholtz was born in Potsdam, southwest of Berlin and educated at the Gymnasium where he displayed a keen interest in physics. He was not able to pursue his penchant for physics immediately, as economic necessity led him to study medicine (with an army scholarship) at Berlin. There he came under the influence of Johannes Müller, and formed his life-long friendship with Emil du Bois Reymond (1818–1896). Helmholtz completed his medical studies in 1842. His dissertation was based on microscopic studies of the nervous system, and he was able to demonstrate that nerve fibres originate in the ganglion cells. Thereafter he took up a post as a surgeon in the army, based at Potsdam, while maintaining his association with Müller in Berlin. During this period Helmholtz provided the empirical and mathematical evidence to support the principle of conservation of energy. However, he was opposed to the vitalism espoused by his teacher, and in 1847, together with his contemporaries du Bois Reymond, Brücke, and Carl Ludwig (1816–1895), he pledged to account for all living processes in terms of physics and chemistry. On release from the army in 1848 he took up an academic career, initially teaching anatomy to art students in Berlin. In 1849 he received the call to the chair of physiology from the University of Königsberg (now Kaliningrad), situated on the Baltic, where he remained for six years. This was a productive period for Helmholtz: he measured the duration of nerve conduction, invented the ophthalmoscope, and initiated his studies of colour vision. He accepted the call to Bonn in 1855, where he occupied the chair of anatomy and physiology. In 1858 he accepted the prestigious appointment to the professorship of physiology at Heidelberg. His tenure in Heidelberg witnessed the culmination of his work on sensory physiology, and after 1867 his energies were directed increasingly towards physics. He was appointed to the chair of physics in Berlin in 1871, was ennobled in 1883, and became director of the specially created Physical–Technical Institute at Charlottenburg in 1888. During his tenure in Berlin he received many awards from scientific bodies throughout Europe.

Ewald Hering was born in Altgersdorf, a small village in Saxony. He was educated at the Gymnasium at Zittau and studied medicine at the University of Leipzig, graduating in 1858. He remained in Leipzig for seven more years where he pursued an academic rather than a medical career. His experiments in vision commenced soon after graduating, and he maintained an interest in vision research throughout his life. One of his early influences was Rudolf Hermann Lotze (1817–1881) and his concept of retinal local signs. Hering was appointed professor of physiology at Joseph's Academy (Josephinum), Vienna in 1865, but his tenure at Vienna was fraught because Brücke, who occupied the chair in physiology at the university, was a close friend of Helmholtz's. In the late 1860s Ewald Hering worked with Breuer in Vienna on the regulation of respiration, although this was not the principal interest of either physiologist. Hering moved to Prague, to succeed Purkinje, in 1870, and finally returned to Leipzig in 1895; he was a colleague of Mach while at Prague. Despite his teaching commitments, Hering was a very productive and ingenious researcher (see Baumann, 2002). Among his many contributions to the study of eye movements was an improved version of Helmholtz's bite bar (Fig. 4.7, right).

The initial battle-ground between Helmholtz and Hering was binocular vision, but it broadened later to encompass eye movements and colour vision. The critical issue was whether retinal local signs were adaptable or fixed and how they served stereoscopic vision.

The Empirical Theory regards the local signs (whatever they really may be) as signs the signification of which must be learnt, and is actually learnt, in order to arrive at a knowledge of the external world... The Innate Theory, on the other hand, supposes that the local signs are nothing else than direct conceptions of differences in space as such, both in their nature and their magnitude. (Helmholtz, 1873, p. 275)

In many ways, Hering's approach was much closer to that of Helmholtz's mentor, Johannes Müller, who considered that identical retinal points were innate. Hering was more concerned with binocular than monocular eye movements. He made the distinction between eye movements in distant vision (with the axes parallel and horizontal) and near vision (with convergence and depression or elevation of the eyes). He did however conduct experiments, like those described by Helmholtz, in which the orientations of line afterimages were determined in a variety of eye positions in distant vision. A vertical line afterimage was formed in the primary position of the eye and then its orientation was determined in secondary and tertiary positions (Fig. 4.8)

Hering found, as Volkmann had before him, that this situation did not apply to near vision:

In symmetric convergence postures, the mid-vertical sections are inclined at the upper end, more outward or less inward than Listing's law stipulates, and that this deviation grows on the one hand with an increase of the angle of convergence, on the other with the lowering of the visual plane, and at the most to about 5°. Furthermore with asymmetric convergence, the relative position of both retinas to one another, and therefore the divergence of mid-vertical or horizontal sections does not differ markedly from that with equally symmetric convergence. (Hering, 1942, p. 133, original italics)

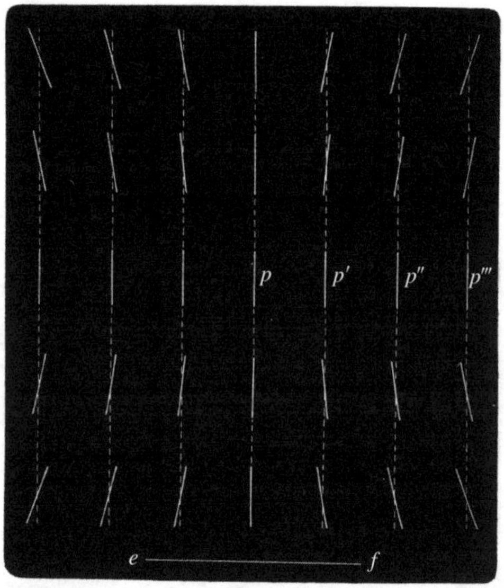

Figure 4.8

The diagram from Hering (1879*a*) showing 'what apparent positions an originally vertical after-image may take in distant vision on a vertical plane with the various postures of the visual line, provided that the visual line in its primary position strikes the vertical plane perpendicularly at the point *p* ... Thus Figure 47 pictures the changes of position which the after-image experiences while the gaze travels in any given direction over the plane.' (Hering, 1942, p. 126)

For Hering, the two eyes moved as a single unit and this union was not dependent upon learning or association, as Helmholtz maintained. Hering stated this point repeatedly and he referred to the yoked actions of the two sets of eye muscles. His diagrams reflected this too; the motions of each eye were referred to those of an imaginary eye between them. In the context of visual direction the locus from which objects are seen was called the cyclopean eye. For binocular eye movements he referred to the directions relative to this 'imaginary single eye' as the binocular visual line (see Fig. 4.9).

Fixations occur between movements of the eyes and Hering showed a clear understanding of the functions that such movements served. That is, his concerns were not only with where the eye alights but how it reaches that point. Technical constraints tended to restrict experimental studies to determining the orientation of the eye rather than how it moved. Nonetheless, the purpose of such movements was described as well as the range over which they can occur:

In ordinary seeing the visual point constantly changes its position; for, in order to recognize the outer objects, we must examine one after another, all their separate parts and endeavor to perceive them with utmost acuity. This can be accomplished only by bringing their images upon the two retinal centers. With small objects the mere turning of the eyeballs in their sockets suffices. But if the object of regard is of large dimensions, we resort to turning the head, and if necessary, the upper body, and finally even changing

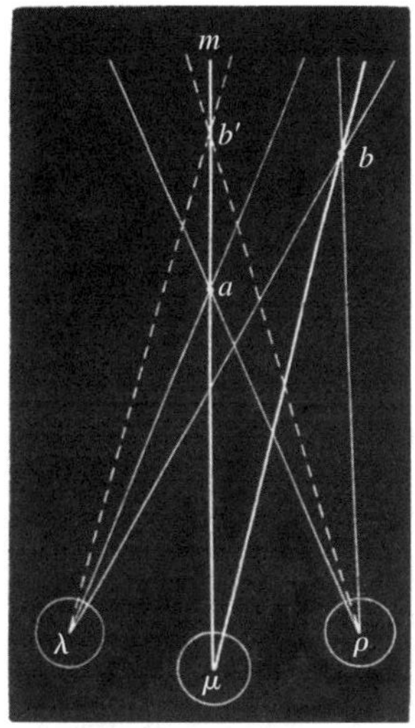

Figure 4.9

Hering's (1879*a*) diagram of binocular eye movements and their relation to the binocular visual line: 'the visual point lies at *a*, the line *μ m* is the visual line of the imaginary single eye accommodating for the point *a*. This accommodation corresponds with the convergence angle *λ a ρ* of the actual visual line. The attention is now drawn to an object at the point *b*, to the right of, and farther than *a*. For the imaginary single eye to see it clearly, a relaxation of the accommodation for the farther distance, and a rotation to the right through the angle *m μ b* would be required.' (Hering, 1942, pp. 154–155).

our location. Rarely do we devote our attention to one spot, even for the duration of a second. Rather does our glance spring from point to point, and in its wanderings it is followed slavishly by the visual point, in whose movements we have greater agility than in any other movement, for no organ is so continuously used as the visual organ. (Hering, 1942, p. 83)

The nature of such movements was studied by Hering (1879*b*) in a short article published in the same year as the long handbook chapter (Hering, 1879*a*), as will be described in Section 4.3.5. Hering employed afterimages again in these studies, but they were not the principal source of evidence regarding the ways in which the eyes moved. Rather, they provided a means of calibrating another technique that he adopted for assessing rapid eye movements and fixations.

The debate between the views of Helmholtz and Hering reverberated throughout the rest of the nineteenth century. This is reflected in Edward Bradford Titchener's (1867–1927; 1901) textbook: most of the experiments were derived from those performed by Helmholtz and Hering, and most of the theoretical issues were referred back to their disagreements. The situation was to change with the development of novel techniques for measuring both eye rotations and fixations. Dodge was at the forefront of these developments, and he was able to integrate the insights derived from research on vertigo with those determined from his own experiments on reading. Dodge (1907) appreciated that fixations are an integral part of vision, as he noted in his extensive survey of them:

> Every complete visual act involves both eye movement and fixation . . . Both eye movement and fixation are means to the attainment of a satisfactory visual impression; and since both are the products of muscular activity, fixation, even if it were absolute, would be only a limiting instance of eye movement, while the study of the latter finds its natural complement in a study of the consequent fixation. The close relationship between eye movement and fixation is reflected in the uncertainty of traditional terminology. The term 'fixation' is frequently used to cover the entire process of visual adjustment, including the antecedent eye movement. In general, however, fixation appears to mean that the point of regard remains relatively unchanged within the visual field. In this sense the point of regard is commonly called the fixation point. It is obviously in this sense that I have used the term. On the other hand it is a commonplace of physiological optics that the globe of the eye is never fixed in the sense that it is free from minute irregular movements. (Dodge, 1907, p. 1)

The 'minute irregular movements' to which Dodge was referring were described in Section 4.2.1, and his measurement of saccades will be discussed in the next section.

4.3 Saccades

As we have seen in the earlier sections of this chapter, numerous studies in the nineteenth century investigated eye movements outside the context of nystagmus. However, an appreciation of the distinction of saccades as a specialized family of movements, or of their importance in vision is absent from most of these works. When eye movements were investigated it usually involved attempts to measure their velocity. For example, Volkmann (1846) recorded the frequency of alternating fixation between two pins throughout 30s. He varied the separation of the pins from 1 to 70° and compared monocular with binocular observation. He concluded that eye movements were slower than finger movements, those with two eyes were slower than with one, and the time required increased with separation. He did not, however, provide a value for the velocity. Lamansky (1869) delivered light flashes in a fixed location at intervals of approximately 5 ms and counted the number of afterimages visible when the eye passed over them. On the basis of these experiments he calculated eye movements velocities of between 720° and 1500° s^{-1}, but the task was said to be very difficult to perform. He also found that horizontal eye movements were faster than vertical.

Helmholtz did describe a discontinuity of eye movements (jerks) in the context of visual vertigo:

> For example, when a person travelling on a train has been looking for some time at objects close to the track outside, and then turns to look at the floor of the carriage, although the latter is at rest relative to his body, it seems to be moving from under him in the same direction as the train. The reason of this is because there is an apparent motion of the objects on the track in the direction opposite to that of the motion of the train. Wherever the traveller tries to focus one of them, he has to jerk his eyes quickly in the direction opposite to that of the motion of the train. . . . But if the passenger gazing out of the coach should happen to fix his attention constantly on a speck on the window, the aforesaid giddiness will not be developed. (1925/2000, pp. 247–248)

This account occurs in the section on 'The direction of vision' rather than that on 'Movements of the eyes'. The term 'jerk' was added by the translator (James Southall); an exact translation of Helmholtz's (1867*a*, p. 603) text would be that 'his eyes moved quickly in the opposite direction to the train' (seine Augen schnell der Richtung des Zuges entgegen bewegen). Helmholtz then addressed visual vertigo from body rotation. When he whirled round with his eyes closed, he did not experience any visual motion afterward if he opened his eyes when the sense of body rotation had ceased (as would be expected). However, if he opened his eyes beforehand, he experienced visual motion but attributed this 'to an illusion about the time when the body itself comes to rest' (1925/2000, p. 248). He did not make the distinction between saccadic and other types of movement and rather appears to hold the view that eye movements are continuous, but with varying velocities. As we have seen in Section 4.2.4, Hering (1879*a*) provided a clearer account of how the eyes move when inspecting objects in a scene, although he did not describe the discontinuous movements with any degree of detail in that publication. Such descriptions are generally associated with Javal's deliberations on the physiology of reading which were published at about the same time. In the literature on eye movements, Javal's name has been intricately linked with the study of saccades.

4.3.1 Javal

Helmholtz's *Handbuch* had an enormous impact on visual science. It introduced a new degree of experimental rigour and provided a unified interpretation of most phenomena discussed. It was translated and published in French in the same year as the complete German edition (Helmholtz, 1867*b*). One of the translators was Louis-Émile Javal (1839–1909; Fig. 4.10, left). Javal was the son of an Israeli banker and studied sciences to become a mining engineer in 1862. However, one year after beginning his engineering career, he returned to academia to study medicine and went on to become director of the ophthalmology laboratory at the Sorbonne and a member of the Académie de Médecine. Javal's main research focus was upon visual deficits; an interest that probably arose because his sister was strabismic and Javal himself was astigmatic.

In the course of his research Javal developed an interest in the visual processes involved in reading, and it was on this topic that Javal published his landmark series of papers (Javal, 1878*a–c*, 1879*a–e*) from which his understanding and even measurement of saccadic eye movements has since been asserted. Javal is now widely credited as being the first writer to use the term 'saccade' to refer to rapid eye movements and is also said to have observed saccades during reading (Huey, 1908; Woodworth, 1938). However it now seems likely that Javal's contribution to the early understanding of saccadic eye movements may be somewhat less

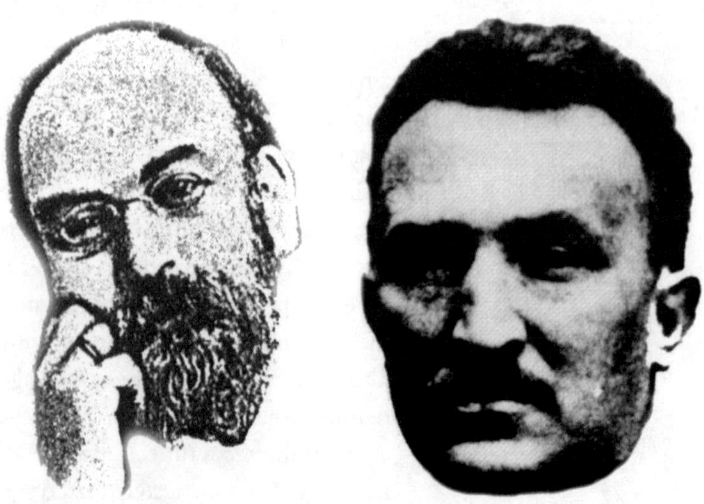

Figure 4.10
Left, Louis-Émile Javal (1839–1909) after a portrait in Taylor (1937). Right, Marius Hans Erik Tscherning (1854–1939) after a frontispiece photograph in Tscherning (1900).

than previously thought (see Tatler and Wade, 2003; Wade et al., 2003). Of Javal's eight papers on reading, only two discussed eye movements in any detail. His main assertions about eye movements during reading, were in fact based upon his own intuitions rather than objective measurement and fell into the same types of pitfall that Porterfield (1759*b*) had made in his descriptions of vertigo—namely a reliance on the subjective impressions of how the eyes moved rather than any measurements of them. Javal (1879*e*) reasoned that the eye made no vertical movements during reading: 'If, during reading, we maintain perfect immobility of the book and the head, the printed lines come to be painted successively on the same parts of the retina, while the spaces between the lines constantly fall upon the same parts of the retina' (p. 246). Thus, Javal seems to have been of the opinion that the eye glides smoothly along the line during reading; an assertion that would appear unlikely given Javal's popular accreditation as the discoverer of saccadic eye movements in reading. He wrote that: 'gaze glides along a line slightly higher than the centre of the characters. The reason for this is easy to see: if gaze simply glides horizontally, complicated and useless movements are avoided, and the chosen position of the horizontal is determined by the structure of the typographic characters' (Javal, 1878*c*, p. 251).

While these examples suggest that Javal may not have possessed as keen an awareness of the saccadic nature of eye movements as history has bestowed upon him, he did recognize the necessity to measure eye movements objectively and made several attempts to do so. Javal (1878*c*) tried to examine eye movements during reading by observing the movements of an afterimage, but found that the technique was difficult to apply because of the contrast between the letters, the page, and the afterimage. He also considered attaching a feather to the eye so that movements could be recorded on a smoked drum, and he attempted (unsuccessfully) to measure the deflections of light from a mirror attached to his eye.

> It does not appear impossible to me to be able to carry out the same demonstration in the context of an objective experiment, which would consist of reading by a one-eyed person whose bad eye has retained good mobility, to which one could attach a feather for registering its movements on a smoked cylinder; I am certain that one would thus note the absence of vertical movements of the eye during reading. (Javal, 1878*c*, p. 250)

Javal did mention saccades in a footnote on the penultimate page of the final article of his series in 1879. However, this was a reference to work by his colleague Lamare, rather than by Javal himself:

D'après des recherches entreprises par M. Lamare dans notre laboratoire, l'œil subit même plusieurs saccades dans le courant de chaque ligne, environ une par 15 à 18 lettres de texte, il est probable que, chez le myope à chacune de ces saccades de l'œil répond une variation brusque de l'accommodation. (Javal, 1879*e*, p. 252)

which translates as follows:

Following the research of Mr. Lamare in our laboratory, the eye makes several saccades during the passage over each line, about one for every 15–18 letters of text. It is probable that in myopes the eye reacts with a rapid change in accommodation with every one of these saccades.

It seems likely that it is from this footnote that Lamare's work has become mistakenly attributed to Javal. Certainly Javal did use the term 'saccade' in his final article in 1879, both in the above footnote and on the preceding page, where he referred to saccades when describing rapid changes in accommodation during reading:

Considering our specific ideas about the mechanism of accommodation, it is not surprising that the series of saccades imprinted to the choroids by the ciliary muscles of myopes have the effect of augmenting their disability. (Javal, 1879*e*, p. 251)

Or, in its original French:

D'après nos idées particulières sur le mécanisme de l'accommodation, il n'est pas étonnant que la série de saccades imprimées à la choroïde par le muscle ciliaire des myopes ait pour effet d'augmenter progressivement leur infirmité.

This and the footnote on the following page of this article are the earliest uses of the term saccade to describe eye movements that we know of and Javal therefore deserves due credit for first using the term. While Javal did use the term 'saccade', it was at the time an unremarkable French word, in common usage, meaning 'jerk' or 'twitch'. That the term came to be adopted widely was due not to Javal but to later researchers.

4.3.2 Lamare

Later, in his book on reading and writing, Javal (1904, 1906) noted that an error had been made regarding saccade size and a revised value of ten to twelve letters between saccades was adopted. Javal was referring to the initial investigations by Lamare, who published an account of his experiments in 1892. Javal's book was based on the essays that were published in 1878–1879; the first edition appeared in 1904, and a revised and corrected second edition was published two years later. The second edition was translated into German (Javal, 1907). The chapter in the book most concerned with eye movements (entitled 'On the mechanism of reading') described and essentially reprinted the article by Lamare (1892). Javal commenced the chapter: 'Lamare established, in an important work conducted in my laboratory, that the horizontal movements of the eyes during reading are by no means continuous, but proceed by saccades' (1904, p. 127). Thus, Javal was not making a claim for his own research but was assigning the credit to Lamare.

Lamare (1892) described several methods he applied to study the number of such saccades along a line of text. The first method was based on counting: he counted the number of letters he could read in one minute and divided that by the estimated number of pauses made. The average value he arrived at was ten letters per saccade. He then tried to determine, during fixation, the extent of letter recognition in the periphery. The third method involved counting the number of distinct movements the eye made along a line. It was in this context that he described how the discontinuous eye movements can be observed in a reader, or felt by placing a finger over the closed eye when reading with the open one: 'An assistant can *see* these movements. He can *feel* them with a finger over the lid of a closed eye' (Lamare, 1892, p. 357, original italics). Lamare was not satisfied with using observation or touch to count the eye movements and so constructed apparatus that could record the movements and pauses. It was during the description of this apparatus that Lamare first used the term 'saccade' in his article: 'on n'a qu'à l'ajouter au nombre des *saccades* entendues depuis la commencement de la ligne' (p. 357, original italics):

> The method that gives the best results is one by which the movements are heard via a drum with an ebonite membrane in the centre and to which a small tube is attached; the tube is in contact with the conjunctiva or eyelid and is connected to both ears by rubber tubes... The apparatus yields distinctive sounds which an assistant can count and add, and note for each line.

> The return movement of the eyes to the beginning of a line gives a longer and louder noise that is easy to recognise; one counts the number of *saccades* from the start of the line to be able to *note* the number of divisions that occur in a line. (Lamare, 1892, p. 357, original italics)

By noting the number of letters on a line, Lamare was able to calculate the average size of saccades; concluding that about ten letters must be read in each pause (which Lamare refered to as *sections*) between the eye movements. A crucial and insightful aspect of this paper was to compare the number of letters read per fixation for text displayed at different distances. Lamare found that: '*Regardless of the DISTANCE at which one reads from the same text* (from 0.30 m to 1 m), *the number of letters per section DOES NOT VARY*' (Lamare, 1892, p. 361, original italics and capitals). For the last few pages of the article, Lamare invited a discussion of his work, feeling that his results were neither complete nor supported by theory: 'Although the results of this work are incomplete and do not support any theory, they may be useful to those who wish to pursue this interesting work, and I place my calculations, notes and diagrams at your disposal' (Lamare, 1892, p. 361).

After this generous statement, there followed in the article a series of comments by colleagues, each responded to by Javal. This discussion illustrates that even though Lamare's article was published some thirteen years after Javal's report of Lamare's work, the issue of the nature of eye movements during reading was still much in debate. M. Armaignac took issue with some of Lamare's results arguing that: 'This very interesting work brought to our attention by reading our colleague, appears to me to be based upon a very debatable foundation and, consequently, the conclusions that he draws are not, I believe, accurate' (Armaignac in Lamare, 1892, p. 361). M. Armaignac felt that the work that he had conducted over the previous twelve years, showed that people read whole words and therefore Lamare's assertions about the number of letters read per fixation was misguided. Javal's response to this was to re-state the importance of Lamare's work, especially that regarding the effect of varying the distance at which text was read, and to highlight the implications of Lamare's work to Javal's own primary interest in myopia. He suggested that myopes make fewer saccades when reading and that this suggested that they may have an advantage over those with normal vision when reading at certain distances. Javal's re-centring of the debate onto myopia was reflected in the comments and replies in the rest of the article.

As we have seen, Lamare was recording the number of saccades during reading a line of text, not their extent. Inferences about the latter could be made as an indirect calculation based on the number of letters on a line and on the assumption that the saccades were equal in length. It would appear that Lamare's research on eye movements during reading has been overshadowed by Javal's description of it. Citations of Lamare's work have not been consistent. Very few subsequent researchers have referred to Lamare's experiments, but among those who have is the Danish ophthalmologist, Tscherning.

4.3.3 Tscherning

Marius Hans Erik Tscherning (1854–1939; Fig. 4.10, right) was a student of Peter Ludvig Panum (1820–1885) before going on to train in ophthalmology under Edmung Hansen Grut (1831–1907). During this time, Tscherning recorded the frequency of myopia in men being examined for military service in Denmark. Of the 7564 men examined in his doctoral research, Tscherning found that myopia was more prevalent in those from Copenhagen (9.6%) than in those from rural communities (2.2%). Tscherning's interests in myopia overlapped significantly with those of Javal, and Javal invited Tscherning to visit him at the Sorbonne. Tscherning took up the position of Javal's assistant and remained at the Sorbonne for the next 26 years. He became director when Javal retired because of the onset of blindness due to glaucoma. For more details on the life and works of Tscherning see Norn and Jensen (2004).

Whereas Javal had translated Helmholtz's *Handbuch*, Tscherning translated and annotated Thomas Young's papers on optics and the eye (Young, 1894). This could have been the spur to Tscherning's interests in the movements of the eyes. In his *Optique physiologique* (Tscherning, 1898, 1900), he included a section on 'Les mouvements saccadés des yeux'. This section was translated as 'Jerking movements of the eyes', and the English word used for saccades was jerks in Weiland's translation:

> It seems as if the eye should be kept motionless in order to obtain an impression, at least an impression which can be perceived with some distinctness. If, in a railroad train which is going quite fast, we fix a point on the window,

> the landscape appears confused, the images of its different parts succeeding one another too quickly on the retina to be perceived distinctly. Observing the eyes of any one who is looking at the landscape, we see that they move by jerks. The eyes of the person observed make alternately a rapid movement in the direction of the train to catch the object, and a slower movement in the opposite direction to keep the image of the object on the *fovea*. Then they again make a rapid movement with the train to catch a new object, and so forth. (Tscherning, 1900, p. 299, original italics)

Tscherning did not cite Javal in the context of eye movements in his *Optique physiologique*, but he did give a brief account of Lamare's experiments:

> The eyes are, therefore, in perpetual motion which is made by jerks: they fix a point, make a movement, fix another point, and so forth. While reading, the eyes also move by jerks, four or five for each line of an ordinary book. *Lamare* constructed a small instrument, formed from a point which is supported on the eye across the upper eyelid, and which is fastened to the ears of the observer by rubber tubes. With this instrument each movement of the eyes causes a sound to be heard. We hear four or five slight sounds during the reading of one line, and a louder sound when we begin to read a new line. (Tscherning, 1900, p. 299, original italics)

The translation of Tscherning's description of Lamare's method differs slightly from the one we have made from Lamare's (1892) article; the distinction relates to the French word 'tige'; it could be a pointer or a tube. Since Lamare's method is based on hearing the sounds made by rapid movements of the eye, it seems to us more likely that a tube was applied to the eyelid or conjunctiva rather than a pointer or rod.

4.3.4 Origins of the term 'saccade'

In attempting to discern who first described the saccadic nature of eye movements in situations other than vertigo, an important issue is to consider the origin of the term 'saccade' itself. The word saccade derives from the old French *saquer* or *sachier* meaning 'to pull' and at the time of Javal, translated as 'jerk' or 'twitch'. It was first used by Rabelais in the 16th Century to refer to certain rapid movements of a horse during dressage (see *Trésor de la langue française*, 1990). Thus at the time that Javal first referred to 'saccadic' eye movements in reading 'saccade' was an unremarkable French word in common usage. That the term came to be more generally adopted as a specialized term for describing a particular family of rapid eye movements, was due not to Javal and Lamare, but to later researchers. For example, its adoption by English writers followed a suggestion by Dodge (1916), although his statements regarding its origins were enigmatic: 'German and Scandinavian writers are commonly using the descriptive class term "saccadic" to denote the rapid eye movements for which we have only the arbitrary name of "type I". I am not sure with whom the term originated, but it seems worth adopting' (pp. 422–423). Dodge was not intentionally trying to conceal the origin of the term, but he did not say who the German and Scandinavian writers were, nor did he cite Javal.

Javal did not provide a thorough description or measurement of saccadic eye movements in his series of papers in 1878 and 1879. Furthermore, at the time that Javal and Lamare referred to eye movements as saccadic this was a common French term meaning 'jerky'. In considering the historical origins of the discovery and measurement of saccades, we must therefore look further than Javal and Lamare and consider any researchers contemporary to them who used terms equivalent to 'saccadic' to describe the discontinuity of eye movements. Key figures in the early work describing the discontinuity of eye movements in reading and everyday vision include Hering, Crum Brown, and Dodge; the contributions of these researchers will now be considered.

4.3.5 Hering

It is evident from Section 4.2 that much of the nineteenth century research on eye movements in Germany was concerned with the geometry of eye position following a movement, rather than the kinetics of the movements themselves. Both Breuer (1874) and Mach (1875) observed the movements of afterimages following body rotation. Breuer carried out a series of experiments in which he demonstrated the fast and slow phases of nystagmus and the absence of vision during the rapid return movements. Mach improved on the method by generating an afterimage from observing a flaming magnesium wire: 'After stopping, the afterimage moves slowly across the objects clockwise, interrupted by jerklike movements in the opposite direction. The objects then move counterclockwise' (Young, et al., 2001, p. 84). The translation of Mach's description uses the term 'jerklike' for the rapid returns of the eyes; the German word used was 'ruckweise'.

Afterimages were also employed by Hering (1879*b*) to study eye movements, but in a radically different way to Mach and Breuer. Hering accepted that the movements between real images and afterimages reflected the movements of the eyes, and used this as a source of evidence to support a novel method of measurement. He used two rubber tubes, rather like a miniature stethoscope, placed on the eyelids to listen to the sounds of the ocular muscles. With this technique he observed: 'Throughout one's observations, one hears quite short, dull clapping sounds, which follow each other at irregular intervals' (p. 145). He found that these 'clapping' sounds were evident when observers read lines of text but disappeared if they were instructed to fixate a stationary target. The sounds were attributed to contractions of the oculomotor muscles accompanying eye movements. Hering provided evidence for this conclusion by comparing the occurrences of clapping sounds with the movements of an afterimage: 'every clapping sound corresponds to a displacement of the afterimage' (p. 145). Thus, Hering described the discontinuity of eye movements and recognized the class of rotations that we now refer to as saccadic. He was amongst the first to offer a description of the discontinuity of eye movements outside the context of vestibulo-ocular reflexes.

Hering's experiment is significant not only because he compared afterimage movement to the sounds of muscular movements, but also because he applied the technique to reading: 'One can observe the clapping sounds very clearly during reading. Although the eyes appear to glide steadily along the line, the clapping sounds reveal the jerky movement of the eyeball' (p. 146). Hering's report of his experiments was published in the same year as Javal's brief footnote regarding Lamare's initial studies. Indeed, the method that Lamare (1892) finally employed to listen to the sounds from eye movements bears a striking similarity to that employed earlier by Hering in 1879.

Another system similar to Hering's, involving an eye attachment, was developed by Ahrens (1891). He placed an ivory cup on the cornea and attached a bristle to it, so that movements of the eye could be registered by the displacements of the bristle on a revolving smoked drum. He was not able to obtain any detailed recordings of eye movements, but his method was adopted by Delabarre (1898) and Huey (1898, 1900) to record eye movements during reading (see Section 4.5.1).

4.3.6 Crum Brown

Crum Brown (Fig. 4.11, left) made significant advances to the study of eye movements and vertigo, which were discussed in Section 3.7. He continued his studies of eye movements, and in 1878 he provided illustrations of nystagmus occurring during and after body rotation (Fig. 4.11, right). In 1895 he delivered the Robert Boyle lecture at Oxford University; it was reported briefly in *Nature* (Crum Brown, 1895*a*) and more extensively in book form (Crum Brown, 1895*b*). In the book, Crum Brown gave the graphic description of eye movements in general:

We fancy that we can move our eyes uniformly, that by a continuous motion like that of a telescope we can move our eyes along the sky-line in the landscape or the cornice of a room, but we are wrong in this. However determinedly we try to do so, what actually happens is, that our eyes

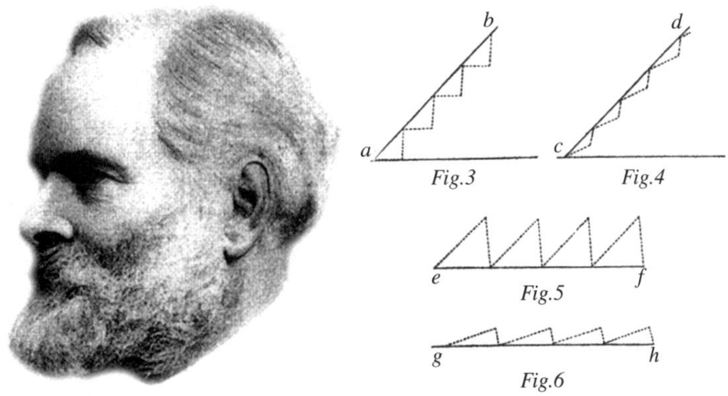

Figure 4.11
Left, Alexander Crum Brown (1838–1922) after a portrait in Walker (1923). Right, representations of eye movements during and after body rotation: 'When a real rotation of the body takes place the eyes do not at first perfectly follow the movement of the head. While the head moves uniformly the eyes move by jerks. Thus, in the diagram, *Fig.* 3, where the abscissæ indicate time and the ordinate the angle described, the straight line *ab* represents the continuous rotatory motion of the head and the dotted line the continuous motion of the eye. Here it will be seen that the eye looks in a fixed direction for a short time, represented by one of the horizontal portions of the dotted line *ab*, and then very quickly follows the motion of the head, remains fixed for a short time, and so on. After the rotation has continued for some time the motion of the eye gradually changes to that represented by the dotted line *cd* in *Fig.* 4. The eye now never remains fixed, but moves for a short time more slowly than the head, then quickly makes up to it, then falls behind, and so on. At last the discontinuity of the motion of the eye disappears, and the eye and the head move together. If now the rotation of the head be stopped (of course the body stops also) the discontinuous movements of the eyeballs recommence. They may now be represented by the dotted line in *Fig.* 5. The intermittent motion of the eyes gradually becomes less, passing through a condition such as that shown by the dotted line in *Fig.* 6, and at last ceases.' (Crum Brown, 1878, p. 658).

move like the seconds hand of a watch, a jerk and a little pause, another jerk and so on; only our eyes are not so regular, the jerks are sometimes of greater, sometimes of less, angular amount, and the pauses vary in duration, although, unless we make an effort, they are always short. During the jerks we practically do not see at all, so that we have before us not a moving panorama, but a series of fixed pictures of the same fixed things, which succeed one another rapidly. (Crum Brown, 1895*b*, pp. 4–5)

Here, Crum Brown offered an eloquent description of eye movements in which he demonstrates an understanding not only that the eyes move in a series of jerks, but also that these vary in size, and that vision only occurs during the intervals between these jerks. Crum Brown used the term 'jerk' to describe these movements, the English equivalent of Javal's 'saccades'. Porterfield (1737) gave a similar, though less precise, description when he referred to 'the quick and almost continual Motion of the Eye, whereby it is successively directed towards all the Parts of the Object in an Instant of Time' (p. 186).

Crum Brown went on to describe an afterimage method for demonstrating these discontinuous eye movements:

That the eye jerks in the way now stated can be made plain by means of a simple experiment. If we have in the field of view a bright object, such as an incandescent electric lamp, and after running our eyes over a scene before us, we see secondary images [afterimages] of the bright object. Now, if the eyes moved continuously from one position to another, we should see between the two secondary images of the bright object corresponding to these two positions, a bright band composed of an infinite number of images each infinitely near its two neighbours. But we see no such band, but a finite number of sharp individual images, each of which corresponds to the position of the eyes during a pause between jerks . . . This habit of jerking the eyes from one position to another, as fast as the light, well-poised globes can be swung round by the quick-working, straight-fibred muscles which move them, may be an innate habit, or it may have been acquired by our looking at things and turning quickly from one object of interest to another; at all events, it is now the way in which we alone can move them, unless we fix them on a moving object. (1895*b*, pp. 5–6)

Crum Brown's afterimage method was cited by Dodge (1903), who wrote: 'The effort to move the eyes slowly from one point of regard to another always results in one or more complete stops, of which, however, the subject is almost never directly conscious. The simplest method of convincing one's self of this fact is the method of Brown' (p. 311).

4.3.7 Dodge

Raymond Dodge (shown again in Fig. 4.12, upper right) began his academic career as an aspiring philosopher. After being rejected by Harvard and Columbia Universities, Dodge moved to Halle in Germany, feeling that learning German was essential for success as a philosopher. Soon after arriving at Halle, Dodge attended a seminar by Benno Erdmann (1851–1921; Fig. 4.12, upper left) on the psychology of reading. Dodge became fascinated with the problem of designing apparatus that would improve the study of reading, a task that Erdmann considered to be impossible. Hence Dodge's initiation into psychology was in the form of addressing this technical problem, which he solved in the development of the Erdmann-Dodge tachistoscope. Dodge's prowess as an engineer of experimental apparatus was echoed throughout his academic career. Indeed, he is probably best known as a key figure in the development of photographic eye movement recording devices, paving the way for instruments that

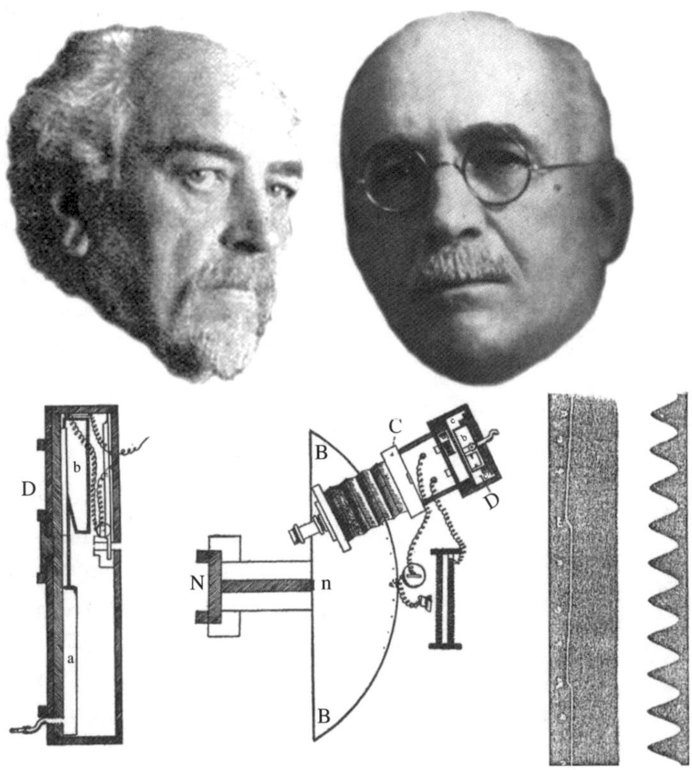

Figure 4.12
Upper left, Benno Erdmann (1851–1921). Upper right, Raymond Dodge (1871–1942) after a portrait in Murchison (1930). Lower left, the photographic apparatus used by Dodge and Cline (1901) to record eye movements. Lower right, their first published trace of an eye movement (from Dodge and Cline, 1901).

serve as vital components of eye movement research and have been of fundamental importance to the progress and direction of eye movement research. However, Dodge's abilities extended far beyond the construction of ingenious experimental devices. It was in the employment of such equipment and of simple observational approaches that he excelled.

Dodge's studies offered insightful and timely observational techniques that expanded upon the state of research at the time. After leaving Halle, he took up a teaching post at Ursinus College, Pennsylvania, which he held only briefly before moving to Wesleyan College. It was there that Dodge spent the majority of his academic career and carried out much of his seminal research. Perhaps one of his most significant contributions was the exploration of the relationship between eye movements and visual perception, in studies conducted in the early years at Wesleyan. Prior to Dodge's research, studies that attempted to relate the detailed metrics of eye movements to the perception of visual stimuli were rarely undertaken.

Dodge's explorations of the relationship between eye movements and perception arose primarily from a chance observation when conducting experiments, with Erdmann, on vision during reading (Erdmann and Dodge, 1898). They had been using mirrors to observe subjects' eye movements while reading text. When looking into the mirrors themselves Erdmann and Dodge

> chanced on the observation that when the head was held perfectly still we could never catch our own eye moving in a mirror. One may watch one's eyes as closely as possible, even with the aid of a concave reflector, whether one looks from one eye to the other, or from some more distant object to one's own eyes, the eyes may be seen now in one position and now in another, but never in motion. (Dodge, 1900, p. 456)

Until these reports by Erdmann and Dodge, it was generally thought that that eye movements were themselves an integral part of the processes of visual perception. It was believed that perception continued during eye movements and that the continuous movement of gaze over an object would be sufficient for its perception (see Chapter 6). Erdmann and Dodge, however, recognized that this was not the case. Critically, they appreciated the errors and pitfalls of self-observation when describing eye movements and perception, in the same way that Wells had distrusted Porterfield's recourse to subjective experience over

100 years earlier. Consequently, they employed an assistant to observe their eye movements, or to be observed.

It was this understanding of the problems of self-examination that led Dodge to make some crucial observations about the true nature of the saccade-and-fixate oculomotor strategy and its relation to perception. Dodge realized that in many situations where we feel that our eyes are moving continuously, at slow speeds, the reality is that we are making a series of small rapid eye movements separated by fixation pauses. Moreover, two observations led Dodge to propose that visual perception was suspended during the eye movements themselves. The first was the simple but elegant self-observation while looking at one's own eye in a mirror, described in the quotation given above (from Dodge, 1900). The second piece of evidence derived from experiments in reading whereby if a subject looked directly from one end of a line of text to the other, without any intervening fixations pauses (verified by an observer watching the reader's eyes) then the subject could not perceive the text in the middle of the line. This inability to read the middle of the line occurred in spite of the fact that the eye travelled over this region of text during its movement from one end to the other. Using these two pieces of evidence, Dodge proposed that there was no visual perception during eye movements, only during fixation pauses and that the impression that we have of visual perception during eye movements is merely an illusion. Dodge's ideas about the nature of perception within eye movements will be addressed in Chapter 6.

When he returned to America, Dodge continued to refine techniques for measuring rapid eye movements during reading. Dodge and Cline (1901) developed a photographic method in order to overcome problems associated with lever techniques that were attempted by other researchers (see Sections 1.3 and 4.5). Initially they attempted to photograph the eye itself, but the light source needed to be intense, and the margin between the iris and pupil was difficult to define. They found:

> Satisfactory results were first obtained when, after considerable experimentation, we hit upon the plan of utilizing the eccentric surface of the cornea as a reflector. Instead of photographing the eye directly, we photographed the movement of a bright vertical line as it was reflected from the surface of the cornea. Such lines give clean-cut records permitting considerable magnification in reading, while the amount of light needed is comparatively small. (Dodge and Cline, 1901, pp. 148–149)

Using this technique they developed the 'Dodge Photochronograph', which was used in numerous studies by Dodge and colleagues and provided key early insights into the metrics of eye movements (e.g. Diefendorf and Dodge, 1908; Dodge, 1903, 1904; Dodge and Cline, 1901). Crucially, Dodge (1903) classified five types of horizontal eye movements. Type I movements correspond to what were later called saccades, and they have the following characteristics:

> 1. Eye movements of the first type are fundamentally reactions to eccentric retinal stimulation, and are dependent on the tendency, developed during the first month of infancy, to move the eyes so that the point of interest will be seen with the visual centre of the retina. 2. Their velocity is practically uninfluenced by voluntary effort. While their duration shows a slight individual variation under similar circumstances, it varies in direct proportion with the angle of movement. 3. They are primarily not periods of perception, but rather interuptions of vision, whose sole function is to move the line of regard to an eccentric point of interest. (Dodge, 1903, p. 316)

The other types of eye movements were pursuit, compensatory, reactive compensatory, and convergence. Dodge's contribution to our understanding of saccades and fixations, and to their relation to perception, is a very significant one. His photographic eye tracking technologies had an immediate influence on the development of eye tracking devices and following the description of the Dodge Photochronograph, variations on the photographic theme were played in a variety of laboratories (see Taylor, 1937). Today's eye trackers owe much to the prioneering work of Dodge at the turn of the twentieth century. Dodge's legacy is not just a technological one. His ideas and experiments represented somewhat of a change in the emphasis of eye movement research, highlighting the discrepancy between eye movements and visual experience. Chapter 6 will deal in more detail with the implications of Dodge's work relating eye movements, perception and cognition in vision, and the research questions it defined.

4.4 Did Javal discover saccades?

Having considered the work of Lamare, Hering, Crum Brown, and Dodge, it is clear that several researchers contemporary with Javal were describing eye movements as discontinuous and 'jerky'. Furthermore, Javal referred to eye movements as 'saccadic' only in a footnote describing work carried out by Lamare. In his article

(Javal, 1879*e*) and later in his book (Javal, 1904, 1906) Javal did not himself attempt to take credit for the work describing saccadic eye movements and was explicit in attributing this work to Lamare. Why then should it be that Javal has been acclaimed as the originator of a description that he himself did not make or claim credit for? An understanding of how this might have happened comes from considering early citations of Javal's work in English and subsequent perpetuation of this mis-accreditation by later researchers.

Huey (1898) appears to have been the first writer in English to cite Javal's work, although it was not with reference to eye movements but to accommodation while reading. In a later article, Huey (1900) elaborated on Javal's description of eye movements during reading, and indicated that he had corresponded with Javal, who had sent 'to me personal papers bearing on his researches' (p. 284). Huey also made reference to Lamare's studies: 'Lamare, working with Javal, finding that the movement of the eye in reading was not continuous, but by little jerks (*par saccades*), devised the following method for counting these' (p. 285, original italics). Huey then gave a brief account of Lamare's auditory method of detecting eye movements. Javal was not cited in Huey's (1901) second article on reading.

Several years later, in a book regarded as a classic of psychology, Huey (1908) provided an historical account of research on eye movements and reading. It is in this book that Huey established Javal as the founder of research in this area:

> As you watch the reading [of another person], you notice, too, that the eyes do not move continuously from left to right along the line, but proceed by a succession of quick, short movements to the end, then return in one quick, usually unbroken movement to the left. You find all this very evident. And yet most of those who have studied the eye have curiously failed to note that the movement was discontinuous; and up to 1879, when Professor Javal called attention to it, I find no mention of the fact in the literature. Indeed, I have not myself seen mention of these reading movements until 1898, except in the writings of Javal and some other French authors who took up his discovery, and in a paper published in 1895 by Professor Alexander Brown, of Edinburgh. It is a curious instance of the failure of scientists to make first-hand observations except along certain lines that have become habitual. (Huey, 1908, pp. 15–16)

It is possible that Huey's description of observing the eyes of a reader have been attributed to Javal, because of the juxtaposition of the statements above. Alternatively, the account might have derived from their correspondence. Huey is one of the few writers to cite Crum Brown's (1895*a*,*b*) work, which mentioned the discontinuous movements that occur during scanning a scene, but Crum Brown did not apply them explicitly to reading.

Huey (1908) implied that the experiments reported by Javal had been conducted by Javal, and Lamare was not cited. Moreover, Huey later noted:

> Professor Javal, of the University of Paris, seems, as has been said, to have been the first to note the actual character of the eye's movements in reading. He concluded that there was a pause about every ten letters, and thought that this was about the amount that could be seen clearly at one fixation. He found that after reading he had after-images of straight gray lines corresponding to the parallel lines of print, and concluded that the eye's fixation point did not leave the line as it moved forward in reading . . . While not all of Professor Javal's observations are conclusive, he deserves more than does anyone else the credit for making the initial discoveries in this field, and for initiating a considerable number of later studies. (1908, p. 18)

It is perhaps this last statement, assigning credit to Javal, that has lead others, on the basis of Huey's writing, to accord Javal the honour of having conducted the experiments. Moreover, giving the number of letters between saccades as ten suggests that Huey was basing his assessment on Javal's (1904, 1906) book, rather than the article of 1879.

Taylor (1937) also surveyed early research on eye movements and reading, and his view of this history was somewhat more circumspect than that by Huey: 'Apparently Javal and Lamare were the first to observe and record the fact that, during the act of reading, the eye moves across the page in a series of short fixations' (Taylor, 1937, p. 47). Moreover, Taylor provided a footnote with the quotation (in French) from Javal (1879*e*, which we have given in French and in translation in Section 4.3.1), giving the number of letters between saccades as 15–18. It would seem that Huey's statements have been used by others to support the view that Javal conducted the first experiments on discontinuous eye movements during reading. For example, Woodworth (1938), in the chapter on eye movements in his influential textbook noted:

> The most important single fact, it is true, was discovered by Javal (1878) without any more special technique than simply watching the eye of a school child who was reading. His very eminent predecessors had assumed the truth of the common belief in 'sweeping the eyes over a scene or along a line of

> print.' He found, not a steady sweep, but a series of little jumps with intervening fixation pauses. The eye moved, as he said, 'par saccades,' from which expression comes the name *saccadic* now applied to this class of quick eye movements. (Woodworth, 1938, p. 577, original italics)

Woodworth did not provide an exact reference to the paper in which this was reported, and we have been unable to find use of the term 'par saccades' in Javal's essays on reading, but it was used by Huey (1900). Woodworth did cite Huey's (1908) book. Later in his chapter on reading Woodworth observed: 'Javal (1878) by watching the reader's eyes, found that they moved along the lines not with a smooth, steady movement, but in a series of jumps or "saccades" separated by fixation pauses' (1938, p. 715). Woodworth (1923) had written an earlier work in which eye movements were described briefly: he did not cite Javal or Huey, but gave an account of Dodge's photographic studies. Two varieties of eye movements were said to occur which Woodworth referred to as jumps and pursuit.

Vernon (1931) in her textbook on reading further reinforced this sentiment: 'The first attempts at observing and measuring eye movements were made by methods of direct observation. Thus Javal in 1878 observed eye movements during reading by reflection from a mirror' (p. 1). In his *Text-book of ophthalmology* Duke-Elder (1932) stated that Javal made observations of eye movements using a telescope in 1878. We have not been able to find such a description in the articles by Javal, and the page numbers given by Duke-Elder do not correspond to Javal's articles. It is also claimed that the method was improved by Erdmann and Dodge (1898), but they did not cite Javal. Duke-Elder's textbook in its many editions is taken as an authoritative source of historical accuracy, and it has been used as such in subsequent histories of ophthalmology (e.g. Albert and Edwards, 1996). It is unfortunate that origins of eye movement measurements did not display the scholarship that marks the book otherwise. As another example, when he discussed complex movements in reading, Duke-Elder wrote:

> It might be imagined that in reading and writing the eyes moved slowly and continuously backwards and forwards over the lines. That such a smooth regular motion does not occur was first shown by Javal (1878–79). The eyes move forward in very short rapid jerks (*saccadic movements*) and after each advance there is a *fixation pause* during which the eyes remain relatively at rest, suffering only the fine constant fixation tremor; and only the backward

sweep of the eyes from the end of one line to the beginning of the next is regular and uninterrupted. (Duke-Elder, 1932, p. 610, original italics)

4.4.1 The discoverers of saccades

When contemporary texts on eye movements do address the history of their measurement they tend to rely on Huey's (1908) account, but Huey was not precise about the attribution of Lamare's method as described by Javal. Saccadic sweeps in nystagmus were described and measured before they were investigated in the context of reading. Hering and Lamare deserve the credit for demonstrating the pattern of eye movements during reading. The descriptions of Lamare's experiments by Javal, and the account of Javal's writing by Huey, seem to have resulted in the discovery being associated with Javal rather than Lamare. Hering's and Lamare's initial investigations demonstrated the discontinuities of eye movements but not their velocities. That the French description of 'saccades' for this class of eye movements was adopted, appears to be due largely to a suggestion by Dodge in the early twentieth century.

Following the discovery of discontinuous eye movements, their significance in perception became a central issue. This could only be assessed when methods of measuring the eye movements could be related to the ensuing perception. Reading provided the ideal domain for such enquiries. In this context, the name given to the rapid eye movements is not as important as the relationship between them, fixations, and comprehension. Javal played a minor roll in establishing the links between eye movements and reading. The contributions of Lamare, Hering, Crum Brown, and Dodge, on the other hand, stand out as milestones pointing towards a more exact understanding of the nature of eye movements and the functions they served. Not until Dodge's development of photographic techniques for recording corneal reflections could the significance of saccades and fixations for perception be established. They allowed more accurate measures of the velocities of saccades and the durations of fixations to be made and paved the way for later eye movement recording technologies.

4.5 Developments after Dodge

After Dodge's development of his photographic eye tracker and his seminal researches, there followed something of a revolution in eye movement research and a proliferation of new experiments in this field. Other researchers developed similarly easy-to-use and effective eye trackers and research extended beyond the domain of reading (which had been central to much of the eye movement research at the end of the nineteenth century). Now researchers began to consider whether the newly described saccade-and-fixate strategy applied to tasks other than reading, and it was soon realized that this was the case. As eye movement research encompassed more varied task domains, so the research questions also evolved. A key component of the early twentieth century eye movement research was the consideration of the link between eye movements and cognitive processes including visual experience, aesthetics and illusions. It is to those researchers who played central roles in this early twentieth century evolution of eye movement research, that we now turn our attention.

4.5.1 Delabarre and Huey

While Lamare, Hering, Crum Brown, and Dodge are key figures in the origins of descriptions of the discontinuity of eye movements, Edmund Burke Delabarre (1863–1945) and Edmund Burke Huey (1870–1913; Fig. 4.13, upper) deserve credit as being among the first to construct successful devices for recording the characteristics of eye movements. The possibility of recording a reflection from a mirror attached to the eye on a photographic plate had been entertained by Javal (1878*c*) and Delabarre (1898) returned to it, but he was not successful in developing the technique. In its stead, Delabarre attached a lever to a plaster eye-cup, and the eye movements were registered on the smoked drum of a kymograph: 'Slow movements could thus be recorded with great accuracy. But in the case of the more natural rapid movements, the tendency of the lever and the elastic fibre to continue vibratory movements of their own after those of the eye had ceased led to some results difficult to interpret' (Delabarre, 1898, p. 573).

In the article in *The American Journal of Psychology* following that by Delabarre, Huey (1898) also examined the movements of the eyes in reading. He noted that: 'the most casual observation showed that the eye moved along the line by little jerks and not with a continuous steady movement' (p. 583). He then went on to record eye movements with a similar system (illustrated in Fig. 4.13, lower left) to that used by Delabarre. Both methods

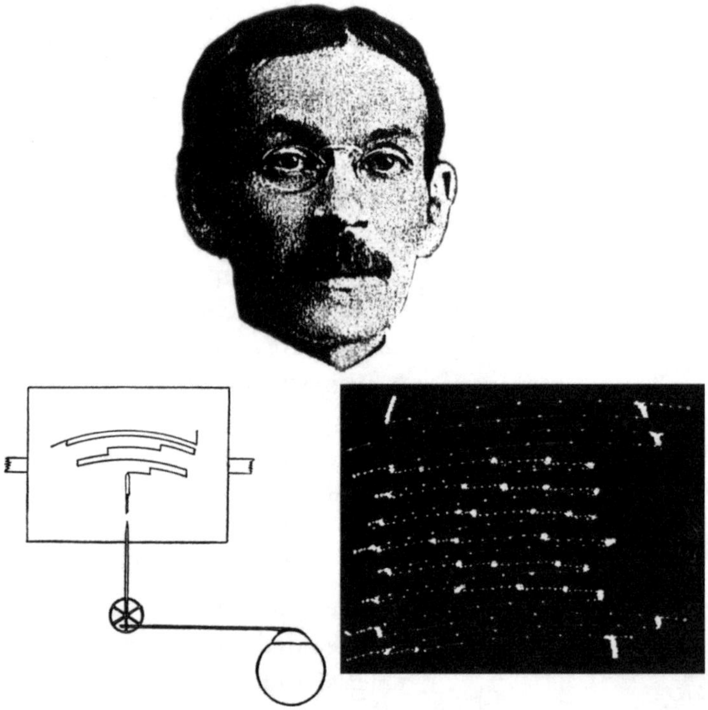

Figure 4.13

Upper, Edmund Burke Huey (1870–1913) after a portrait in Taylor (1937). Lower left, Huey's (1898) technique for recording eye movement during reading. A lever was attached to a plaster eye-cup and moved a pen over a rotating smoked drum. The initial records shown are for calibration across the lines, followed by jerks and pauses during reading. Lower right, a record of eye movements during reading using the lever device (from Huey, 1900). The tracing on the smoked drum was photographed and then engraved. 'The curve shows the movements of the eye in reading six lines, preceded and followed by two free movements of the eye each way, in which it was swept from one end of the line to the other, the beginning and end alone being fixated' (Huey, 1900, p. 290).

used plaster-of-Paris eye-cups, which required the eye to be anaesthetized with cocaine. Huey refined the technique and was able to register discontinuous eye movements during reading. His record is shown in Fig. 4.13, lower right. Huey also refined the controls necessary for eye movement recording. The head was stabilized by head clamps and an individual bite-bar; a calibration recording was made initially, with the eye moving from one end of the line to the other; he also used a time marker. Like Lamare (1892), he remarked that: 'By reading the same matter at different distances from the eye, the number of jerks was shown to be a function of the matter read rather than of the arc described by the eye's rotation' (p. 585).

When describing their methods for measuring eye movements photographically, Dodge and Cline (1901) cited only two studies, before Huey's experiment, that addressed the question of the angular velocity of eye movements—those of Volkmann (1846) and Lamansky (1869). Huey's records were acknowledged as a 'material advance', but the problems of any lever system were evident because of the additional force that was applied to the eye. It was also the case that the system involved some overshoot that could not be estimated accurately; this can be seen in the calibration traces in Fig. 4.13 (lower). While later variants of the lever devices were attempted (see Section 1.3.2), and while the idea of contact lens eye trackers was developed in different ways in later years (see Section 1.3.2), lever devices such as Huey's were somewhat superseded by photographic eye tracking devices (see Section 4.3.7).

4.5.2 Stratton

George Malcolm Stratton (1865–1957; Fig. 4.14, upper) established the Psychological Laboratory at the University of California in 1899 and became president of the American Psychological

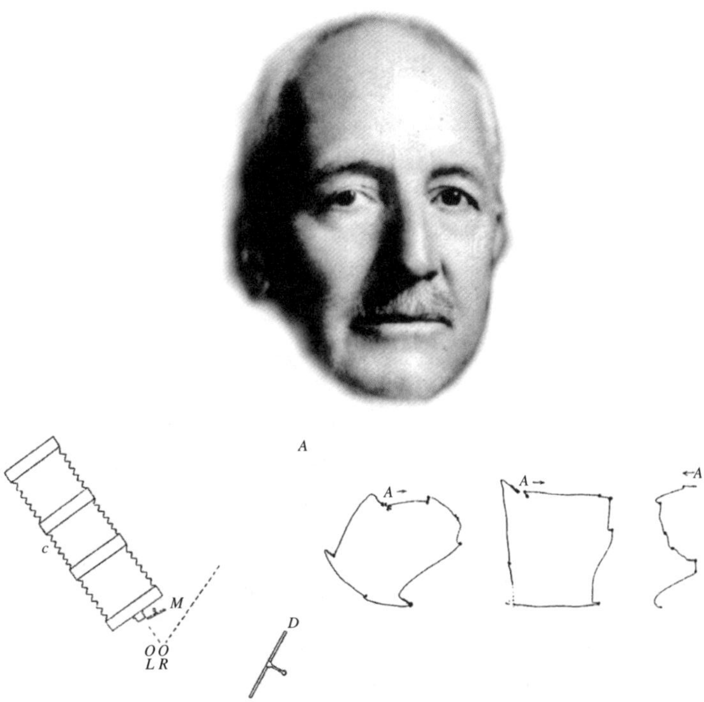

Figure 4.14
Upper, George Malcolm Stratton (1865–1957) after a photograph kindly supplied by the University of California, Berkeley. Lower left, Stratton's camera for recording eye movements, and lower right, records for tracking a circle, square, and an S shape (both from Stratton, 1902).

Association in 1908. In spite of his undeniably significant contribution to psychology—not least from his experiments on inverted vision—Stratton features only rarely in biographies of psychologists (but for more details see Wade, 2000c). Stratton also employed a photographic technique to examine eye movements, the apparatus for which is shown in Fig. 4.14, lower left. He was one of the first researchers to apply the work that contemporary researchers were conducting on eye movements during reading to the question of eye movements when viewing patterns (Stratton, 1902, 1906). This was an important new direction for eye movement research and served to highlight the importance of saccades outside the context of reading. Like his contemporaries, Stratton was surprised by the discontinuity of eye movements: 'The eye darts from point to point, interrupting its rapid motion by instants of rest. And the path by which the eye passes from one to another of these resting places does not seem to depend very nicely upon the exact form of the line observed' (Stratton, 1902, p. 343).

The above quote highlights a key aspect of Stratton's work: he demonstrated that the path taken by the eye during saccades did not appear to relate to the form of the pattern viewed. Stratton (1906) returned to this issue of the relationship between patterns and eye movements in a later article, which opened by saying that: 'our pleasure in graceful curves could not be due to the ease and smoothness of the eye's own motion in viewing these curves. For the ocular movement itself, when photographically recorded, is found to be interrupted and jerky and most unlike the figures we enjoy' (Stratton, 1906, p. 82). The article went on to consider the Wundt-Lamansky law (that vertical and horizontal eye movements follow straight paths, whereas diagonal movements are curved); whether eye movements can explain simple visual illusions (see Chapter 5); and whether eye movements can explain the aesthetics of symmetry. Stratton found no evidence for eye movement explanations of the Müller-Lyer, Poggendorff, or Zöllner illusions:

> If some special form of the eye's movement is the cause of a particular illusion, such a movement must be present on every occasion when the illusion is felt. But in the actual records we find plenty of instances where the movements which have been supposed to produce a given illusion are present when the illusion is absent, and absent when the illusion is present.

One can hardly believe, then, that the supposed causal connection really exists. (Stratton, 1906, p. 93)

In his investigation of the eye movements of observers while looking at a variety of symmetrical and non-symmetrical figures, Stratton was again surprised by what he found when he examined the photographic negatives recorded:

In examining the negatives one is struck by the almost grotesque unlikeness between the outline observed and the action of the eye in observing it. For the most part the eye moves irregularly over the figure, seeking certain points of vantage from which the best view of important features may be obtained. And these positions are marked by the eye's momentary resting there. (1906, p. 94)

Again, the path taken by the eye during movements did not relate precisely to the form of the figure being viewed (Fig. 4.14, lower right), but Stratton also observed that the positions fixated did not show any clear and consistent relationship with the figure:

Now these points of rest are evidently of more consequence to the observer than the path by which the eye reaches them; indeed the form of any single path between two stops usually bears no observable resemblance to the outline which the subject was taking in, and which in many cases he believes his eye to be accurately following. But even these points of rest are not so arranged as to supply of themselves a rough sense of the form perceived, after the manner of an outline pricked disconnectedly in paper. The points of the eye's rest in the records are usually too few and too inexact to give any such clear and connected perception of the form as the observer regularly and readily obtains. (Stratton, 1906, p. 94)

The phrasing of the article suggests some degree of despair in Stratton's reports of the lack of correspondence between the eye movements and the figure being observed. The degree of surprise and disbelief evident in this article highlights the fact that the saccade and fixate behaviour of the eye was still very much a new aspect of vision research. This continued to surprise and intrigue researchers even nearly 30 years after Javal's report of Lamare's work and Hering's article describing saccadic eye movements. Not only was there no clear relationship between the eye movements and form of the figure viewed, but there was also no clear relationship between the symmetry of the figure viewed and the symmetry of the eye movements made when viewing it: 'As regards the question of the symmetry of the movements of the eye, in some instances the negatives displayed a rude balance. But it must be said that even the most symmetrical of these records can be called so only by courtesy... The more frequent records have not even this rough approximation to symmetry' (Stratton, 1906, p. 94).

Stratton's work is also significant in that it attempts to bridge the gap between visual phenomena (illusions), cognition (aesthetic judgements), and the underlying perceptual mechanisms (eye movements). Thus, both Stratton and Dodge defined new directions for eye movement research, highlighting the discrepancy between cognition and perception in vision. Stratton explicitly states the inadequacy of eye movements as an explanation for aesthetic judgements: 'The sources of our enjoyment of symmetry, therefore, are not to be discovered in the form of the eye's behaviour. A figure which has for us a satisfying balance may be brought to the mind by most unbalanced ocular motions' (1906, p. 95). It is clear from Stratton's closing remarks in his article on eye movements and symmetry that he appreciated the gulf between perception and cognition and that he was aware that his work was defining new questions in vision that would be addressed in the future:

> The discussion of the present experiments has been intentionally confined to the point of showing, not that they disprove any muscular theory whatever, but that they tend to make eye-muscles appear a trifle ridiculous when one compares their actual performances with the marvels which have been attributed to them. The mythology of the eye-muscles will some day make an interesting paragraph in the history of delusions in psychology; and we shall not be long, I expect, in gaining the facts which will permit this mythology to be recognized and narrated. (Stratton, 1906, p. 96)

Stratton would perhaps be interested to see the volume of literature still devoted to understanding the link between eye movements and cognition and that a century after his statement, this link remains largely unknown; we are as yet not in a position to write that 'short paragraph' explaining Stratton's 'mythology'.

4.5.3 Judd

Charles Hubbard Judd (1873–1946; Fig. 4.15, upper left) considered that his interest in science arose in no small part as a result of his strict religious upbringing (Judd, 1932); his curiosity was aroused by the discrepancy between this and the scientific texts he read at high school. After graduating from Wesleyan University in 1894, Judd moved to Wundt's laboratory in Leipzig from where

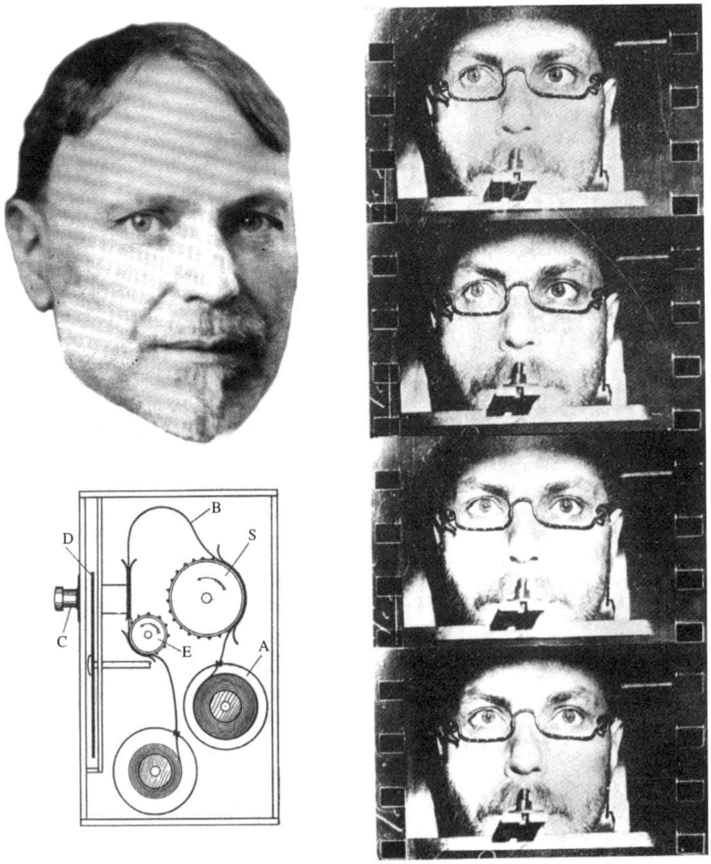

Figure 4.15

Upper left, Charles Hubbard Judd (1873–1946) after a photograph in Murchison (1932). Lower left, his Edison kinetoscope movie camera used in his experiments to record eye movements and, right, a sequence of stills showing records of Judd's eye movements (both from Judd et al., 1905).

he gained his PhD after only two years. Shortly afterwards Judd translated Wundt's *Grundriss der Psychologie* (1896) into English (Wundt, 1897). He worked initially on geometrical illusions (Judd, 1899) and was dismissive of interpretations based on angle expansion and perspective. Rather he favoured what he called the movement hypothesis: 'The more intense the sensation of movement, the greater will be the estimation of the distance; conversely, the less the intensity of the sensations of movement, the shorter the estimated distance' (Judd, 1899, p. 253). He did not equate the hypothesis with actual movement nor did he, at this stage, provide any measurements of the extent of eye movements.

Judd's eye movement research was conducted during his time at Yale, where he became director of the Psychological Laboratory. He was impressed by the work of Dodge and Stratton, but felt that the eye trackers used by both were somewhat limited in the range of tasks to which they could be applied: Dodge's eye tracker was designed for recording movements only along a straight line (as occurs in reading) and Stratton's lacked temporal resolution and required a dark room in which the photographic plate was exposed during experimental recording. Judd developed a 'kinetoscopic' eye tracker (Fig. 4.15, lower left) in which a small fleck of Chinese white, which had been affixed to the cornea, was photographed; eye movements could thus be discerned in two dimensions, and did not require a dark room (Judd et al., 1905). While Judd's eye tracker offered specific advantages over previous photographic devices, it was still somewhat limited in its temporal resolution, typically operating at about 8 to 9 frames per second (cf. Dodge's 100 Hz Photochronograph). Fig. 4.15, right, shows frames recorded by the kinetoscope camera; the subject pictured in this figure is Judd himself. One impressive feature of Judd's eye tracker was that it allowed binocular recordings to be taken.

Having developed this new photographic eye tracker, Judd and colleagues went on to use it to investigate eye movements between simple targets (McAllister, 1905) and the role of eye movements in the Müller-Lyer illusion (Judd, 1905*a*), the Poggendorff illusion (Cameron and Steele, 1905) and the Zöllner illusion (Judd and Courten, 1905). In the first of these reports (McAllister, 1905) observers were asked to alternate fixation between two targets. The nature of these targets was varied comprising different arrangements of dots and lines. McAllister found that, 'From the records of Mr. LaBlanc . . . it can be said that the character of the fixation of a point in the visual field is in many cases modified by the character of the figure and the direction of the lines surrounding it; also by the character of the figure from which the eye moves in order to fixate the point' (1905, p. 37).

Similar results were found for other participants: the details of fixation and the eye movements between the fixation targets varied according to the nature of the targets. However, large individual differences were found in the precise patterns of eye movements, although the implications of these differences were not considered in any great detail. McAllister found that the eye was not stationary during periods of fixation, undergoing constant drift (see Chapter 6) and concluded that: 'The image of a point fixated does not fall upon any particular point of the retina, but may fall upon any point of a considerable area of the retina, around about, and including the *fovea centralis*. The same elements of the retina are not stimulated during any successive periods of fixation of a point, except merely by chance' (McAllister, 1905, pp. 52 and 53).

When comparing the two eyes during inspection of the targets, McAllister noted that while the two eyes generally behaved similarly, they were not identical; rather they showed some lack of coordination in the details of their movements.

In his investigation of the Müller-Lyer illusion, Judd (1905*a*) found that there was some evidence for there being differences in the eye movements when looking at the overestimated and underestimated regions of the illusions, and also that practise influenced eye movements:

> The positive outcome of our researches consists, therefore, in the exhibition of a consistent tendency on the part of five subjects to show restricted movements in looking across the underestimated Müller-Lyer figure and freer movements in looking across the overestimated figure. One of these subjects who performed a series of adjustments with sufficient frequency to overcome the illusion showed a marked change in the character of the movement. (Judd, 1905*a*, p. 78)

In the case of the Poggendorff illusion, eye movements again correlated with the experience of the illusion (Cameron and Steele, 1905). However, this was not the case for the Zöllner illusion: 'The usual fact... is that the eye movement, and consequently the sensations from these movements, are in the wrong direction to account for the illusion' (Judd and Courten, 1905, p. 137). It is interesting to note that Stratton and Judd appeared to disagree in their investigations of the role of eye movements in visual illusions. While Judd offered eye movement explanations for the Müller-Lyer and Poggendorff illusions, Stratton, as we have seen, proposed that no such explanations were possible.

Judd's interest in interpreting the results of the studies discussed above was in addressing his interest in the relationship between movement and perception (Judd, 1905*b*). Judd sought to use his results to dismiss the notion that perceptions might arise directly from movements themselves; rather he stressed the importance of visual information from the retina both in forming perceptions and in coordinating the movements: 'When the eye moves toward a point and the movement does not at first suffice to bring the point in question on the fovea, the retinal sensations which record the failure to reach the desired goal will be a much more powerful stimulus to new action than will any possible muscle sensation' (Judd, 1905*b*, p. 218).

While much of Judd's discussion of his eye movement studies focused upon the discussion of their relation to theories of movement sensation, he did also notice that the pattern of eye movements was likely to be influenced by the instructions given to the observers during the experiments:

> we must recognize that the actual movements executed are in no small sense responses to the verbal stimuli which the subject receives in the form of general directions. The subject reacts to the demands imposed upon him by the general situation . . . The whole motive for movement is therefore not to be sought in the figures themselves. The figures guide a movement which is initiated by outside stimuli. (Judd, 1905*b*, pp. 216–217)

The recognition that eye movements were not entirely directed by the stimulus being viewed echoed the opinion expressed by Stratton at the same time, but it was not investigated in any great depth by either Judd or Stratton. A more thorough treatment of this question was not conducted until some years later when Judd's former doctoral student, Buswell, conducted an impressive series of eye movement studies.

4.5.4 Buswell

Guy Thomas Buswell (1891–1994; Fig. 4.16, upper) became interested in psychology after reading Munsterberg's *Psychology and industrial efficiency* (1913) while at college. Buswell's undergraduate years at the University of Chicago were first interrupted when he left for three years to earn enough money to continue his studies, and then again when he was drafted into the Army Signal Corps during World War I. In 1917, he returned to the University of Chicago where he completed a PhD under the supervision of Judd. Buswell's initial research interests were eye movements during reading and the processes involved in learning and teaching arithmetic (Buswell, 1920, 1922, 1926, 1937; Judd and Buswell, 1922). Buswell moved from Chicago to Berkeley in 1949. He became professor emeritus in 1958 and was elected into the Reading Hall of Fame in 1974. Buswell died at the age of 103 in 1994.

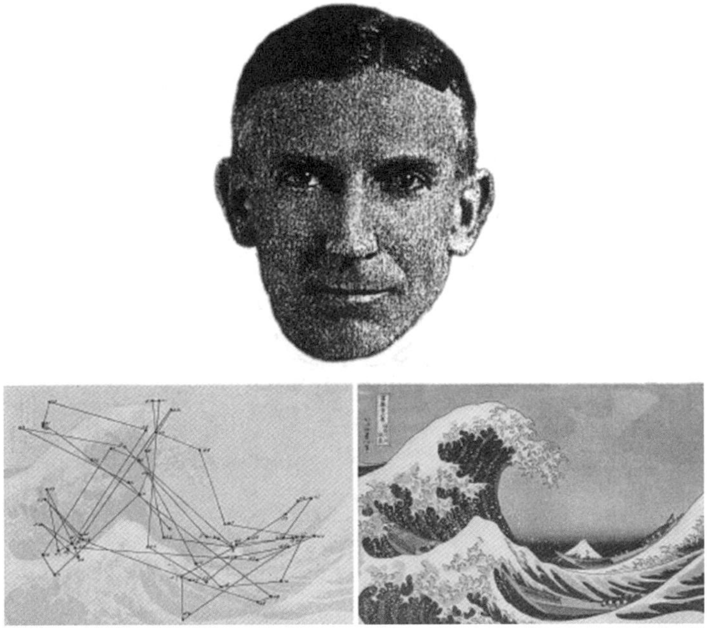

Figure 4.16
Upper, Guy Thomas Buswell (1891–1994) after a portrait in Taylor (1937). Lower left, eye movement record of one subject viewing 'The Wave' painted by Hokusai. Each black circle represents a fixation made by the observer. The lines indicate the saccades that moved the eye from one fixation to the next. Each fixation point is numbered in sequence from the start of viewing. Lower right, Hokusai's 'The Wave', from which the eye movements shown on the lower left of this figure were recorded (after Buswell, 1935).

While Buswell's work on reading is probably his most renowned work, it was from his study of eye movements when viewing pictures that one of his key contributions to eye movement research arises. The latter work was published in his impressive monograph *How people look at pictures* (Buswell, 1935). In the monograph, Buswell reports eye movement data recorded from 200 participants each viewing multiple pictures, such that his data comprised some 1,877 eye movement records each containing a large number of fixations. This volume of eye movement data is impressive by modern standards, but particularly so given the technology at the time and the need to transform manually the horizontal and vertical position of the eye indicated in the eye movement records into precise locations on the pictures viewed (see Fig. 4.16, lower left and Fig. 1.12, right). This work was the first to explore in a systematic way eye movements of observers while viewing complex pictures, rather than text or simple patters, and represented somewhat of a revolution in eye movement research. Using complex images and scenes has become a central aspect of modern eye movement research and is an important part of understanding eye movements in everyday vision.

Buswell's monograph explores a wide range of issues regarding the eye movements made while viewing pictures, including some surprisingly modern concerns: he looked at the overall distribution of fixations on pictures; he compared the first few fixations on a painting to the last few; he compared the durations of fixations made early in viewing to those made near the end of viewing; he looked at how fixation duration changed with viewing time; he compared the consistency between different observers when viewing the same picture; and he looked at the influence of instructions given to observers upon their eye movements when viewing a picture.

By making density plots of where all participants fixated when viewing pictures, Buswell showed that not all locations and objects in pictures are fixated, with particular 'centres of interest' where fixations are concentrated. He also appreciated that there could be quite large individual differences in where people fixate when viewing pictures:

> The positions of the fixations indicate clearly that for certain pictures the center or centers of attention are much more limited than in other pictures. The fact that the density plots represent composite diagrams from a great many different subjects obviously results in a wider distribution of fixations on account of the varied interests of different individuals in looking at the same picture. However, the density plots do give a rather clear indication as to what parts of a given picture are likely to prove most interesting to a random selection of subjects. (Buswell, 1935, p. 24)

The issue of individual differences in the patterns of eye movements was explored in detail in a section at the end of the second chapter. The differences that were present in the locations fixated by individuals when viewing each image were also reflected in the durations of the fixations, with a large variation between observers in their average fixation duration on each picture. Buswell's investigation of individual differences extended to exploring differences between artistically trained individuals and those without training; between children and adults; and between Western and Oriental participants. In all cases, differences between the groups were small: 'The average differences between the groups were so much less than the individual differences within each group that the results cannot be considered significant' (Buswell, 1935, p. 131). Differences were found in the eye movement data that emerged over the course of viewing a picture for some time. The regions fixated in the picture were more consistent between observers for the first few fixations than for the last few on each picture. Buswell also found that fixation duration increased over the course of viewing a picture for some time.

Buswell devoted a chapter of the book to looking at the influence of the characteristics of the picture upon where is fixated. This work is very reminiscent of that conducted some years earlier by Stratton (see Section 4.5.2) although he did not cite Stratton's work. In places Buswell appears to argue that eye movements do tend to follow lines in pictures:

> In the main the eyes followed the lines of the figure, with the occasional interruptions for examining details of the decoration. Picture 23 [of a chaise longue] furnished an excellent example of the way the eye follows the main lines in a piece of furniture of this type. Record after record showed a clear tendency to follow the lines of the couch back and forth laterally, and then to make movements down to the feet at each end. In some cases the shape of the couch could almost be traced from the lines connecting the successive fixations of the eye. (p. 108)

This is contrary to Stratton's suggestion that eye movements do not appear to be particularly influenced by the form of the figure being viewed. However, other aspects of Buswell's data suggest less concordance between eye movements and the characteristics of the picture. When Buswell showed participants more basic designs and patterns he found that: 'The effect of different types of design in carrying the eye swiftly from one place to another is apparently much less than is assumed in the literature of art . . . The writer should emphasize that the data from eye movements are not to be considered as evidence either positively or negatively for any type of artistic interpretation' (p. 115).

Like Stratton, Buswell felt that the pattern of eye movements was insufficient to explain our visual experience and so highlighted the need to appeal to cognitive explanations of vision, rather than purely perceptional.

Perhaps the most often overlooked aspect of Buswell's work was his investigation of how different instructions given to observers prior to viewing an image can influence the eye movements made during viewing. For example, when presented with a picture of Chicago's Tribune Tower eye movements were first recorded while the participant viewed the picture 'without any special directions being given. After that record was secured, the subject was told to look at the picture again to see if he could find a person looking out of one of the windows of the tower' (Buswell, 1935, p. 136). Very different eye movement records were obtained in these two situations, demonstrating that cognitive factors such as the viewer's task can have a strong effect upon how a picture is inspected. Such descriptions of influences played by high level factors upon eye movements are not typically associated with Buswell, but rather it is Yarbus who is generally regarded to be the first to have offered such an observation (Yarbus, 1967).

Buswell's impressive monograph illustrates the rapid changes that were taking place in eye movement research in the first half of the twentieth century. Understanding of saccadic eye movements was rapidly increasing, as was the technology with which they could be measured; with these changes came both new questions about vision and the ability to address them in increasingly realistic viewing conditions and with increasing flexibility and precision. Buswell's book discussed a wide range of issues regarding the relationship between eye movements and visual experience and these questions have been reflected in much of the eye movement research that followed.

5

Visual motion illusions and eye movements

5.1 Introduction

It was noted in previous chapters that interest in eye movements often derived from an appreciation of specific visual phenomena. Binocular single vision provided the stimulus for examining convergence and binocular eye movements (Chapter 2). The apparent rotation of the visual world in vertigo stimulated enquiry into eye movements that accompanied it (Chapter 3). The realization that distinct vision is restricted to a small region of the retina led to speculations about scanning eye movements (Chapter 4). The converse was also the case: visual phenomena involving motion have often been interpreted in terms of eye movements. Long before their characteristics had been established by experiment, eye movements were employed to explain a variety of visual phenomena. Prominent amongst these were visual illusions.

The second half of the nineteenth century was the era of illusions. Many of the illusions graced by the names of their discoverers derive from this period. Helmholtz (1867*a*) did describe a few spatial illusions, but not many. The avalanche descended in the later decades when the likes of Ponzo, Poggendorff, Mach, and Müller-Lyer described their eponymous phenomena. These illusions have an important place in the history of psychology, because they were amongst the factors that led Wundt to establish his Psychological Institute at Leipzig in 1879—he could not envisage how illusions could be accounted for in physiological terms, and so they, along with consciousness, required a separate discipline. Wundt took as his yardstick the proximal stimulus (the retinal image)—and he could not accept that, say, two linear extents that produced equivalent retinal extents could yield perceptual inequality due to physiological processes. Wundt (1898) sought to determine correlates with illusions, and the one most favoured at that time was in terms of eye movements, although other higher level alternatives were also entertained.

Thus, illusions were studied in the late nineteenth century because they were not amenable to the extant physiology—hence their place in psychology. They also fostered the use of two-dimensional stimuli in perceptual experiments. They were interpreted in terms of eye movements, which was why Stratton conducted the experiments described in Section 4.5.2. For instance, if one component of the Müller-Lyer illusion appears longer than another then the eyes might move over a greater extent for the longer part. The situation is one of equating perceived size with the magnitude of an eye movement. Such a theory was espoused by Wundt (1898) and others. Eye movement theories of geometrical illusions did have the virtue of being open to test. Stratton (1906) was one of the first to submit them to such scrutiny. It is clear from his report that they failed the test. Another way of testing the eye movement theory was to present the patterns tachistoscopically, so that the eyes were not able to move over the displayed parts. The illusions persisted despite such brief exposures. Accordingly, eye movement interpretations were generally abandoned (see Robinson, 1972). Illusions involving visual motion were not open to such ready rebuttal, and so eye movement interpretations could be sustained for longer.

Visual motion illusions are compelling and some have been investigated for many centuries. In the first instance, interpretations of the motion illusions are often associated with eye movements. This reflects a desire to link an objective expression of motion (of the eyes) with a subjective experience of motion. If the two are correlated then it is assumed that the perception has been accounted for. That is, if motion of a stationary stimulus over the retina (as a consequence of eye movements) is equated with perceived motion then the latter is accounted for by the former. Motion with respect to the eye (or the retina) is taken as the most basic interpretation of motion perception, and it does not require any understanding of subsequent processes (like those in the visual pathways or brain). It reflects a concern with aspects of perceptual experience (motion perception) and associated changes that can also be experienced subjectively or observed in others (eye movements). This approach has a long history, and it is examined with respect to induced motion, motion aftereffects, visual vertigo, autokinetic effect, stroboscopic motion, and visual vection.

Relating motion illusions to eye movements requires some means of determining each of the component phenomena. Little in the way of even approximate measurement was involved for either component in the initial studies describing them. An illusion was typically considered to occur if there was some mismatch between observations of the same object at different times. For example, if the moon appears stationary at one time and moving at another (when clouds pass over it) then the motion in the latter case can be considered as illusory. This conclusion is based on an assumption of object permanence. That is, an object will be, and will be perceived to be, constant over time; if this does not occur, then either the object has changed or its perceived properties have undergone some modification. Motion illusions were amongst the first to be described because the perception of displacement over time is generally precise and accurate. Thus, the detection of a change in the apparent stability of the moon would have been compelling, as would the apparent upward motion of rocks after viewing descending water. These phenomena involve the perception of motion in one part of the visual field relative to others. Visual vertigo results in the motion of all visible objects, whereas the autokinetic effect occurs when a small object is visible without any background. Vection represents the converse of vertigo: displacement of the whole scene with respect to the observer results in apparent motion of the body and not the scene.

As noted in previous chapters, movements of the eyes can be determined subjectively, from their displacements within the orbit, or by observing the eyes of others. The former technique was initially employed, often with the assistance of applying a finger lightly on the eyelid in order to determine whether an eye is moving. It was less common to make observations of other eyes, and so emphasis was placed upon the subjective aspects of eye movements. Afterimages were enlisted to examine eye movements more precisely in the context of some visual motion illusions. The relationship between illusions and eye movements is examined with respect to several visual motion illusions; although visual vertigo was discussed in Chapter 3, it will be returned to briefly here.

5.2 Induced motion

Induced motion refers to the apparent visual movement of a stationary object, usually in the opposite direction to the real movement of other objects. It can be produced with a wide range of stimulus configurations, and it occurs with linear and rotary motions in the frontal plane and with motion in depth. Induced motion is a contrast effect in the motion domain: if several objects move together and another remains stationary, then the latter will appear to move in the opposite direction. Stimuli that are used to induce motion in contemporary research are shown in Fig. 5.1.

Some of the stimuli were described several centuries ago, but most have been introduced in the twentieth century. Despite this apparent modernity, what seems to be a clear description of induced motion was given over two thousand years ago by Euclid (Fig. 5.2) in his *Optics*. He wrote:

> *If, when certain objects are moved, one is obviously not moved, the object that is not moved will seem to move backward.* For, let B and D move, and let G remain unmoved, and from the eye let the rays fall, ZB, ZG, and ZD. So B, as it moves, will be nearer

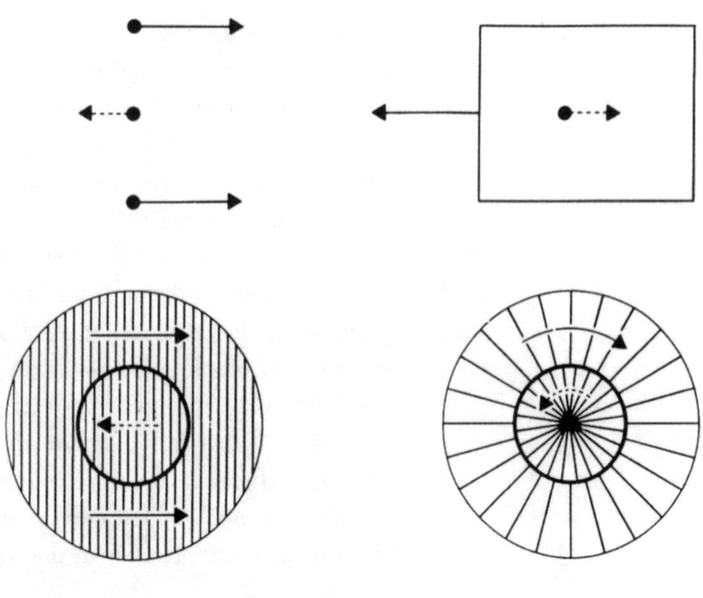

Figure 5.1
Stimuli that are used to induce movement in a stationary target in modern laboratory studies. In all cases the physically moving parts are shown by solid lines and the dashed lines indicate the induced motion of the stationary components. Upper left, two moving dots; upper right, dot and rectangle; lower left, annular movement of a grating; and lower right, rotary motion of a radial annulus. (Adapted from Wade and Swanston, 2001)

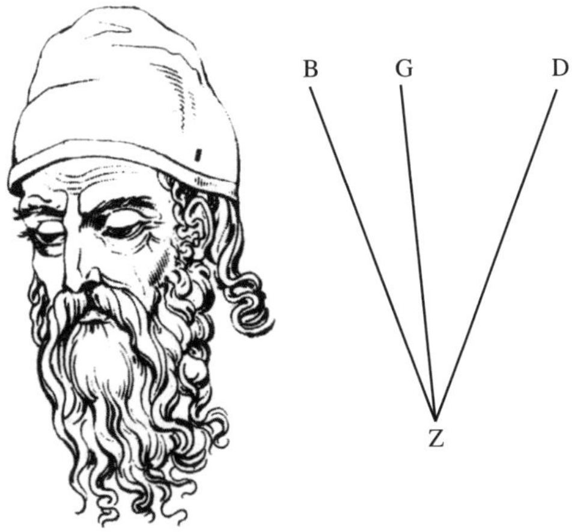

Figure 5.2
Left, Euclid (ca. 323–283 BC) after an engraving in *The historic gallery of portraits and paintings*. Vol. 7. (1811) London: Vernor, Hood, and Sharpe. Right, his diagram of induced motion (after Burton, 1945).

to *G*, and *D*, receding, will be farther away; therefore, *G* will seem to move in the opposite direction. (Burton, 1945, p. 371, original italics)

This account is rather puzzling, since it flies in the face of Euclid's geometrical account of vision. That is, Euclid sought to provide a theory of space and motion perception that reduced these phenomena to projective geometry: size perception was equated with visual angles and motion perception was associated with optical displacements. One possible explanation is that Euclid was assuming that the eyes followed the moving objects. Support for this interpretation derives from the fact that the quotation above is sandwiched between two others that are concerned with eye movements, and both define the perceived motion in terms of the optical geometry. For example:

If, when several objects move at unequal speed, the eye also moves in the same direction, some objects, moving with the same speed as the eye, will seem to stand still, others, moving more slowly, will seem to move in the opposite direction, and others, moving more quickly, will seem to move ahead. (Burton, 1945, p. 371, original italics)

Therefore, if the eye was following the two moving objects, the stationary one would move in the opposite direction with respect to the eye, and this would, according to Euclid's theory, account for the perceived motion.

There is no such doubt about the description given two centuries later by Lucretius of a naturally occurring instance of induced motion: 'when the winds carry scattered clouds across the sky in the night time, then the shining stars seem to glide against the clouds and to pass above them in a very different direction from their true one' (1975, p. 311). A distinction is implied between the real and apparent motion of the stars, presumably because the stars appeared to remain stationary when the clouds were not visible. Similarly, Ptolemy in the second century noted the phenomenon with regard to water flowing past a stationary boat:

> When a boat is stationary on a calm river flowing without waves, a passenger who does not look at the distant land (but only at the water) thinks that the boat is moving quickly and that the water is still. . . . Since the water appears stationary, the motion must be seen as coming from the boat. However, if the water, land, and boat are observed at the same time, and if we are aware that the land is stationary, we will see the water in motion. (Lejeune, 1956, pp. 78–79; see Smith, 1996, for an alternative translation)

Ptolemy's account displays an appreciation of the relativity of motion perception with respect to the frames of reference that are in operation.

Perhaps the most common and compelling instance of induced motion is when moving clouds partially obscure the moon rather than stars, as Alhazen noted: 'Sight therefore perceives the moon as moving behind the swiftly moving cloud because it correlates a part of the moon with successive parts of the cloud' (Sabra, 1989, p. 261). This observation has been repeated and reported many times in the last millennium, as it provides one of the most readily visible instances of induced motion in the natural environment. For example, Porterfield (1759*b*) described the natural occurring instance and gave a generalization from it: 'If two or more Objects move with the same Velocity, and a third remain at rest, the Moveables will appear fixed, and the Quiescent in Motion the contrary Way. Thus, Clouds moving very swiftly, their Parts seem to preserve their Situation, and the Moon to move the contrary Way' (p. 424). This is equivalent to the situation represented in Fig. 5.1, upper left.

Such examples of induced motion were discussed generally in eighteenth century books on optics and vision. For example, a clear link between such perceived motion and unconscious eye movements was made by Joseph Harris (1702–1764; 1775) in his book on *Optics*:

> If two or more objects, having the same apparent velocity, move all the same way; an object at rest, by which they pass, may appear to move the contrary

way, whilst the objects in motion may seem at rest. For no motion among themselves is perceivable, since their images upon the retina keep the same distances from each other; and if the spectator insensibly moves his eye, so as to keep these images in the same place, the image of the object at rest will pass successively over them, after the same manner as if that object had been in motion the contrary way. (Harris, 1775, p. 106)

Thus, after two thousand years, Harris adopted much the same interpretation of induced motion as Euclid. However, he added two additional features. On the one hand, he remarked that the physically moving objects appear stationary. The other feature that is made explicit in Harris' account is that the pursuit movements were 'insensible' or unconscious. Harris also applied the concept of unconscious inference to binocular single vision: 'And it is very certain, that in at least abundant of cases, the visive faculty is assisted by a kind of reasoning, drawn from former experience, tho' perhaps unattended at the time we use it' (1775, p. 111). The concept of unconscious inference was to have wide currency in the nineteenth century: it was adopted and amplified by Wheatstone (1838) in the context of stereoscopic vision, and it provided a cornerstone for Helmholtz's (1867*a*) theory of vision (see Finger and Wade, 2002).

Experimental studies of induced motion commenced rather late, considering this rich history. Induced motion was referred to as motion contrast by German researchers in the early twentieth century, and it was often linked to the motion aftereffect. For example, von Szily (1905) fixated a point in the centre of a stationary disc while a surrounding pattern of striped lines moved laterally—the disc appeared to move in the opposite direction, which was motion contrast. The stimulus situation is like that shown in Fig. 5.1, lower left. However, von Szily noted that when the disc was viewed subsequently, relative to a stationary background, it appeared to move in the same direction as the background had done formerly. This observation was confirmed by Basler (1910), who added many subtle variations to stimulus and observation conditions.

Motion can be induced with a simple arrangement consisting of a pair of moving and a single stationary stimulus (usually dots), as was described by Porterfield (1759*b*). This was one of the situations examined by Duncker (1929); under these conditions the physically stationary dot is seen as moving in the opposite direction. A more compelling stimulus for inducing motion in a stationary dot is to displace a surrounding frame (see Fig. 5.1, upper right). Ehrenstein (1925) presented a diamond-shaped frame in two successive positions with respect to an enclosed stationary dot; the dot appeared to move in the opposite direction to the displacement. Duncker (1929) also used a moving rectangular frame surrounding a stationary dot. Under these circumstances the rectangle can be moved below its detection threshold and still induce motion in the dot. The possibility that the inducing motion resulted in unconscious eye movements was still entertained, and both psychophysical and physiological tests of this hypothesis were examined. In addition, Duncker described the rotation induced in a stationary radial pattern by rotation of a patterned annulus or surround, as in Fig. 5.1, lower right. The eye does undergo torsion as a consequence of surround rotation, but it is of limited extent and so is unlikely to be the basis of induced rotation. Evidence from measures of eye torsion confirms this conclusion—stimuli that modulate the degree of torsion that can be measured do not influence the magnitude of induced rotation reported (Wade et al., 1991). Another psychophysical technique involves inducing motion in opposite directions simultaneously (Gogel, 1977); it is difficult to argue that the eyes can move in opposite directions simultaneously. Finally, direct measures of eye movements and linear induced motion fail to demonstrate their dependence (Levi and Schor, 1984).

A more subtle version of the eye movement hypothesis is that it is either uncompensated eye movement signals or tendencies for the eyes to move that are correlated with the induced visual movement. These have the same problems in dealing with apparent rotations, motions in depth, and opposite linear motions as do simpler eye movement interpretations: eye movements would result in displacements of all contours rather than some specific ones. Accordingly, the perception of motion in a stationary stimulus induced by a larger moving one is unlikely to be explained by any correlated movements of the eyes.

5.3 Motion aftereffect

Induced motion is an example of simultaneous motion contrast, whereas the motion aftereffect reflects successive motion contrast. Having observed a moving stimulus for some time, a stationary

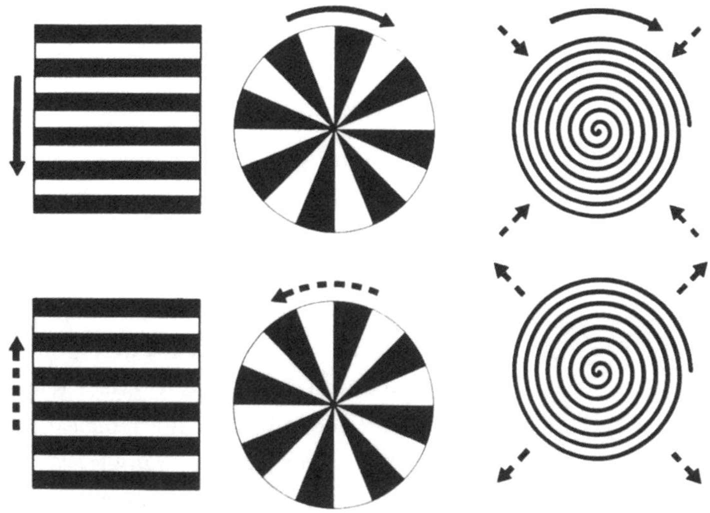

Figure 5.3

Laboratory stimuli that are used to produce motion aftereffects. In each of the three cases the physical motion is shown at the top (solid lines), and the motion perceived in a stationary pattern is shown at the bottom (dashed lines). Left, linear motion of a grating; centre, rotation of a sectored disc; and right, rotation of a spiral. The physically stationary patterns are initially seen as stationary. During the physical motion the movement is perceived as shown by the solid arrows, but the spiral also appears to contract. Following about 30 s adaptation the stationary patterns appear to move in the directions indicated by the dashed lines. (Adapted from Wade and Swanston, 2001)

one appears to move in the opposite direction. Stimuli of the type used to investigate the motion aftereffect in the laboratory are shown in Fig. 5.3. They bear a strong resemblence to those employed for induced motion.

The motion aftereffect has a less even history than that for induced motion (see Wade and Verstraten, 1998), but similar interpretations have been applied to it. Aristotle described the phenomenon, but he did not relate it specifically to eye movements, nor was his description unambiguous regarding the direction of perceived motion: 'When persons turn away from looking at objects in motion, e.g., rivers, and especially those which flow very rapidly, they find that the visual stimulations still present themselves, for the things really at rest are then seen moving' (Ross, 1931, p. 459b). The description given by Lucretius was more precise, and implicated the motion aftereffect with induced motion:

When our spirited horse has stuck fast in the middle of a river, and we have looked down upon the swift waters of the stream, while the horse stands

> there a force seems to carry his body sideways and pushing it violently against the stream, and, wherever we turn our eyes, all seems to be rushing and flowing in the same way as we are. (Lucretius, 1975, p. 309)

Thus, when Lucretius was surrounded by flowing water and looking down at it the horse seemed to be moving against the current. This is an instance of induced motion. When he looked at the bank of the river it seemed to be moving in the same direction as the induced motion—that is, opposite to the flowing water.

Unlike induced motion, the motion aftereffect seems to have drowned in the waters of antiquity. Indeed, it did not resurface until the nineteenth century, when Purkinje's acute vision was directed to it, although some earlier observers came very close to describing it. For example, Willis (1672) might have been referring to this phenomenon when he discussed vertigo. In his Oxford lectures he stated that: 'Vertigo may also be caused by the sight of a mobile object such as running water because the spirits concerned with vision are caught up in this similar movement' (Dewhurst, 1980, p. 114). The stimulus was appropriate but the report is not precise enough to link it with the motion aftereffect. In the second edition of *Zoonomia* Erasmus Darwin similarly described the vertiginous effects of viewing rotating and translating motions, but did not mention any aftereffects: 'Thus some people become dizzy at the sight of a whirling wheel, or by gazing on the fluctuations of a river, if no steady objects are at the same time within the sphere of distinct vision' (1796, p. 233). Therefore, the visually disturbing aspect of viewing moving patterns was clearly apparent, but its carry over to stationary patterns subsequently seen was not noted.

Purkinje (1820) described the aftereffect that follows observation of a variety of motions such as rotation and translation, and he related these to eye movements. His article was principally about vertigo, to which the motion aftereffect was linked:

> Another form of visual vertigo can be demonstrated if one observes a passing sequence of spatially distinct objects for a long time, e.g., a long parade of cavalry, overlapping waves, the spokes of a wheel that is not rotating too fast. When the actual movement of the objects stops there is a similar apparent motion in the opposite direction. (1820, pp. 96–97)

Purkinje's initial interpretation was elaborated in 1825: eye movements generated by moving objects continued when stationary ones were subsequently observed. He described the consequences of observing a parade of cavalry for over an hour and then viewed the houses behind them.

> While the eye did strive to fixate on each individual row of militia during observation, it moved unconsciously in the same direction as the parade; this movement was repeated so often that it became habitual, and continued when the parade had passed. The eye attempted to fixate on the stationary objects in a similar manner to the motion it had become accustomed to fixating, and therefore glided unconsciously over them in the usual direction, so that the objects appeared to slide away in the opposite direction. (Purkinje, 1825, pp. 60–61)

An unconscious eye movement explanation is explicitly adopted: the eyes pursue the moving objects and continue to do so with respect to stationary ones observed later.

Robert Addams (ca. 1800–1875) independently rediscovered the motion aftereffect following fixation on part of a descending waterfall (see Fig. 5.4), and it later became known as the waterfall illusion (Thompson, 1880). His interpretation is essentially similar to Purkinje's:

> I conceive the effect to be owing to an involuntary and *unconscious* muscular movement of the eyeball, and thus occasioning a displacement of the images on the retina. Supposing the eyes to be intently gazing at any point in a transverse plane passing through a vertically moving body, they will naturally and even irresistibly tend to follow the motion of that body; nor can the muscular

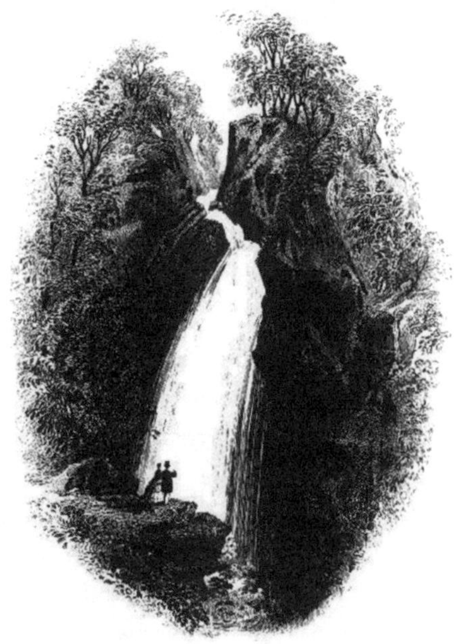

Figure 5.4
A nineteenth century engraving of the Falls of Foyers (reproduced by kind permission of Mike Swanston). Addams would have observed the waterfall from the platform shown. The River Foyers runs into Loch Ness, in northern Scotland.

apparatus of the eye maintain a stable equilibrium when the sight is fatigued and bewildered with a rapid change of moving forms before the eye. Now in the case of the descending water, the eyes, being directed to a particular part in a horizontal section of it, cannot be prevented moving downwards through a small space: every new form in the moving scene invites the eyes to observe, and for that reason to follow it; but the voluntary powers are engaged to raise the axes of the eyes again to the section. This depression of the axes below the *intentional point of sight* seems to be repeated three or four times per second, whilst looking at the water-fall. Then, when the eyes are suddenly turned upon the rock, the muscles, having been brought into a kind of periodic contraction, will perform at least one of these movements after the exciting cause ceases to act; and thus the axes of the eyes, by moving downwards, will occasion a motion of the image of the rock over the retina in a direction from above downwards, and consequently the object giving that image will *appear* to move the contrary way, that is, upwards, agreeably to observation. (Addams, 1834, pp. 373–374, original italics)

Both Purkinje and Addams describe what would now be called optokinetic nystagmus. The description by Addams is much more precise than that by Purkinje, as it refers to the cyclical nature of the movements and the frequency with which they occur. Moreover, Addams was explicit in relating involuntary eye movements and retinal displacements, which, he suggested, were the basis for the phenomenon. Addams proposed a way of producing the motion aftereffect 'by mechanical means, such as by a rapid unrolling of pieces of calico having some pattern or markings on them' (1834, p. 374); this is equivalent to the stimulus depicted in Fig. 5.3, left. He also observed that the motion aftereffect could be produced by head movement relative to a stationary pattern.

The involvement of eye movements could have been excluded at an early stage, because of the stimuli that can produce motion aftereffects, but the conclusion was not made. Joseph Plateau (1849; Fig. 5.5) rediscovered the motion aftereffect yet again, in the course of conducting experiments using the phenakistoscope (or stroboscopic disc). This was a simple instrument which presented slightly different pictures to the eye in rapid succession. Plateau (1836, 1849) had been studying the effects of rotating patterns on the perception of motion and noticed that motion was visible in stationary objects following prolonged exposure to motion. He introduced the stimulus employed most widely throughout the second half of the nineteenth century for the study of motion aftereffects. It can be seen in Fig. 5.5, and it consisted of a black disc with a white Archimedes spiral on it; it became called

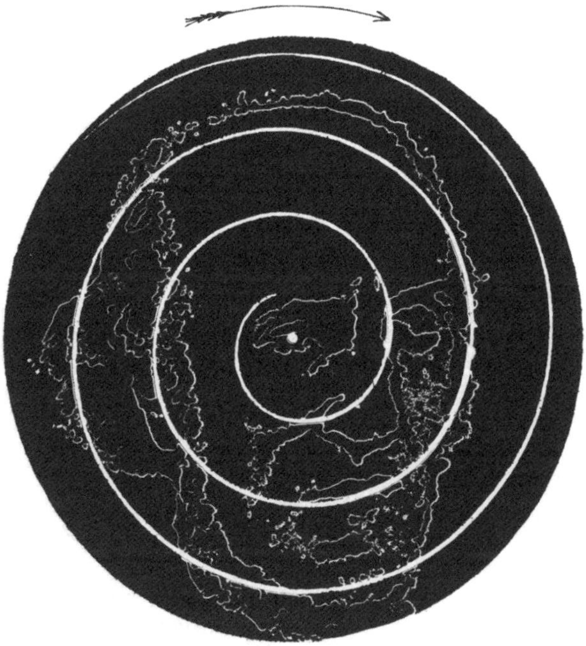

Figure 5.5
Plateau spiral. Plateau's portrait is embedded in the spiral pattern he used for inducing the motion aftereffect (from Wade, 1995).

the Plateau spiral. Rotating spirals, like that shown in Fig. 5.3, right, continue to be used in studies of motion aftereffects, and they are often referred to as spiral aftereffects. Plateau described what he saw in the following way:

> If the disc rotates in the direction indicated by the arrow, and one looks at it with the eyes fixed on the centre for a time sufficiently long, but not long enough to tire the eyes, then one immediately directs the eyes to another object, such as the face of a person, for example, one experiences a singular effect: the head of the person appears to shrink for some time. If the disc is turned in the opposite direction, the resulting effect is opposite: it is as if the head of the person appears to expand. (Plateau, 1849, p. 257)

That is, the visual motion is radial, either centrifugal or centripetal, which would be difficult to match with any eye movements, as was recognized by Plateau. As Holland (1965) remarked: 'The spiral of Plateau sounded the death knell for the eye-movement theory' (p. 89), but it was clearly not heard by many. This was the case even though Plateau's article was rapidly translated into German (Plateau, 1850).

Despite his awareness of Plateau's work, Helmholtz (1867*a*), also adopted an eye movement interpretation of the motion aftereffect, although he did not describe formal experiments on the phenomenon. He suggested that: 'The requisite movements of the eyes are not much understood, and so they have not been noticed by Plateau and Oppel, who carried out observations on these phenomena' (Helmholtz, 1925/2000, p. 248). Reference was made to Oppel because he had conducted studies of motion aftereffects (Oppel, 1856).

There is a logical difficulty of accounting for the phenomenon in this way: any after-movement of the eyes would affect all contours in the visual field, rather than being restricted to regions exposed to prior motion. Motion aftereffects are generally restricted to the regions of the retina that have been exposed to motion. Mach (1875) pointed to the problems associated with eye movement interpretations and the difficulty they would have in accounting for radial motion seen in the spiral aftereffect. He drew attention to the shortcomings of Helmholtz's analysis:

> Plateau and Oppel already assumed that the motion aftereffects of images result from processes in the retina. To explain them by eye movements, as Helmholtz later attempted, could be ruled out on the basis of evidence from details of older experiments. Since eye movements can only shift the visual field as a whole, the following is sufficient proof against the eye movement hypothesis. The illusory enlarging spiral causes a shrinking of objects towards a certain central point after the spiral stops. (Young et al., 2001, pp. 59–60)

One of Mach's students (Dvorak, 1870) had shown that concentric counter-rotating spirals produce aftereffects that are centrifugal and centripetal at the same time. Moreover, Kleiner (1878) rotated a central sectored disc (like that shown in Fig. 5.3, centre) in the opposite direction to two adjacent ones, and reported oppositely directed motion aftereffects that were visible simultaneously. Linear motion in two directions simultaneously was examined by Sigmund Exner (1849–1926; Fig. 5.6, left). Horizontal and vertical gratings were moved vertically and horizontally, respectively, behind a circular aperture. Exner (1887) reported that the motion seen during adaptation was in a diagonal direction, with a motion aftereffect in the opposite diagonal. Exner (1894) presented a model to account for motion aftereffects based upon eye movement centres. Exner's model (Fig. 5.6, right) was expressed in terms of influences on eye muscles, but it could be interpreted more generally. The symbols *a*–*f* denote units receiving input from retinal receptors, which will be stimulated in succession, dependent on the direction of motion. Prolonged

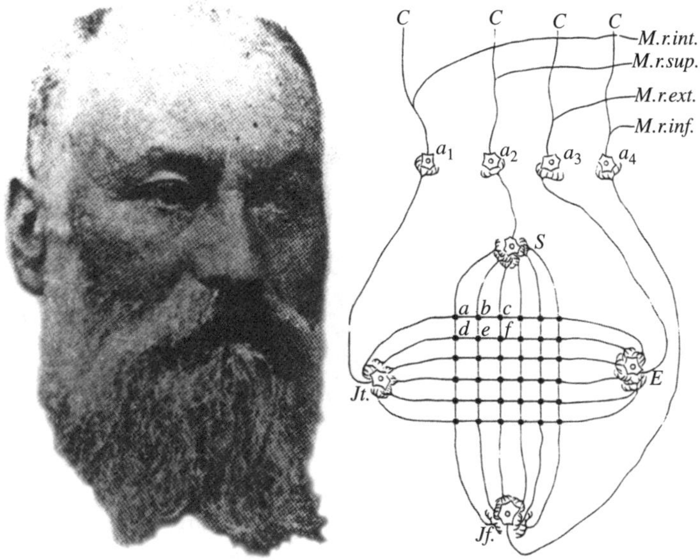

Figure 5.6

Left, Sigmund Exner (1849–1926) after a portrait in Pagel (1901). Right, Exner's model for eye movement centres and motion aftereffects: 'Schema for a centre of optical motion detection. *a–f* and the analogous points are the locations at which the fibres from the retinal elements enter the centre. The cells S, E, Jt, and Jf represent centres to which each and every point of excitation arrive and where they can be summated. The time required by the excitations to reach there from any one of these points would be approximately proportional to the distance given in the diagram. a_1–a_4 are centres which are closely related to, or perhaps identical with, the nuclei of the external eye muscles (only four are shown in the schema: M. rectus internus, superior, externus, and inferior). C are fibres to the cortex, the organ of consciousness.' (Exner, 1894, p. 193).

stimulation in a given direction (e.g. *a–c*) will lead to the fatigue of the summation cell E, but not of Jt; this imbalance will be displayed when a stationary stimulus is subsequently viewed.

Exner also influenced Adolf von Szily (1848–1920; Fig. 5.7, left) who made several important discoveries concerning motion aftereffects in two articles (Szily, 1905, 1908). He demonstrated the aperture effect both for the perception of real motion and for the motion aftereffect it generates. This was achieved by presenting horizontally moving vertical gratings behind a rectangular window placed at an angle to the horizontal. Motion was perceived in the direction of the long axis of the rectangle and the motion aftereffect was in the opposite direction. He also examined the effects of motion over the retina produced by object movement and eye movement. That is, he compared motion aftereffects with

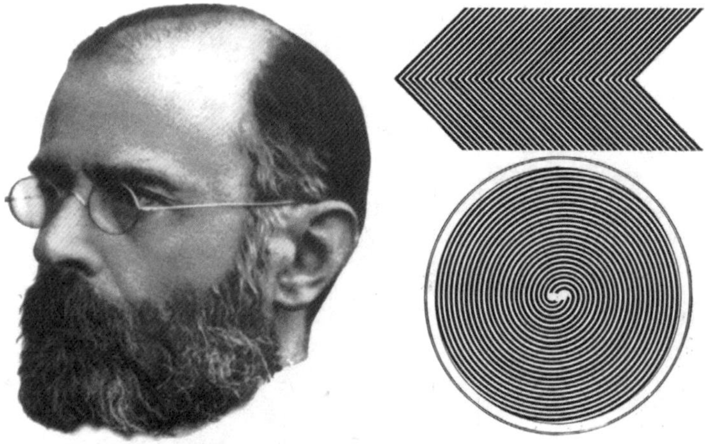

Figure 5.7
Left, Adolf von Szily (1848–1920) after a portrait in Küchle (1982). Upper right, his stimulus for examining the influence of stimulus and eye movements on motion aftereffects; lower right, his stimulus for generating rotations in opposite directions for each eye (both from von Szily, 1905).

moving contours relative to a stationary eye to those with eye movements relative to stationary contours like those shown. The whole stimulus (Fig. 5.7, upper right) could be moved sideways or the eye could move slowly across the stationary contours. The motion aftereffects were said to be equivalent.

Von Szily examined binocular interaction by exposing each eye to oppositely directed rotations of a spiral pattern (Fig. 5.7, lower right). He achieved this by viewing oppositely directed rotations alternately or by placing a Dove prism in front of one eye and viewing the rotating spiral with both eyes. Rivalry was seen during adaptation; no motion aftereffect was visible when both eyes viewed a static test pattern, but motion aftereffects in opposite directions could be seen when each eye was used alone. Since the eyes cannot rotate in opposite directions at the same time, this provided further evidence against the involvement of eye movements in motion aftereffects. In an article a few years later, Szily (1908) confirmed that exposure of the whole visual field to motion did not yield a motion aftereffect. This he examined with a vertically striped cylinder rotating around the head. The result was in accordance with earlier observations by Mach (1875) and Aitken (1878).

Many of von Szily's experiments were repeated and confirmed by Wohlgemuth (1911) in his masterly review of motion aftereffects. For example, he was able to induce motion aftereffects in opposite directions in the two eyes; when both eyes viewed the stationary test pattern the aftereffects engaged in rivalry, but each motion aftereffect could be seen when the other eye was closed.

Adolf Wohlgemuth (1911) classified the previous interpretations into physical, psychical, and physiological. Eye movement explanations were considered to be physical. Wohlgemuth devoted most attention to the physiological interpretations, particularly that advanced by Exner (1894). Exner's model has been acclaimed by Dierig (1994) as the first representation of a neural network, although Alexander Bain (1818–1903) had presented one some 20 years earlier (see Wilkes and Wade, 1997); Bain's was a forerunner of Hebb's (1949) model. Exner's model was expressed in terms of influences on eye muscles, but it could be interpreted more generally. Wohlgemuth (1911) raised certain problems with it, and modified it slightly by incorporating inhibition as well as excitation (see Wade and Verstraten, 1998).

Eye movements can be discounted experimentally because the motion aftereffect occurs with stabilized retinal images (Drysdale, 1975*b*; Sekuler and Ganz, 1963) and eye rotations are not correlated with the rotary aftereffect (Seidman et al., 1992). It is clear that motion can be seen in an isolated stimulus following prolonged pursuit (Chaudhuri, 1991), and that this can be attributed to after-nystagmus. Moreover, as Szily (1905) and Basler (1910) demonstrated, the motion aftereffect can be induced in a stimulus that has not itself moved over the retina. This has been conformed by Swanston and Wade (1992) and Wade et al. (1996).

5.4 Visual vertigo

Visual vertigo will be returned to briefly here because it provides a good example of a phenomenon that is amenable to interpretation in terms of eye movements. The early nineteenth century studies of motion aftereffects were stimulated by the investigations of visual vertigo, although the phenomenon had long been known. The dizziness and giddiness caused by alcohol, looking down from heights, as well as a variety of ailments have been recounted since antiquity (see Chapter 3). There were also descriptions of the visual effects of body rotation: Lucretius described it as a children's game, and Ptolemy related vertigo to prior exposure to visual motion.

Research on post-rotational visual motion commenced in earnest in the eighteenth century, largely as a consequence of Porterfield's (1759*b*) association of eye movements with visual

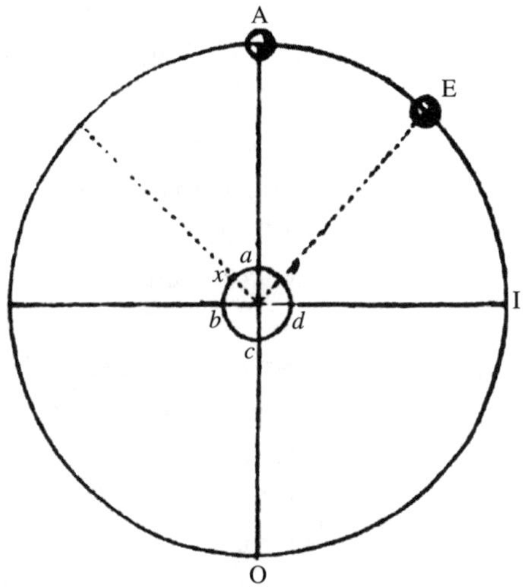

Figure 5.8

Porterfield's diagram representing the interaction between eye movements and vertigo: 'let *abcd*... be the Eye moving round, according to the Order of the Letters *a*, *b*, *c*, *d*, and let A be an Object at rest seen by that Eye: When the Eye moves from *a* to *b*, if we attend to, and are sensible of the Velocity with which it moves, we will attribute the change of Situation of the Object intirely to the Motion of the Eye, and will therefore conceive the Object at rest, as it truly is: But if we are entirely unattentive to the Motion of the Eye, and imagine that it is absolutely at rest, the Object A will then seem to move the contrary Way, with a Velocity proportional to its Distance, so as to describe an Arch similar to that described by the Eye in the same time, that is, in the Time the Eye moves round from *a* to *b*, the Object will seem to move from A to I.... But if, when the Eye is absolutely at rest, it be imagined to turn round from *b* to *x*, with the Velocity *bx*, all Objects, as A, will appear to move the same Way in the Order of the Letters AEI; and consequently will appear to continue their Motion for some Time after the Eye ceases to move' (Porterfield, 1759*b*, pp. 427–428).

motion. Porterfield sought to accommodate this visual vertigo within his broad analysis of visual motion. In modern terminology he was suggesting that it was the signals for eye movements, rather than the eye movements themselves, that generated the post-rotational visual motion. Porterfield provided an illustration (Fig. 5.8) to support his analysis.

Porterfield went on to list a range of motion phenomena, including the lucid definition of visually induced motion given in Section 5.2. Vertigo was the final visual phenomenon discussed in his book, and he argued that the eyes did not move when the body stopped rotating. The evidence was subjective: Porterfield was not aware of any movements of his own eyes and so he was convinced that they remained stationary following rotation.

Wells (1792, 1794*a*,*b*) demonstrated that the eyes did move following body rotation, and that the visual motion was of the whole visual field rather than a part of it. Erasmus Darwin (1794) was reluctant to implicate eye movements in visual vertigo, but his description of tracking, and never catching, a peripheral afterimage necessarily involved eye movements. However, Darwin believed that the peripheral afterimages were produced during rotation. In addition to Wells' criticisms of this position, Darwin had a doughty opponent in Thomas Brown (1778–1820), who subjected Darwin's *Zoonomia* to detailed scrutiny. Initially Brown, an eighteen-year-old student at Edinburgh University, wrote to Darwin praising the book and promising a lengthier appraisal. Darwin appreciated the praise but was disparaging about the appraisal, so much so that Brown's biographer (Welsh, 1825) forbore to reprint Darwin's response. Following more congenial correspondence, Brown committed his thoughts to print. In his critique of almost 600 pages, Brown (1798) dissected Darwin's structure chapter by chapter. Brown attacked Darwin's spectral theory of vertigo by drawing attention to its inconsistencies. Brown observed that the objects that appeared to move following body rotation were those that were in front of the eyes, not those that had been passed during rotation. In order to produce a clear afterimage Brown rotated his body while looking at a book held in front of him; when rotation ceased he did not experience any afterimage of the book. When he rotated his body with his eyes open and then stepped into a darkened room he did not experience any visual vertigo. On the other hand, when he rotated in one room (with his eyes open) and then stepped into another lighted room, it was the objects in the latter that appeared to rotate. Finally, he bandaged his eyes during body rotation and removed the cover after rotation ceased, only to experience visual motion once more. For these reasons Brown rejected Darwin's theory and adopted one rather like Porterfield's. Nowhere in his critique of Darwin did Brown mention Wells' experiments.

Purkinje (1820, 1825) repeated some of Wells' experiments, in ignorance of the fact. Indeed, Purkinje's assessment of eye movements were not as precise as the afterimage method adopted by Wells. Purkinje concluded that the basis for the visual vertigo was oscillatory movements of the eyes 'which can be detected by gently touching one's own eye or by observing someone else's eye' (1820, p. 95). Very few writers in English were cited by Purkinje. Darwin was mentioned in his first work on vertigo (Purkinje, 1820), and in his second book on subjective visual phenomena he did note: 'Had Porterfield established the movements of the eyes in vertigo, he would not have formulated his interpretation' (1825, p. 60). As was described in Chapter 3, Purkinje used a mechanically rotating device for generating vertigo. This was more precise than rotating the body actively, but most of his observations were made as a consequence of his own body rotation. We know this because he made a 'magic disc' for simulating visual motion from a sequence of still images (like Plateau's phenakistoscope). One of the sequences he produced was of his own body in rotation (Fig. 5.9), so it remains possible to observe Purkinje in the process of generating vertigo.

When Müller (1840, 1843) was considering the same issue, his views differed little from those expressed by Porterfield, even though he was aware of Purkinje's work on vertigo:

> Sometimes the object appears to move when both object and eye are fixed. This is the case in the vertigo produced by moving our body round on its axis; surrounding objects then, when our body and eyes cease to move, appear to perform a circular motion in the opposite direction to that in which our head had moved. Some remarkable observations, by Purkinje, seem to show that these apparent motions are owing to an impulse to motion in the determinate direction imparted to the brain; for the direction of the apparent rotation of objects maintained a constant relation to the head, although the position of the head were changed after its own movement was remitted. With these phenomena of apparent motion we must not confound others dependent on spectra left by strong impression on the retina . . . The

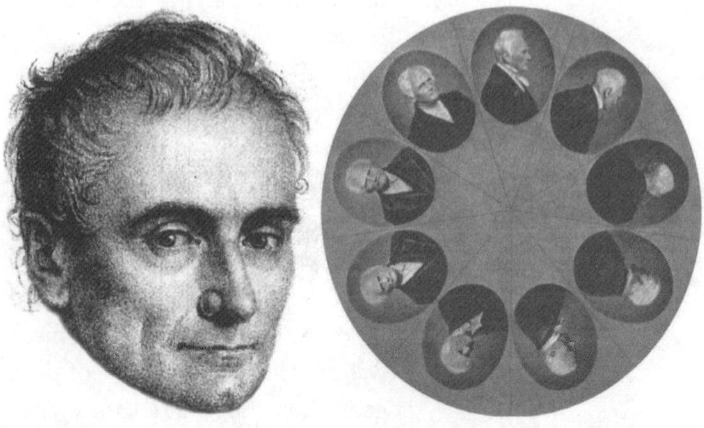

Figure 5.9

Left, Jan Evangeslista Purkinje (1787–1869) after a frontispiece illustration in Vol. 3 of his *Opera omnia*. Right, a sequence of pictures of Purkinje during spinning made for his magic disc or phorolyt for producing apparent motion (after Psotníčková, 1955).

sensations of rotatory movement of objects produced by turning the body on its axis are quite independent of the previous impressions on the retina; for they can be produced by moving round with the eyes closed. (Müller, 1843, pp. 1178–1179)

Müller was clearly unaware of Wells' experiments on vertigo, and he believed that the eyes remained stationary following rotation. This rendered the dependence of the direction of the visual motion on the orientation of the head particularly puzzling. The situation was to change with an understanding of vestibular function, evidence for which was derived from the direction of eye movements following body rotation. Mach (1875) provided support for Wells' conclusions, although Wells was not mentioned by him. Mach also generated an afterimage prior to rotating his body, and noted its apparent motion when rotation ceased. Breuer (1874) obtained a similar result, and Crum Brown (1878) gave graphic depictions of eye movements during and following body rotation. Mach summarized his many experiments on vertigo in the following way: 'We see that the phenomena of visual vertigo can be explained by eye movements, which are induced by reflexes stemming from movement sensations' (1875, p. 90). Subsequent research on vertigo has tended to be in the context of medicine (e.g. Baloh and Honrubia, 1990; Brandt, 1991; Brandt et al., 2004; Furman and Cass, 2003). It has a more specific application to aerospace medicine, because vertigo can have such a disruptive influence on astronauts.

Thus far there is one phenomenon (visual vertigo) that correlates eye movements with visual motion, and two (induced motion and motion aftereffects) which do not. As would be expected of a phenomenon that is related to eye movements, visual vertigo involves a rotation of the whole visual world, rather than a part of it.

5.5 Autokinetic motion

Yet another motion phenomenon relates to the apparent movement of stars at night. In 1799 the great German naturalist, Alexander von Humboldt (1769–1859, Fig. 5.10, left), recorded that when he observed certain stars they appeared to wander about haphazardly in the night sky:

Here is the place, at least in passing, to mention another optical phenomenon which I observed only once in all my mountain climbing, which occurred

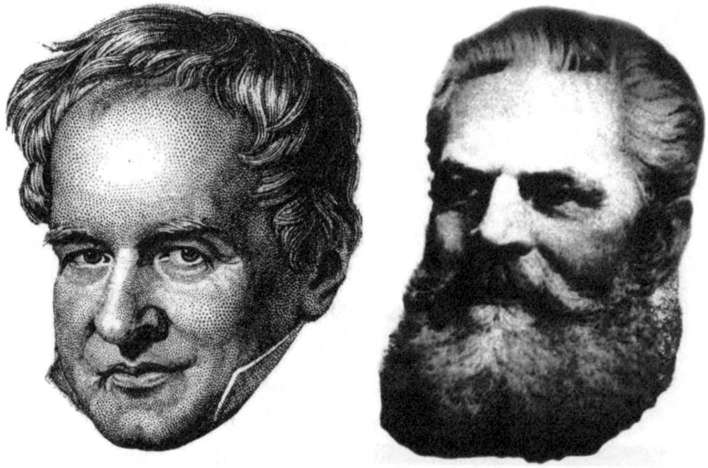

Figure 5.10
Left, Alexander von Humboldt (1769–1859) after an engraving in *The world's great men* (1854). London: The London Publishing Company. Right, Hermann Aubert (1826–1892) after an illustration in Polyak (1957).

before sunrise on 22 June 1799 on the slopes of the Pics of Tenerife. In the Malpays, at a height of 10,700 feet above sea level, I saw with my naked eye low-lying stars in a wonderful wandering motion. Illuminated points rose upwards, moved sideways and fell back to their original positions. The phenomenon lasted 7 to 8 minutes and came to a halt long before the appearance of the sun above the horizon. The same motion could be seen through a telescope; there remains no doubt that it was the stars themselves that moved. (Humboldt, 1850, p. 73)

The observation was made during a scientific voyage to South America, and it is clear that Humboldt genuinely believed that the stars did undergo the rapid motions that he perceived. He even called the phenomenon 'Sternschwanken' or star wandering. Exner (1896) remarked that the same observation was made from the same spot independently some 50 years later by Prince Adalbert von Preussen. Other observers were able to see the phenomenon too, though they did not all describe the haphazard movements in a similar way. A debate arose about the precise basis for the star movements, and its subjective nature was determined by Schweizer (1857, 1858), an astronomer in Moscow; his work has been summarized by Exner (1896) and Holt-Hansen (1962). Schweizer made many observations on the phenomenon, both under naturalistic conditions and in the laboratory. His evidence that the visual motion was subjective rather than objective derived from a simple study, in which he and a colleague observed Sirius together and compared their reports of the motion paths:

By this means a new fact was established that *at one and the same moment* the appearance was different for each of us. Sometimes I saw the star rise while

Herr Bredichin saw it fall; at times it appeared stationary to me while the other observer caught sight of it in rapidly advancing movement; at yet other times the star described a circle for me while for Herr Bredichin it rose or fell in a slanting direction. (Schweizer 1857, p. 443, original italics)

As there was no consistency in the motions of the same star seen at the same time by different observers, it became clear that it was a perceptual rather than a physical phenomenon. The phenomenon is not confined to stars in the sky, and Schweizer (1857) simulated the conditions with artificial stars in a darkened room. If you look at a stationary and very dim light in an otherwise totally dark room it will appear to wander about haphazardly, like the stars that Humboldt observed. Schweizer noted that the movements in a horizontal direction were more pronounced than those in the vertical. He also saw the motion with a black spot on a white wall, and vice versa; after a short time the spot moved in various directions but always returned to the original point. This was referred to as 'Punktschwanken' to distinguish it from Sternschwanken. 'Scheinbewegung' or apparent motion was applied to the movement of a faint light in a dark room (Exner, 1896). Adams (1912) suggested that they should all be included under the rubric autokinetic sensations.

Most early reports noted that there is a latency of some seconds before the autokinetic motion is seen, and thereafter the amplitudes can be considerable. There was, however, much debate about the pattern and velocity of the motion seen. Charpentier (1886) described the motion as radial and slightly curved with a low velocity; the amplitude could be over 30°. Carr (1910), on the other hand, reported slow and irregular motions in the central visual field but the velocity was estimated as up to $20° s^{-1}$ when the eyes were fatigued.

Hermann Aubert (1826–1892, Fig. 5.10, right) was initially unaware of Charpentier's experiments when he independently rediscovered autokinetic motion in 1887, and both failed to cite Schweizer's studies. Some years earlier, Aubert (1865) imposed some degree of order on a wide range of visual phenomena, particularly those involving motion. For example, he measured the thresholds for detecting uniform and relational motions. When a target moved in isolation its motion could be detected when it reached a velocity of about $0.3° s^{-1}$. When a patterned background was visible the threshold was approximately

$0.03° s^{-1}$. Since isolated stimuli have higher thresholds for motion they can only be seen to move when they undergo quite large displacements. Thus, there is clearly an influence of the visible reference frame in motion perception, but that was not considered to be the sole factor. Aubert returned to the examination of motion phenomena in the 1880s, and rediscovered the apparent motion of a static light in a dark room; he gave it the name autokinetic sensation (Aubert, 1887).

As with the phenomena mentioned above, eye movement explanations were the first candidates for the autokinetic sensations, but experimental investigations failed to find a simple link. Carr (1910) adopted an afterimage technique to examine this by comparing the movements of the afterimage with those of a spot of light. The afterimage remained relatively stable, even during quite large apparent movements of the spot. Using direct recordings of eye movements, Guilford and Dallenbach (1928) found that the direction and amplitude of the movements did not correlate with those of autokinetic motion. However, there were some aspects of the phenomenon that could be related to the direction of eye movements. For example, autokinetic motion is in the same direction as prior eccentric fixation (Carr, 1910), that is, following fixation to one side of the median plane. The direction of autokinetic motion can also be related to the physiological position of rest of an eye (Levy, 1972)—the position that is assumed by the eye in repose. Nystagmic eye movements have been induced by rotary and caloric stimulation, and these produce similar apparent motions of an isolated light (Skolnick, 1940). As with visual vertigo, the apparent motion was associated with involuntary rather than voluntary eye movements.

In the autokinetic effect there is no stimulus motion, so the perceived movement must be caused by some internal process, probably related to actual or suppressed movements of the eyes (Levy, 1972; Post and Leibowitz, 1985). An assessment of these interpretations can be found in Howard (1982) and Mack (1986).

5.6 Stroboscopic motion

All the aspects of motion perception discussed above are instances of apparent motion. That is, physically stationary objects are perceived as moving. Stroboscopic motion refers to perceiving motion from a rapid sequence of spatially separated static stimuli. It differs from real motion, in which objects change their location over time. The logic of applying eye movement interpretations is much the same as with the previous phenomena: if the eyes move between the two stationary stimuli then there could be motion over the retina. It was with the invention of instruments like the stroboscopic disc (Plateau, 1833; Stampfer, 1833) that motion perception was rendered experimentally tractable. Since the 1830s, stroboscopic motion—the apparent motion between briefly presented stimuli—has been one of the most intensely studied areas of motion perception. However, the history of the devices that could synthesize motion from a series of static pictures is more extensively documented in chronicles of film and photography (see Hecht, 1993; Herbert, 2000; Mannoni, 2000) than in histories of vision.

In antiquity, Lucretius gave an account of what appears to be apparent motion, although it occurred in the context of discussing dreams:

> When the first image perishes and a second is then produced in another position, the former seems to have altered its pose. Of course this must be supposed to take place very swiftly: so great is their velocity, so great the store of things, so great the store of particles in any single moment of sensation, to enable the supply to come up. (1975, p. 337)

Plateau (1878) remarked that Lucretius had come very close to appreciating the nature of apparent motion. No further reference to this phenomenon is encountered until the nineteenth century. Apparent motion is dependent upon visual persistence, and so it is not surprising that the impetus to examine it derived from a description of a phenomenon linking the two (see Wade, 2004*a*; Wade and Heller, 1997). Peter Mark Roget (1779–1869) is best known for his *Thesaurus* but he retained a life long interest in vision. In 1825, he described the pattern of spokes moving behind a palisade and suggested that this could provide an accurate means for measuring the duration of visual persistence. Roget's account spurred his friend, Michael Faraday (1791–1867, Fig. 5.11, left), to pursue the topic of persisting visual images; he was fuelled by this 'optical deception', and noted another instance of it with counter-rotating cog wheels. Faraday enunciated the principle upon which all the subsequent devices were based: 'The eye has the power, as is well known, of retaining visual

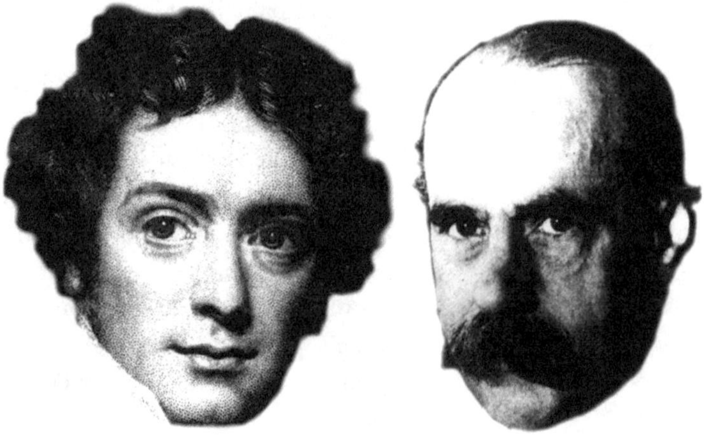

Figure 5.11
Left, Michael Faraday (1791–1867) after an engraving in Taylor (1846). Right, Max Wertheimer (1880–1943) after an illustration in Runes (1959).

impressions for a sensible period of time; and in this way, recurring actions, made sufficiently near to each other, are perceptibly connected, and made to appear as a continuous impression' (1831, p. 210). This statement was to prove the stimulus for both Plateau's and Stampfer's experimental enquiries into stroboscopic motion. Plateau's (1833) phenakistoscope or fantascope was almost identical to Stampfer's (1833) stroboscopic disc—both presented a short sequence of slightly different figures intermittently to the eye, and both were eagerly adopted by the public as instruments of amusement.

Later in the nineteenth century, Exner (1875) explored the phenomenon of stroboscopic motion by using light sparks produced by electrical discharges. The time interval and spatial separation between the two sparks could be controlled, and Exner found that two slightly separated sparks, one appearing more than 50 ms after the other, appeared as a single light moving from one location to the other. On the basis of this observation, Exner contended that motion was a fundamental sensation that did not require combined elements of location and time. Bowditch and Hall (1881) were to reach a similar conclusion on the basis of their experiments on motion aftereffects: 'We cannot resist raising the question whether we may not be here very near the quale of real, pure sensation' (pp. 300–301).

Max Wertheimer (1880–1943, Fig. 5.11, right) built upon these phenomena of motion seen following successive stimulation of two spatially distinct stimuli, and he gave them a new interpretation

(Wertheimer, 1912). When the interval between the two stimuli was around 100 ms the visual motion was optimal. He argued that the perceived motion was a Gestalt that could not be divided into smaller units. In furthering this theory, he examined the possibility that eye movements could be involved in stroboscopic motion. Wertheimer presented several arguments against the implication of eye movements. First, the duration of tachistoscopic exposure was shorter than that required to initiate an eye movement. Second, a fixation point remained stable during apparent motion; this applied to an afterimage too. The strongest evidence derived from an experiment in which apparent motion was produced simultaneously in opposite directions. Wertheimer also demonstrated that there was no perceived distinction between apparent motion between two spatial locations and real motion.

Stroboscopic motion, like induced motion, can occur in different directions at the same time. This renders any interpretation in terms of eye movements difficult to sustain. Stroboscopic motion can also occur simultaneously from a central point in radial directions, and so the arguments against the involvement of eye movements that applied to the motion aftereffect are pertinent here too.

5.7 Vection

When an observer is surrounded by a cylinder of vertical stripes, rotation of the cylinder initially results in optokinetic nystagmus: the eyes follow a particular edge and then make a ballistic return to approximately straight ahead and the cycle is repeated. If the rotation continues at a constant angular velocity then, after around 30 s, the cylinder no longer appears to rotate and the body feels as if it is rotating in the opposite direction. The apparent rotation of the body is referred to as vection (Tschermak, 1931) and it is also called visually induced self-motion. Vection can be induced in the three dimensions of space and it is often distinguished by the axis of rotation—as in linear or circular vection.

The methods for inducing self-motion might seem to be modern but the techniques were long in use by artisans before they were put under experimental scrutiny. These perceptual

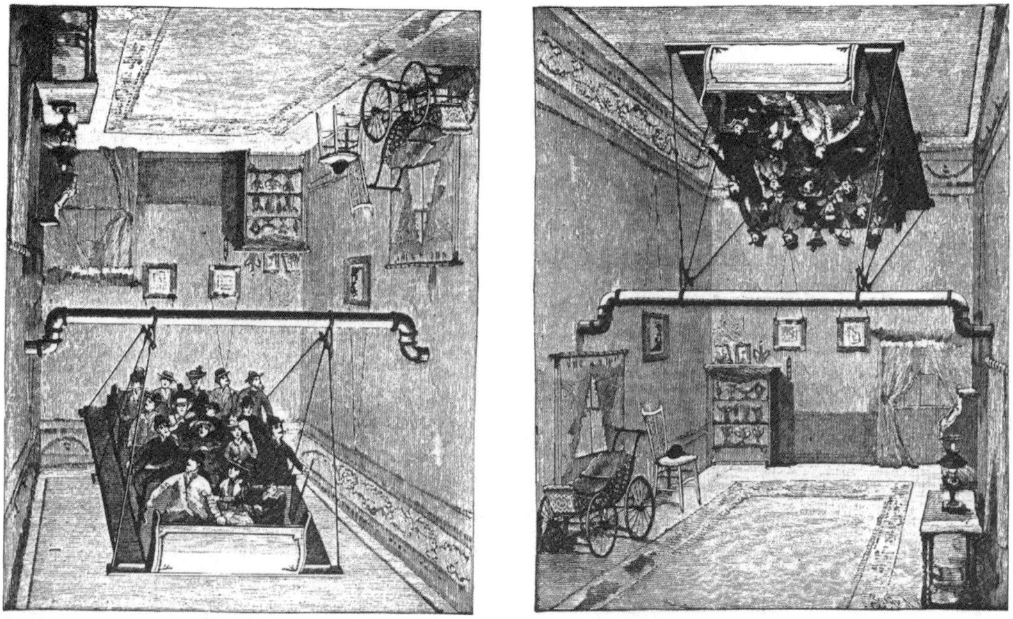

Figure 5.12
An illustration of a haunted swing from Hopkins (1898). The caption for the left picture is 'True position of the swing'. That for the right is 'Illusion produced by a ride in the swing'. The two illustrations are the same apart from their orientation.

effects that have a venerable but veiled past because they have been associated with financial gain. This applies to fairground phenomena, many of which embody an understanding of illusions that was far in advance of the contemporary visual science. Many fairground attractions involve abnormal patterns of motion, both vestibular and visual. One that is based on vection is called the haunted swing; it consists of a platform on which an individual sits or stands and then experiences considerable self-motion although little physical movement occurs (Fig. 5.12). The visible room surrounding the person is not anchored to the ground, but rotates around them. This induces the impression of self-motion in the opposite direction to that of the room; such impressions are intensified when allied with an unstable platform on which the hapless individual sits or stands. In the late nineteenth century it was engagingly described thus:

Those who are to participate in the apparent gyrations of the swing—and there may be quite a number who enjoy it simultaneously—are ushered into

> a small room. From a bar crossing the room, near the ceiling, hangs a large swing, which is provided with seats for a number of people. After the people have taken their places, the attendant pushes the car and it starts into oscillation like any other swing. The room door is closed. Gradually those in it feel after three or four movements that their swing is going rather high, but this is not all. The apparent amplitude of the oscillations increases more and more, until presently the whole swing seems to whirl completely over, describing a full circle about the bar on which it hangs. To make the thing more utterly mysterious, the bar is bent crank fashion, so that it seems demonstrably impossible for the swing to pass between bar and ceiling. It continues apparently to go round and round this way, imparting a most weird sensation to the occupants, until its movements begin gradually to cease and the complete rotation is succeeded by the usual back and forth swinging, and in a few seconds, as the children say, 'the old cat dies.' The door of the room is opened and the swinging party leave. Those who have tried it say the sensation is most peculiar and the deception perfect. The illusion is based on the movements of the room proper. During the entire exhibition the swing is practically stationary, while the room rotates about the suspending bar. (Hopkins, 1898, pp. 91–94)

The history of the haunted swing, like those of other fairground illusions, is itself mysterious. Since there was advantage in keeping the trick secret, very few records of their construction were made. Thus, in contrast to science in which information is shared, the fairground illusions were guarded secrets. A report of the haunted swing did appear in the second volume of *Psychological Review*: Wood (1895) experienced its joys at the Midwinter Fair in San Francisco, where the swing could hold 'forty or more persons'. His report was more analytic than that by Hopkins (1898):

> The swing proper was practically at rest, merely being joggled a trifle, while the room itself was put in motion, the furniture being fastened down to the floor, so that it could be turned completely over. The illusion was good, though the absence of centrifugal force, and the fact that the swing did not move with uniform acceleration as it descended, would indicate to a careful observer that he was not swinging freely. The curious and interesting feature however, was, that even though the action was fully understood, as it was in my case, it was impossible to quench the sensations of 'goneness within' with each apparent rush of the swing. The minute the eyes were shut the sensation vanished instantly. Many persons were actually made sick by the illusion. I have met a number of gentlemen who said they could scarcely walk out of the building from dizziness and nausea. (Wood, 1895, pp. 277–278)

It is clear that the haunted swing could induce vertigo, and experimental interest in the phenomenon derived from studies of vertigo, which also involves apparent body as well as visual motion. Vertigo can be induced by rotating the body with respect to a stationary world whereas vection is produced by rotating the visible world around a stationary body. Vertigo can be thought of as vestibular–visual interaction because the visual world rotates as a consequence of vestibular stimulation (from turning). Vection, on the other hand, involves visual–vestibular interaction because the motion of the visual world results in a stationary body feeling as if it is moving. Vection has also been described in the context of stimuli that have been used generate motion aftereffects. Vection has often been studied with a stationary central stimulus and a large moving surround; this is essentially a stimulus for induced motion, and some early experimental studies of the latter described vection (see Duncker, 1929). Finally, vection has been associated with motion sickness (Dichgans and Brandt, 1973).

In discussing vertigo (Chapter 3) it was noted that Ptolemy, Willis, Erasmus Darwin, and Purkinje all described how moving patterns can produce feelings of body motion. For example, Darwin wrote:

> Thus in a room hung with a paper, which is coloured with similar small black lozenges or rhomboids, many people become dizzy; for when they fall, the next and the next lozenge succeeds upon the eye; which they mistake for the first, and are not aware, that they have any apparent motion. But if you fix a sheet of paper, or draw any other figure, in the midst of these lozenges, the charm ceases, and no dizziness is perceptible.—The same occurs, when we ride over a plain covered with snow without trees or other eminent objects. (1796, pp. 232–233)

The descriptions were insightful but mainly anecdotal. The onset of experiments to study vection was dependent upon having equipment suitable for inducing it and in framing questions appropriate to it. The former was provided by Mach (1875) who was able to modify his rotating frames (Fig. 3.8) to this purpose:

> Consider a horizontal circular wooden disk of $1\frac{1}{2}$ m diameter placed above the head of the observer that can be rotated about an axis that passes near the observer's head. Around the rim of that disk we attach a $\frac{1}{2}$ m broad paper stripe covered on the inside with equidistant vertical lines. The observer therefore sits inside a hollow, turning, lined cylinder. When this drum alone is kept turning for a few minutes one quickly notices himself turning in the direction opposite to the drum, along with all those things that are not hidden by the drum. However, on occasion one feels quickly returned to rest with the drum still turning, and the two subjective states alternate frequently. After several repetitions of this experiment it seemed to me as if the peripheral part of the visual field were placed in motion most easily. (Young et al., 2001, pp. 85–86)

Mach acknowledged that the phenomenon was not new, and he related it to the impression of motion that occurs in railway carriages when an adjacent train moves away. He did, however, provide a method for examining it which has become a part of clinical practice. It is not necessary to have such intricate equipment to induce vection. A few years later, John Aitken (1839–1919) achieved the same effect by using a small box suspended over the head. He was investigating the motion aftereffect and wished to determine whether it occurred if the whole retina was exposed to motion:

> Experiments were also made to determine the effect of influencing the whole retina. This was done by looking so closely at the moving band [of vertical stripes] that its image covered the whole retina, but no decided effect was noticed. Experiments were also made with the same object by means of a large box-shaped arrangement, the sides of which were made of tracing paper having vertical bands of black paper 4 cm broad and fixed 4 cm apart. The observer being seated in a chair, the box was let down over him and put in motion, which was continued for some time; the box was then raised, but no appearance of motion in surrounding objects was observed. There were, however, some curious effects produced by the rotation of this apparatus. At certain times, while surrounded by the rotating box, the observer felt as if rotating in the opposite direction. The most certain result, however, was a most disagreeable sickening effect, which continued for some time after the experiment was made. The effect of this rotating apparatus might form an interesting study in connection with the important investigation at present conducted by Professor Alex. Crum Brown on the function of the semicircular canals. (Aitken, 1878, pp. 43–44)

Thus, both Mach and Aitken linked the induced body motion to the vestibular system. Mach was familiar with the effects of body rotation and Aitken was familiar with the researches of his fellow Scot, Crum Brown. The phenomenon was not called vection until much later. The terms linear vection and circular vection were introduced in the 1930s, although detailed studies of vection were not undertaken until the last decades of the twentieth century (see Ebenholtz, 2001).

Mach was sceptical of an interpretation of vection in terms of eye movements, as indeed he was for many motion illusions. This was probably another veiled criticism of Helmholtz, who tried to do precisely that. Mach wrote: 'I have already pointed out the difficulties encountered if one tries to explain all optical illusory movements in terms of eye movements' (1875, p. 88). This scepticism has been borne out for vection: 'Consequently, *vection is basically independent of the direction of eye movements'* (Dichgans and Brandt, 1978, p. 766, original italics).

5.8 Eye movements and visual motion

Eye movements are such an obvious aspect of vision that they have always been of interest. They were remarked upon in antiquity, but determining the characteristics of such eye movements is a more recent preoccupation. Most specifically, their measurement has been rendered independent of the observer. That is, the methods that were used for measuring eye movements in the past (like placing a finger over the eyelid, or observing the eyes of another person) have been improved by more modern techniques. Initially the use of afterimages enabled displacements of the stabilized from unstabilized images to be noted. This method was adopted widely in the nineteenth century. Technical improvements, like tracking Purkinje images or the vessels in the iris, have added precision to the determination of eye movements and eye position. It is perhaps this success in measurement of eye movements that has fuelled the search for precision in understanding visual motion. But is there such a thing as objectivity in the context of motion perception? The movements of the eyes can be measured, as can the extent of perceived motion, but determination of the latter requires the involvement of the perceiver.

In many ways, the development of visual science has reflected a rejection of the subjective experience in human perception. The behaviourist revolution was successful because it concentrated on those aspects that were considered as objective—stimulus and response. Perception has always proved difficult to constrain in this manner. New instruments for stimulus control were invented in the nineteenth century, and these extended the scope of experiments in vision (Wade and Heller, 1997). Moreover, the methods of physics could be applied to the study of vision. The adoption of Fechner's psychophysics was to render responses quantifiable too. Fechner (1860), however, distinguished between an outer and an inner psychophysics. Most attention has been directed to the former.

Behaviourists neglected the study of visual perception, and when it was examined it was in the context of eye movements. The rapid development of photographic methods to measure eye movements during reading in the early twentieth century speaks to this issue (see Chapter 4). It was left to Gestalt psychologists to pursue perception in the early decades of the twentieth century. Köhler (1942) went so far as to speculate on the physiological processes that could mediate perceptual phenomena. When perception did return to the psychological fold, it was aided by more detailed knowledge of physiology. Hebb (1949) sought a synthesis between physiology and perception, and his ideas were rapidly grafted on to the discoveries regarding the properties of single cells in the visual cortex. If eye movements are not correlated with visual motion then perhaps physiological processes are. This approach proved to be remarkably productive in the context of the motion aftereffect. Barlow and Hill's (1963) proposed link between the activity of motion detectors and the experience of the waterfall illusion stimulated a torrent of research (see Wade and Verstraten, 1998).

The subjective dimension of vision has been treated as an oddity rather than a fundamental feature of perception. For example, in the early nineteenth century, certain phenomena were referred to as subjective, as there was little control of the stimuli that gave rise to them. This resulted from Purkinje's (1823*a*, 1825) description of a range of such effects (see Wade and Brožek, 2001). However, even at this stage objections to the use of the term were voiced. Wheatstone (writing under the initials C. W.) noted, in a review of Purkinje's first book, that:

> To distinguish these phenomena from those which arise on the presence of their appropriate external objects, the author [Purkinje] employs the term subjective, which, as denoting this class of phenomena better than any other we are acquainted with, and, to avoid circumlocution, we have purposely retained; it will, however, on consideration, be perceived, that the term is not strictly proper, as, correctly speaking, all phenomena, *as such*, are subjective, *i.e.* in the mind; and were we, without qualification, to admit the classification of phenomena into objective and subjective, we should be unable to determine, with any degree of accuracy, where the objective ends or the subjective begins. (C. W., 1830, p. 102, original italics)

Most of the motion phenomena described above involve the appearance of motion in an object that is physically stationary. They have the characteristics of the phenomena that Purkinje discussed: motion is visible without any corresponding stimulus change. Perhaps this is the source of interest in accounting for them in terms of eye movements which can be measured.

Nonetheless, in all cases the dependence or otherwise of the visual motion illusions on eye movements was established independently of measures of the eyes themselves; psychophysical studies excluded eye movements as the basis for induced motion, motion aftereffects, stroboscopic motion, and autokinetic effect. In the absence of close relationships with eye movements the effects remain in the domain of subjective phenomena, and novel ways of examining them may be needed. Thus, although the issues raised by these motion illusions have been examined in an historical context, they retain contemporary relevance.

6

Perceptual stability and eye movements

6.1 Introduction

A leitmotif of the previous chapters has been that research on eye movements has been guided by an awareness of particular visual phenomena. The principal one is the greater acuity that is found in and around the visual axis relative to more peripheral retinal regions. The same guiding principle has informed studies of visual stability, and it is reflected in the many descriptions of the links between the perception of motion and stability. These are two sides of the same coin, although one side has been examined in much more detail than the other in the history of vision. The issue of stability has been accorded less attention than that of motion. The likely basis for this is the same as that for the early interest in illusions, as indicated in the previous chapter. The assumption of object permanence, which is at the heart of early descriptions of illusions, is also the reason for the neglect of stability. If objects in the world are assumed to be permanent and stable then it is unnecessary to provide an account of their perception as such. Only departures from stability (motion) warrant attention.

As early as the eleventh century, Alhazen distinguished between three conditions under which motion is seen: 'Sight perceives motion in one of three ways: by comparing the moving object with other objects, or with a single object, or with the eye itself' (Sabra, 1989, p. 193). It is the last condition that is of interest in the present context. Alhazen himself expanded on this:

> Sight may perceive motion in any one of these ways even if the eye moves. This happens when sight senses the varying position of the moving object

while sensing that the variation is not due to the eye's motion. There is a difference in condition between the variation in position that happens to that object on account of its own motion and the variation in position that happens to it on account of the eye's motion. Thus, when sight senses the varying position of the moving object, and senses that the variation in the object's position is not due to the eye's motion, it will sense the object's motion. The form of the object may move in the eye as a result of the object's motion, but sight will not perceive the object's motion merely through the motion of its form in the eye. Rather, sight perceives motion only by comparing the moving object to other objects in the way we have shown. For the form of a stationary object may move in the eye while the object is at rest, but sight will not in consequence of this perceive the object to be in motion. For if the eye moves in front of visible objects while they are being contemplated, the form of every one of the objects facing the eye, whether they are stationary or in motion, will move on the surface of the eye as the latter moves. But sight has become accustomed to the motion of the objects' forms on its surface when the objects are stationary, and therefore does not judge the object to be in motion on account of the motion of its form, unless the form of another object occurs in the eye and sight perceives the varying positions of the moving object's form relative to the form of another object, or unless a succession of forms takes place in the eye as a result of the rotary motion. (Sabra, 1989, p. 194)

This is an exceedingly insightful passage. If the term 'form' is replaced by 'retinal image' then it specifies the relationship between perceived motion and stability. Motion over the retina can result in perceived motion but it can also yield stability, provided that there is no relative motion between objects. What makes the analysis even more remarkable is that it was made centuries before the dioptrical properties of the eye had been clarified (see Section 1.1), and before the concept of the retinal image had been established. Moreover, it makes the assumption of object permanence explicit, and hints that it is a consequence of learning.

Following Kepler's (1604) clarification of the image forming properties of the eye, distinctions between the consequences of retinal image motion from object and eye movement became more frequent and were often repeated. For example, Rohault (Fig. 6.5, left) wrote in terms very similar to Alhazen:

Now it is not difficult to conceive, that we know a Body to be in Motion; first, when its Image appears successively applied to different Images of certain Objects, which we do not compare with any other, but imagine to be immoveable; or when we find that we must turn our Head or our Eyes in order to have the Object always at the End of the Line, along which we carry our principal Attention; or lastly, when, if we move neither our Eyes nor our Head, we find it is gone out of that Line. The contrary to all which makes an Object appear to us to be at rest. (Rohault, 1671, from a translation of 1723, p. 257)

More succinct statements were made in the next century by David Hartley (1705–1757; 1749): 'We judge of Motion by the Motion of Pictures on the *Retina*, or our Eyes in following the Objects' (p. 203). Wells (1792) enlarged upon this a little by distinguishing between vision with a stationary or a moving eye:

> If the eye be at rest, we judge an object to be in motion when its picture falls in succeeding times upon different parts of the retina; and if the eye be in motion, we judge an object to be at rest, as long as the change in the place of its picture upon the retina, holds a certain correspondence with the change of the eye's position. (pp. 94–95)

Yet another statement of the same kind was made by Müller (1843): 'We judge of the motion of an object, partly from the motion of its image over the surface of the retina, and partly from the motion of our eyes following it' (p. 1178). These observations make implicit reference to the differential effects of motion over the retina. It can result in either motion or stability, depending upon the motion of the eye. Thus, eye movements were implicated in visual motion and stability. Visual stability during eye movements became an issue of considerable theoretical importance in the nineteenth century. However, the characteristics of eye movements themselves had not been clarified at that stage (see Chapter 4). That is, pursuit eye movements were not distinguished from saccades. Accordingly, much of the nineteenth century research was concerned with stability during pursuit of a moving object or with an eye rotation with respect to a stable scene. The link with saccadic eye movements was to be made in the twentieth century. Accordingly, our discussion of stability will reflect this historical schism. The first section will examine visual stability during pursuit eye movements and the second will survey stability across eye movements.

6.2 Stability during eye movements

The stability of vision has been examined with regard to an aspect of perception that itself has a long history—visual direction. When an object is perceived to move its visual direction changes, and this can occur whether the eye is stationary or follows the object motion. One way of examining the association between eye and image movements is to disturb or sever the link between them. Perhaps the simplest way to achieve this in binocular vision

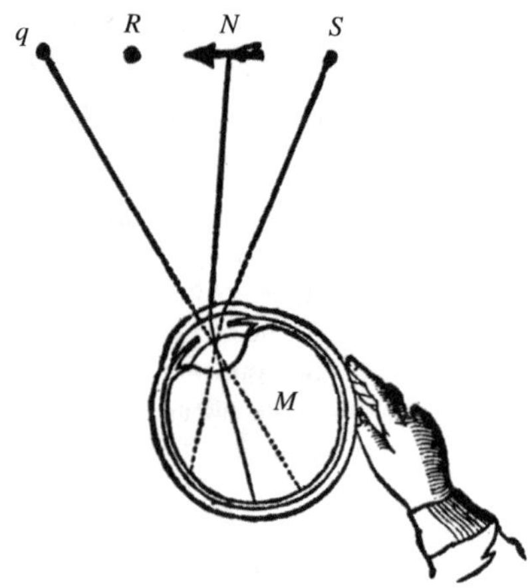

Figure 6.1
Changes in visual direction as a consequence of moving the eye by means of pressure from a finger (from Descartes, 1664/1909).

is to move one eye passively with respect to the other. Aristotle observed that this resulted in one object appearing in two directions: 'if a finger be inserted beneath the eyeball without being observed, one object will not only present two visual images, but will create an opinion of its being two objects' (Ross, 1931, pp. 461b–462a). This observation was frequently repeated and reported. For example, Descartes (1664/1909) both described and illustrated this situation (Fig. 6.1):

> If eye M is turned away by force from object N, and arranged as if looking toward q, the soul will judge that the eye is turned toward R. In this situation rays from object N will enter the eye in the way that those from point S would do if the eye were in fact turned toward R; hence it [the soul] will believe that this object N is at point S and that it is a different object from the one being looked at by the other eye. (Translated in Hall, 1972, p. 65)

Descartes' illustration also represents the passive displacement of a single eye. His *Treatise of man* was not published in his lifetime, and it was initially translated into Latin (Descartes, 1662) and then into French two years later. The Latin version depicts two eyes, with the passive motion of one of them. It is this situation that was given by Rohault (1671), who reflected many of Descartes' views regarding optics and vision. Rohault linked the double vision produced by displacing one eye with the stimulation of noncorresponding retinal points:

> That if we press either of our Eyes with our Finger, so as to make it receive the Image of the Object on a different Part from what it would do by the common Motion of the Muscles; as it is certain, that the Images which are then impressed on the two Eyes, do not fall upon *the Sympathetick Nerves*, nor

reunite in the Brain, so we cannot fail to see the Object double. (Rohault, 1671, from a translation of 1723, p. 256, original italics)

The same point was made by Smith (1738/2004): 'If by squinting or depressing an eye with ones finger, the optick axes are not directed to the same point; in these cases objects appear double: and now it is plain that the pictures are not painted on corresponding places of the retina' (pp. 46–47). Thus, it was widely accepted that the visual direction of an object is not determined by visual stimulation alone, as it also involves information about the position of the eyes—otherwise objects would appear to move with every movement of the eyes.

The topic of visual stability was discussed by Helmholtz (1867*a*) in the section on the direction of vision. He made a distinction between what have become called outflow and inflow theories. The former refers to deriving the eye movement information from efferent (centrally generated) impulses to the eye muscles, whereas the latter reflects use of afferent (sensory) signals from the eye muscles themselves. How this compensation for eye rotation comes about has been a matter of considerable enquiry, the origins of which can be found in the late eighteenth century.

6.2.1 Inflow and outflow

Passively moving the eye is not the only technique that can be employed to investigate visual stability during eye movements. It can also be examined by means of a stabilized retinal image, and the afterimage provided the earliest approach to this. Robert Darwin (1786) made the fortuitous observation that attempting to inspect an afterimage formed in the peripheral retina resulted in its apparent motion in the direction of the eye movement. If the eye remained stationary then so did the afterimage.

If this dark spot [an afterimage] lies above the center of the eye, we turn our eyes that way, expecting to bring it into the center of the eye, that we may view it more distinctly; and in this case the dark spectrum seems to move upwards. If the dark spectrum is found beneath the center of the eye, we pursue it from the same motive, and it seems to move downwards. This has given rise to various conjectures of something floating in the aqueous humours of the eyes; but whoever, in attending to these spots, keeps his eyes unmoved by looking steadily at the corner of a cloud, at the same time that he observes the ocular spectra, will be thoroughly convinced, that they have no motion but what is given to them by the movement of our eyes in pursuit of them. (Darwin, 1786, p. 318)

No theoretical implications were made regarding this by Darwin, unlike Wells (1792), who appreciated fully the import of this and similar observations.

Having looked steadily for some time at the flame of a candle, with *one* eye only, I directed afterward, with both eyes open, my attention to the middle of a sheet of paper, a few feet distant; the consequence of which was, that a spot appeared upon it in the same manner, as if I had viewed the flame with both eyes, though somewhat fainter. My attention remaining fixed upon the sheet, I now pushed the eye, by which the spot was seen, successively upward and downward, to the right and to the left, and in every oblique direction; The spot however never altered its position, but kept constantly upon the middle of the appearance of the paper, perceived by the undistorted eye, though the appearance of the paper to the distorted eye, was always separate from the former, and the sheet consequently seen double... The apparent situation of the spot being... at the same time affected by the *voluntary* motions of the eye, it must, I think, be necessarily owing to the *action* of the muscles by which these motions are performed. (Wells, 1792, pp. 68–70, original italics)

Wells applied his customary acumen to distinguish between the consequences of passively moving an eye (by pushing it with his finger) and actively moving it; the afterimage remained in the same visual direction with passive eye movements but shifted with the voluntary changes of gaze. This was a revolutionary idea. Prior to that time, visual direction had been considered to be the province of retinal location. In short, Wells provided support for outflow theory, although it had not been so named at that stage. Bell (Fig. 6.2, left) confirmed the distinction between the effects of voluntary and involuntary eye movements on afterimage

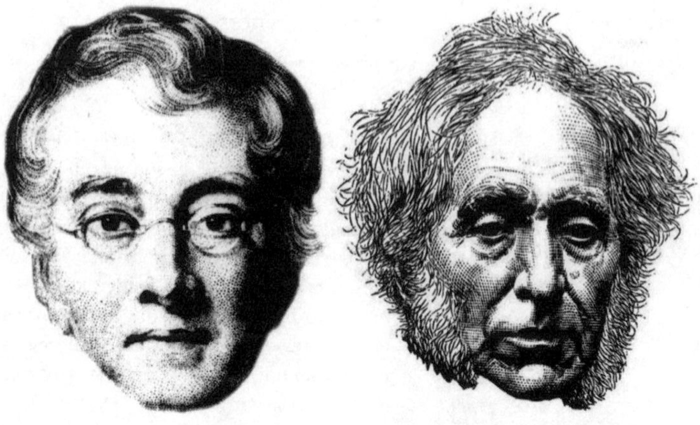

Figure 6.2

Left, Charles Bell (1774–1842) after an engraving in Pettigrew (1840*b*). Right, David Brewster (1781–1868) after an engraving in the *Illustrated London News*, (1868, 52, 189). Despite their many differences, Bell and Brewster were knighted together in 1832.

motion. Although he did not cite Wells' earlier studies, Bell did present an elegant statement of outflow theory:

There is an inseparable connection between the exercise of the sense of vision and the exercise of the voluntary muscles of the eye. When an object is seen, we enjoy two senses; there is an impression upon the retina; but we receive also the idea of position or relation which it is not the office of the retina to give. It is by the consciousness of the degree of effort put upon the voluntary muscles, that we know the relative position of an object to ourselves. The relation existing between the office of the retina and of the voluntary muscles, may be illustrated in this manner. Let the eyes be fixed upon an illuminated object until the retina be fatigued, and in some measure exhausted by the image, then closing the eyes, the figure of the object will continue present to them: and it is quite clear that nothing can change the place of this impression on the retina. But notwithstanding that the impression on the retina cannot be changed, the idea thence arising may. For by an exertion of the voluntary muscles of the eye-ball, the body seen will appear to change its place, and it will, to our feeling, assume different positions according to the muscle which is exercised. If we raise the pupil, we shall see the body placed below us; and all this takes place while the eye-lids are shut, and when no new impression is conveyed to the retina. The state of the retina is here associated with the consciousness of muscular exertion; and it shows that vision in its extended sense is a compound operation, the idea of position of an object having relation to the activity of the muscles... If we move the eye by the voluntary muscles, while the impression [of an afterimage] continues on the retina, we shall have the notion of place or relation raised in the mind; but if the motion of the eye-ball be produced by any other cause, by the involuntary muscles, or by pressure from without, we shall have no corresponding change of sensation. (Bell, 1823, pp. 178–179)

It is most surprising that in this article Bell overlooked Wells' experiments because he was one of the few writers who did cite Wells' work on the motion of afterimages during giddiness from body rotation in an earlier work (Bell, 1803). Wells' *Essay* was not referred to explicitly as, unusually for Bell, no specific reference was cited in this case. Brewster (Fig. 6.2, right), ever an adversary of Bell, raised a pertinent problem relating to passive eye movements—they tend to be translations rather than rotations. Unlike Bell, he did mention Wells' experiments:

When we push up the one eye by the force of the finger, and keep it in its new position, it has not performed an angular movement in its socket, but merely a small vertical ascent, by which, in an upright position of the body and head, it is raised into a more elevated horizontal plane. In this elevated position, the eye can execute horizontal, and even vertical angular movements, and can direct itself to contemplate either one or other of the double images of the objects before it. The consequence of this is that the spectral impression ascends only through a very small space, which it requires nice observation to appreciate, but which increases with the force applied to the eye . . . It is a circumstance not a little remarkable, that it never occurred to Dr. Wells, nor, so far as we know, to any person else, to *press upwards the two eyes at the same time*. When this is done, *the two spectral impressions will be seen to move*, and to rise through spaces so obvious to the dullest perceptions, as to put an end for ever to the extraordinary dogma, that they are capable of being put in motion only by the action of the voluntary muscles. (Brewster, 1826, pp. 267–268, original italics)

Brewster was reluctant to abandon his concept of a retinally defined visual direction. He was continuing in a long tradition that tied visual direction to stimulation of particular retinal locations. For example, Kepler (1611) stated that:

The position of an object is estimated from the direction in which the ray of sight *originally* emerges from the eye, no matter how this direction may be altered by refraction in its path between the eye and the object. For the eye *cannot detect* what happens to the rays outside itself in intervening media, but *assumes* that these proceed in the original direction. (Mach, 1926, p. 44, original italics)

This was elevated to a law by Porterfield (1737), who applied it to account for a range of phenomena from double vision in strabismus to upright perception on the basis of an inverted retinal image. Porterfield described the law and its consequences in the following way:

Every Point on an Object appears and is seen without the Eye nearly in a straight Line, drawn perpendicularly to the Retina, from that Point of it where its Image falls . . . The Judgment we form of Objects being placed without the Eye in those perpendicular Lines, or, which is nearly the same thing, the Judgment we form of the Situation and Distance of visual Objects, depends not on Custom and Experience, but on an original connate and immutable Law, to which our Minds have been subjected from the Time they were first united to our Bodies. (1737, pp. 208 and 215, original italics)

Porterfield provided support for the law from the coloured images that are formed by pressure to the eye applied by a finger, and from the distorted direction in which objects are seen when viewed through a prism. For Porterfield both direction and distance were considered to be innate and not modifiable by experience. It is this principle of visual direction that was attacked by Wells (1792) on empirical grounds. First, it could not predict the diplopia experienced by strabismic individuals after they have aligned an object in each eye separately. Second, it could not account for the apparent direction of afterimages following voluntary movements of the eyes (see Ono, 1981).

If the motions of the eye do play a role in the perception of motion and stability, then some means of compensating for retinal image motion is required. The question was taken up by Müller, who distinguished between the alternative modes whereby the information from eye movements could be utilized:

> If the image upon the retina moves while our eyes and our body are at rest, we conclude that the object is changing its relative position with regard to ourselves. In such a case the movement of the object may be apparent only, as when we are fixed upon a body which is in motion, such as a ship. If, on the other hand, the image does not move with regard to the retina, but remains fixed upon the same spot of that membrane, while our eyes follow the moving body, we judge of the motion of the object by the sensations of the muscles in action to move the eye, or by the currents of nervous energy sent by the sensorium to the muscles. If the image moves over the surface of the retina while the muscles of the eye are acting at the same time in a manner corresponding to this motion, as in reading, we infer that the object is stationary, and we know we are merely altering the relation of our eyes to the object. (Müller, 1843, p. 1178)

Müller was clearly articulating the problem of how the information for eye movement is used—by signals from the eye muscles (afferent or inflow) or signals to them (efferent or outflow). It was this distinction that was examined further by Helmholtz (1867*a*), who assumed 'we know by common experiences that our judgments of the direction of vision are not made by the actually existing position of our eye, when this position is varied by forces other than those of the muscles' (1925/2000, p. 244). He provided evidence for central signals to the eye muscles determining visual stability derived from several phenomena. First, moving one eye passively (by pressing it or pulling the eyelid with the fingers) while observing an object with both eyes produced double images; passive movement of a single open eye resulted in the apparent motion of visible objects. Second, afterimages remained stationary when the eye was moved passively, but they appeared to move when the eye rotated by its own muscular contraction. Third, individuals with paralysed eye muscles experienced apparent motion with attempts to move the eye by using the paralysed muscle. His conclusion was clear: 'These phenomena prove conclusively that our judgments as to the direction of the visual axis are simply the result of the effort of will involved in trying to alter the adjustment of the eyes' (Helmholtz, 1925/2000, p. 275). This statement is very similar to that made earlier by Bell (1823), although neither Bell nor Wells were cited by Helmholtz in this regard.

Mach (1886, 1897) provided a novel twist to the experiment with paralysed eyes, so that it could be performed in an observer whose eyes were not paralysed. He performed the experiment himself in what might be considered as an heroic enterprise:

Let the eyes be turned as far as possible towards the left and two large lumps of moderately hard putty firmly pressed against the right side of each eyeball. If, now, we attempt to glance quickly to the right, we shall succeed only very imperfectly, owing to the incompletely spherical form of the eyes, and the objects will suffer a strong displacement to the right. Thus the *mere will* to look to the right imparts to the images at certain points of the retina a larger 'rightward value,' as we may term it for brevity. The experiment is, at first, surprising. It will soon be perceived, however, that both facts—viz., that by voluntarily turning the eyes to the right, objects are not displaced, and that by the forced, involuntary turning of the eyes to the right, objects are displaced to the left—together amount to the same thing. My eye, which I wish to, and cannot, turn to the right, may be regarded as voluntarily turned to the right and compulsorily turned by an outer force. (Mach, 1897, p. 59, original italics)

James (1890) found it difficult to replicate this effect and suggested an alternative interpretation of the results for this and for paralysed eye experiments:

Take first the case of complete paralysis and assume the right eye affected. Suppose the patient desires to rotate his gaze to an object situated in the extreme right of the field of vision. As Hering has so beautifully shown, both eyes move by a common act of innervation, and in this instance both move towards the right. But the paralysed eye stops short in the middle of its course, the object still appearing far to the right of its fixation point. The left sound eye, meanwhile, although covered, continues its rotation until the extreme rightward limit thereof has been reached. To an observer looking at both eyes the left will seem to squint. Of course this continued and extreme rotation produces afferent feelings of rightward motion in the eyeball, which momentarily overpower the faint feelings of central position in the diseased and uncovered eye. The patient feels by his left eyeball as if he were following an object which by his right retina he perceives he does not overtake. (James, 1890, p. 509)

James was attempting to rescue the afferent or inflow theory from the evidence Helmholtz and Mach raised against it. The innervation in the normally rotating but covered eye was taken to provide the evidence that the object had appeared to move. James' conjecture stimulated Jackson and Paton (1909) to determine how the occluded eye moved in the paralysed eye experiment; they

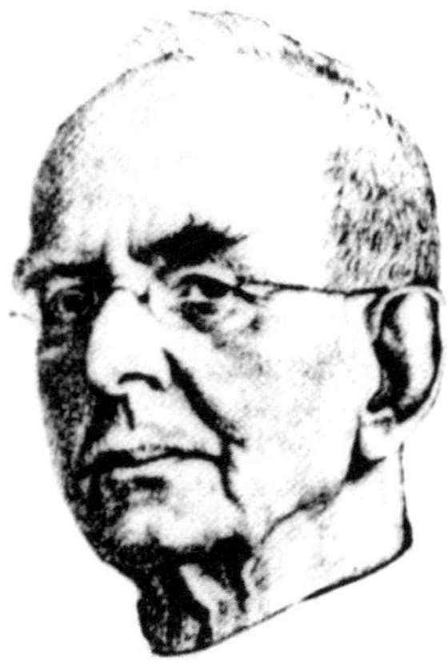

Figure 6.3
Charles Scott Sherrington (1857–1952) after an illustration in Eccles and Gibson (1979).

concluded that it was not sufficient to account for the perceived motion that was reported.

There were other notable supporters of the afferent theory, particularly as more microanatomical details of muscular structure emerged. For example, Charles Sherrington (1857–1952; Fig. 6.3) was able to devote a chapter of a textbook to the muscular sense; he defined it as including 'all reactions on sense rising in motor organs and their accessories' (1900, p. 1002). Six years later, he introduced a novel classification of the senses into extero-, proprio-, and intero-ceptors:

> The excitation of the receptors of the *proprio-ceptive* field in contradistinction from those of the *extero-ceptive* is related only secondarily to the agencies of the environment. The proprio-ceptive receive their stimulation by some action, *e.g.*, a muscular contraction, which was itself a primary reaction to excitation of a surface receptor by the environment. (Sherrington, 1906/2000, p. 130, original italics)

He extended his analyses of muscle systems in reflexes and in the maintaining of an upright posture to the control of eye position and accounted for visual stability during eye movements in terms of afference. One factor that stimulated his interests was:

> The rich supply of afferent nerve-fibres existent in the muscles which move the eyeball invites inquiry as to what may be the contribution which these nerves make to visual reactions. Their reflex function should, like that of other proprioceptives, relate to the adjustment and maintenance of postures. Ocular posturing, such as the adjustment and maintenance of the gaze, is delicate and almost continual throughout the waking day. And the afferent nerves from muscles, as is known of them from other muscular fields, yield besides their purely reflex taxis of local posture and movement, sensory impressions which are the basis of perceptions of postures and movements, in short subserve muscular sense. Muscular sense being, along with vision, touch, and the 'labyrinthine' sense, a chief source when the mind manufactures sensual 'space,' the above is tantamount to saying that the proprioceptive nerves of the eyeball muscles may be expected to contribute to space as perceived with the eye. (Sherrington, 1918, p. 332)

Sherrington's theory was based largely on the logic of the afferent fibres functioning in a manner similar to that of other muscular systems; he provided little experimental evidence to support his views. His theory was roundly criticized by Merton (1961) and by Brindley and Merton (1960); the latter demonstrated that passive movement of both eyes simultaneously by as much as 30° was not perceived, when the conjunctiva was anaesthetized.

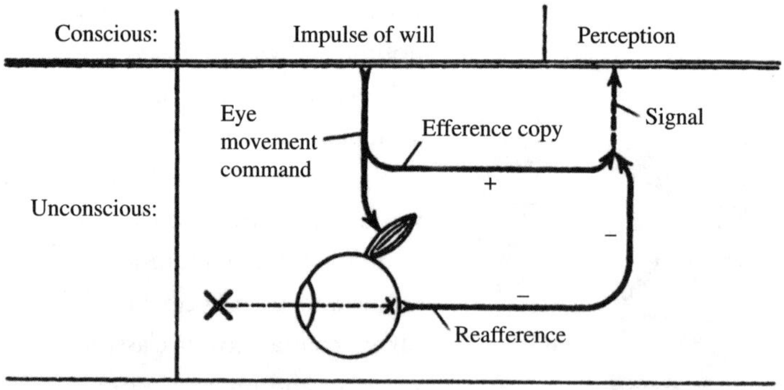

Figure 6.4
Diagram of the reafference principle after Holst (1957).

The principle of retaining some neural copy of commands sent to the extraocular muscles has been extended more broadly by Holst and Mittelstaedt (1950). They coined the term 'reafference' to apply to all sensory stimulation which produces efference as a consequence of self-produced movements (Fig. 6.4). The consensus is that some form of efference copy is used in order to compensate for retinal motion consequent upon eye movements. Reviews of more recent research can be found in Howard and Templeton (1966) and Howard (1982, 2002).

6.2.2 Motion parallax

The concern with efference copies has focused on the perception of stability during eye movements. If the eye is moved with respect to a visual scene then all objects in the scene will move over the retina with a fixed angular velocity. Despite this motion over the retina the scene is seen as stationary. Moreover, the motions of the eyes tend to be rotations with respect to a fixed head. Motion parallax, by contrast, is concerned with relative motions in different directions during translation movements of the eye. Studies have employed more naturalistic scenes and the movements of the eyes have often been due to head movement. The concern has not been the ensuing stability but the depth or motion that is perceived.

One of the clearest descriptions of motion parallax was given by Wheatstone (1838) who related motion parallax to the perception of depth (binocular parallax):

How happens it then, it may be asked, that persons who see with only one eye form correct notions of solid objects, and never mistake them for pictures? and how happens it also, that a person having the perfect use of both eyes, perceives no difference in objects around him when he shuts one of them? To explain these apparent difficulties, it must be kept in mind, that although the simultaneous vision of two dissimilar pictures suggests the relief of objects in the most vivid manner, yet there are other signs which suggest the same ideas to the mind, which, though more ambiguous than the former, become less liable to lead the judgment astray in proportion to the extent of our previous experience . . . A person deprived of the sight of one eye sees therefore all external objects, near and remote, as a person with both eyes sees remote objects only, but that vivid effect arising from binocular vision of near objects is not perceived by the former; to supply this deficiency he has recourse unconsciously to other means of acquiring more accurate information. The motion of the head is the principal means he employs. (Wheatstone, 1838, p. 380)

This is by no means the earliest account of motion parallax, but it does emphasise how motion of the eye through space can give rise to the perception of depth rather than motion. French writers on optics and vision in the late seventeenth century made clear descriptions of motion parallax, without giving it that name. The descriptions occurred in the context of distance (or depth) perception. For example, Rohault (1671) described how distance could be determined from the changes in direction consequent upon the movement of a single eye:

If we make use of but one Eye, we can know the *Distance* of an Object, provided we move from one Place to another; for we have some kind of Memory of the Position of the *Optical* Axis in the first Station, when we really attend to the Position of it in another Station, so that we imagine two *Optical* Axes, though there be indeed but one, and by that means guess at the Distance where they meet; and to this we refer the Object . . . Further, the Interposition of a great many other Objects, between us and the Object we look at, makes us think, that the Distance is greater than otherwise we should . . . It is certain also, that as the Knowledge of the Distance helps us to find out the Bigness, so likewise the knowing of the Bigness helps us to conceive the Distance. Thus, when we know that a Man is about five or six Foot high, when we see him to appear but very little, we conclude him to be at a great Distance. (Rohault, 1671, from a translation of 1723, pp. 252, 254, and 256, original italics)

An even more precise account was given by Phillipe de La Hire (Fig. 6.5, right), who used the term 'parallax' to indicate how near objects can be distinguished in depth (La Hire, 1694). Although his example involved two eyes, the analysis was restricted to the effects from one. The direction of displacement of objects nearer than and farther from the fixated object was clearly specified, and the link between the direction of displacement and the relative depth was duly noted. La Hire was a mathematician and geometer

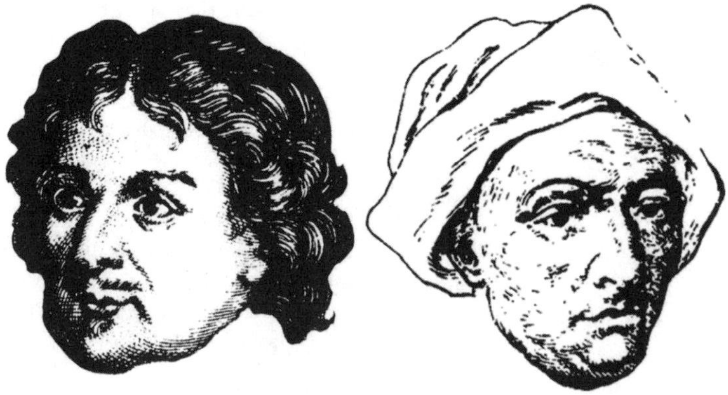

Figure 6.5
Left, Jacques Rohault (1620–1675) after an engraving kindly supplied by the Wellcome Institute, London. Right, Phillipe de La Hire (1640–1718) after an engraving in Augé (1898).

of note, and so it is surprising that this astute description of motion parallax did not throw any light on binocular parallax.

> The parallax of objects is what we use most to recognize distance, but the eyes must change place to recognize which of the two objects is the nearer. For example, if two objects appear near to each other from one position of the eye, when the eye moves to the right the object that thus appears to move away from the other to the right is further away, and the other which remains on the left will be the nearer one. (La Hire, 1694, pp. 236–237)

Natural philosophers like La Hire used the term parallax because it was applied most commonly in the context of astronomy. It referred to the apparent displacement or change in position of celestial bodies when viewed from different positions associated with the rotation of the earth around the sun. In the eighteenth century the concept was also applied to binocular vision, but this did not result in an appreciation of binocular parallax or what Wheatstone (1838) called stereoscopic vision. In his textbook on optics, Harris (1775) linked parallax with depth perception:

> We have other helps for distinguishing the prominences of small parts, besides those by which we distinguish distances in general; as their degrees of light and shades, and the prospect we have round them: Both these, I think, contribute their share to the visibility of such small objects as the pile upon a cloth, etc. And by the parallax on account of the distance betwixt our eyes, we can distinguish besides the front, parts of the two sides of near objects, not thicker than the said distance; and this gives a visible *relievo* to such objects, which helps greatly to raise or detach them from the plane, on which they lie: Thus, the nose on a face, is the more remarkably raised by seeing each side of it at once. These observations, I say, are of use to us in distinguishing the figures of small and near objects; and when the breaks, the prominencies and projections are more considerable, we do not want them. (Harris, 1775, p. 171, original italics)

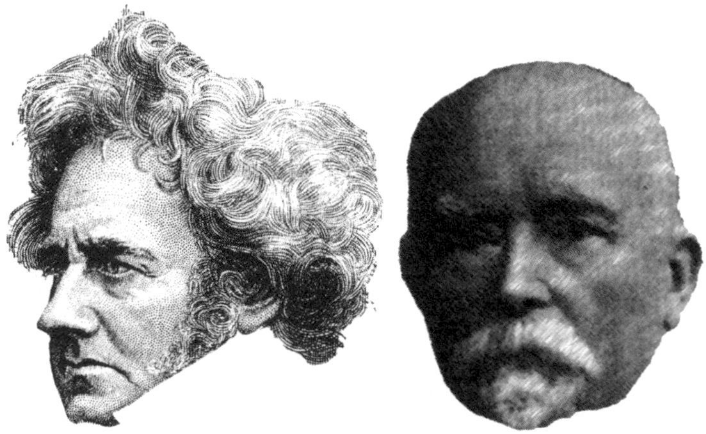

Figure 6.6
Left, John Herschel (1792–1871) after an engraving in *The world's great men*. London, The London Publishing Company, 1854. Right, Benjamin Bourdon (1860–1943) after an illustration in Murchison (1932).

Some connections between binocular and motion parallaxes were emerging towards the end of the eighteenth century. Both had been described, if not understood, and both were seen as an aid to the perception of depth or distance. The linkage of parallax with motion was forged by the astronomer, John Herschel (1792–1871; Fig. 6.6, left). He stated:

> Not only do external objects at rest appear in motion generally, with respect to ourselves when we are in motion among them, but they appear to move one among the other—they shift their *relative* apparent places. Let any one travelling rapidly along a high road fix his eye steadily on any object, but at the same time not entirely withdraw his attention from the general landscape,—he will see, or think he sees, the whole landscape thrown into *rotation*, and moving round that object as a centre; all objects between it and himself appearing to move *backwards*, or the contrary way to his own motion; and all beyond it, forwards, or in the direction in which he moves: but let him withdraw his eye from that object, and fix it on another,—a nearer one, for instance,—immediately the appearance of rotation shifts also, and the apparent centre about which the illusive circulation is performed is transferred to the new object, which, for the moment, appears to rest. (Herschel, 1833, p. 13, original italics)

The situation that Herschel described, viewing a scene through a moving window, is one that is used extensively in present-day illustrations. Not only did Herschel specify the directions of 'parallactic motion' but he also implied that some allowance for this could take place, so that the motion perceived could be attributed to objects or to the observer. Herschel's statements indicate that he was more aware of the subtleties of motion parallax than are many modern writers. The motion with respect to the observer is allocated to depth, motion, or both. Herschel was well acquainted with Wheatstone, and it is not impossible that they discussed issues of parallax, both with regard to astronomy as well as to vision. It was shortly after Herschel's account that Wheatstone (1838) addressed the same problem; he was confronted with the perception of depth by those who did not have recourse to binocular vision. That is, how does an observer with only one eye see depth?

Although several accounts of motion parallax have been given since the time of Wheatstone and Helmholtz, the concept has not received the concerted experimental attention accorded to binocular parallax. One factor that made experiments on motion parallax difficult was the control and measurement of head movement. Despite this, Benjamin Bourdon (1860–1943; Fig. 6.6, right) demonstrated that judgments of the separation between two points at different distances from an observer were made accurately when the head moved, but not when the head remained stationary. Bourdon (1898, 1902) conducted experiments in which two dots were presented, one above the other, at different distances. When viewed with a single eye their relative separations could be determined when the head moved from side-to-side: 'under monocular viewing, head movements represent a better way of judging relative distance than any other cues previously examined' (Bourdon, 1902, p. 287). He also found that judgments were more accurate when the upper point was more distant than the lower one. Partly for this reason Bourdon did not attempt to quantify the role of head (and thereby eye) movement on the estimation of relative depth.

Soon after Bourdon, Leopold Heine (1870–1940; 1905) managed to control the rate of retinal image motion with respect to the head movement. He mechanically yoked his lateral body movement to stimulus movements using a shoulder harness: the closer stimulus physically moved in the same direction and the far one physically moved in opposite direction to head/body movement (see Fig. 6.7, left). That is, the normal relationship between retinal image displacement and head movement was reversed. Under these conditions, the perception of depth was opposite to the actual depth; the near stimulus appeared farther than the far one, which provided convincing evidence that the retinal image motion produced by a head/body movement is a cue to depth

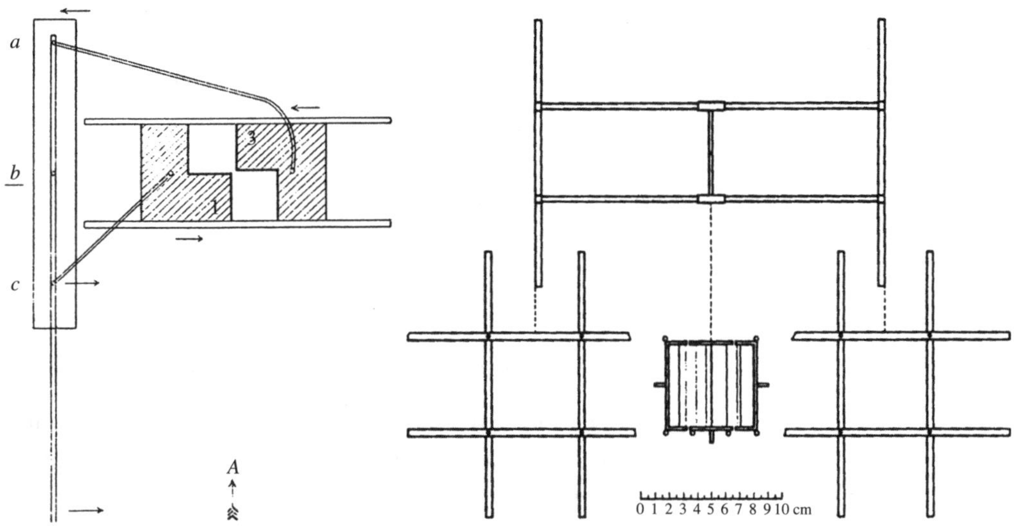

Figure 6.7
Left, Heine's (1905) apparatus for yoking retinal motion to head movement and right, the parallaktoscope of Tschermak-Seysenegg (1939). Both instruments were designed to examine the relationship between lateral head movements and depth perception.

perception. The arrangement is rather like the reversals of retinal disparities achieved with Wheatstone's (1852) pseudoscope. Heine distinguished between seeing depth or motion on the basis of the observer's awareness of the lateral movement. Without 'consciousness' of the lateral body movement the stimuli appear to move; with such awareness, however, depth rather than motion is seen.

Heine (1905) was an ophthalmologist, and his interest in motion parallax was related to the problems encountered when estimating the locations of structures in the eye. Clinical concerns about depth perception in strabismics were the source of Tschermak-Seysenegg's (1939) experiments on what he called 'Parallaktoskopie'. He constructed the device for studying the effects of head or stimulus movement in the perception of depth (Fig. 6.7, right). He found that active head movements produced more reliable impressions of depth than passive stimulus movements.

Early visual scientists were aware of the usefulness of self-generated retinal image motion as a cue to depth and there was a mild but continued interest, which has been recently revived. One reason for the recent upsurge of research is the development of a technique by Rogers and Graham (1979) somewhat similar to that devised by Heine (1905). It consists of electronically yoking dot movements on a computer screen to lateral head movements, and the perception produced is one of surfaces with apparent depth analogous to that produced by the random dot stereograms devised by Julesz (1960). A comprehensive review of research since Rogers and Graham's article can be found in Howard and Rogers (2002).

6.3 Stability and saccades

Towards the end of the nineteenth century a new issue regarding visual stability arose: Namely, how perceptual stability might be explained given the saccade-and-fixate oculomotor strategy that was becoming recognized as a central component of visual behaviour (see Chapter 4). As our understanding of the saccade-and-fixate strategy developed during this period, so it became increasingly clear that understanding the perceptual input to the visual system, a key driving force underlying visual research up to this point, would not be sufficient to explain our visual experience. Our smooth and complete experience could not be explained by the staccato and peripherally blurred visual input supplied by the eye. In order to understand visual experience, accounts would have to include wider aspects of cognition rather than perceptual input alone. Thus, during this period there was a shift in the driving force behind visual psychology from purely perceptual to a more cognitive account of vision.

The debate surrounding inflow and outflow as explanations of visual stability described earlier in this chapter was born of the desire to explain the stability of vision during slow continuous movement. Could these same principles be applied to the rapid saccadic jerks made by the eye? It was initially assumed that perception continued throughout the course of a saccadic eye movement; in part due to the experience that vision is continuous and uninterrupted. As we saw in Chapter 4, even Javal, who is now widely credited as the discoverer of saccadic eye movements, seems to have believed that in reading 'gaze glides along a line slightly higher than the centre of the characters' (Javal, 1878c, p. 251). This notion of gliding movements and continuous sweeps by the eye was a popularly held belief by many researchers at the time. As a result, one

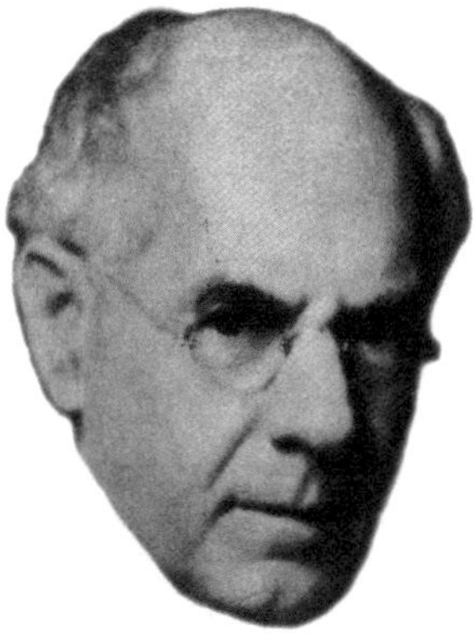

Figure 6.8
James McKeen Cattell (1860–1944) after a portrait in *The American Journal of Psychology*, 1944, **57**, 132.

avenue of concern at this time was to explain how the rapidly moving image arriving at the retina during a saccade could be seen distinctly (Cattell 1900*a*,*b*; see also Dodge, 1900).

James McKeen Cattell (1860–1944; Fig. 6.8) was principal among those researchers attempting to explain how vision remains clear and distinct even during rapid saccadic eye movements. Cattell clearly held the view that perception continued during rapid eye movements, and that during these movements vision remained distinct:

> When black and white surfaces are moved across the retina with the color-wheel at the rate of fifty white stimuli per second, a gray, as every one knows, is seen. When, however, the eye moves so that the line of sight passes over black and white surfaces at the same rate, there is no fusion whatever, the surfaces being seen distinctly side by side. No fusion occurs even when 1,000 stimuli per second fall upon each retinal element. (Cattell, 1900*a*, p. 325)

In this article, Cattell went on to clarify his position on the nature of eye movements as well as his ideas about perception within them; he was clearly not a keen supporter of the recent work suggesting that the eye might employ a saccade and fixate strategy, preferring the traditional notion of continuous movement:

> The fact that we see clearly and side by side objects over which the line of sight moves rapidly is evident. I have no doubt that the explanation I have given is correct—namely, that the visual mechanism is sufficiently sensitive to respond to more than 1,000 stimuli per second, and that we perceive a series of time changes on the retina as a spatial continuum because for our reactions it is in fact a spatial continuum. The only other possible explanations seems to be that the moving eye makes a series of jumps, seeing at each stop a distinct field, or that the distinctness of the field is an illusion, being really a memory image. But these suggestions are invalid. It can readily be observed that the eye does move continuously over the field. (Cattell, 1900*a*, p. 328)

In a footnote to his arguments against the new idea of saccades and fixations, Cattell attempted to explain the observation that movement is not a continuous sweep of the eyes when reading a line of text:

> In reading a line of printed text the eyes do stop as they sweep over the page. This, however, is not because there is any blurring of the letters with the moving eyes, but owing to the limited amount that can be simultaneously perceived and the time it takes to perceive it. (Cattell, 1900*a*, pp. 328–329)

Some researchers, however, did not accept the intuitive notion that perception continued throughout a saccade. Erdmann and

Dodge's (1898) accidental discovery that one cannot observe one's own eyes during saccades, suggested that vision might be disrupted during saccades. Dodge went on to clarify his position in an article in 1900:

> If one fixates the beginning of a line on this page, for example, the words in the middle of the line will be altogether illegible. The same will be true when the right end of the line is fixated, although the general character of the line is seen from both fixation points. If we look quickly from one end of the line to the other, it will seem as though we saw the letters and words during the movement, but an analysis of what was seen will show that we have not seen a particle more than we saw from one fixation point or the other. (Dodge, 1900, pp. 456–457)

One of the problems faced at this time by those trying to explain visual stability in the context of saccades was, as has often been the problem in eye movement research, the error of introspection. Dodge (1900) highlighted this issue in his article on *Visual perception during eye movement*, when explaining the demonstration suggested in the quotation above:

> It will be clear that when the eye moves as rapidly as possible from one fixation point to the other nothing new is seen; but it will seem that, when the eye moves more slowly, the entire line is seen very distinctly. If the observer takes the precaution to have some one watch his eyes, as recommended, he will find that what in self-observation passes for a slow movement of the eyes is in reality broken by one or more clearly defined full stops. (Dodge, 1900, p. 457)

In this statement Dodge is very likely making reference to Cattell's work on perception during eye movements, in which Cattell proposed that when moving the eye at a speed of $45° s^{-1}$, vision was distinct even though the movement was continuous (Cattell, 1900*a*). From his work with Erdmann, Dodge went on to suggest that vision was suppressed during saccades. In the same issue of *Psychological Review* as Dodge's article on vision during eye movements appeared, a response by Cattell was also published (Cattell, 1900*b*). In this response, Cattell accepted Dodge's finding that vision was fused during rapid eye movements despite it being completely contrary to Cattell's own suggestions in his article published earlier in the year and in which he dismissed the notion of fusion within eye movements:

> Professor Dodge finds that there is fusion when objects are exposed only when the eye is moving. It would follow from this that the hypothesis

discussed in my paper, but there rejected, must be accepted or at least considered. This is, that there is clear vision only in the pauses of movement, there being no peripheral perceptions while the eye is moving and the apparent distinctness of the field of view being an illusion. (Cattell, 1900*b*, pp. 507–508)

While Erdmann and Dodge appear to be the first researchers to have systematically employed objective experiments to investigate the nature of perception during saccadic eye movements, they were not the first to suggest that vision may be suspended during rapid eye movements. Over a century before their work, Wells observed that:

My conclusion from this experiment [on visual vertigo] is, that, although the eye during it moves forwards and backwards, still the two motions are not exactly similar, but that in one the picture travels slowly enough over the retina to allow me to attend to the progression of the paper; while in the latter the passage of the picture is so rapid, that no succession of the paper's apparent places can be observed. (Wells, 1794*b*, p. 906)

In his descriptions of nystagmus, Breuer (1874) expressed the opinion that there is no visual awareness during the rapid phases of nystagmic eye movements. He argued that during rotation the eyes lag behind the head in order to maintain a steady retinal image; then they make rapid jerky motions in the direction of head rotation. When the body rotation ceases the eyes rotate in the same direction as prior head rotation, and the visual world appears to move in the opposite direction interspersed with rapid returns. He stated that there is no visual awareness during these rapid returns. This is a clear reference to saccadic suppression, although he did not use the term saccade. Similarly, in his description of jerk-like eye movements, Crum Brown observed that 'During the jerks we practically do not see at all, so that we have before us not a moving panorama, but a series of fixed pictures of the same fixed things, which succeed one another rapidly' (Crum Brown, 1895*b*, p. 5). In spite of these earlier suggestions by Wells, Breuer, and Crum Brown, it was not until Dodge's work at the start of the twentieth century that the question of what was seen during a saccade was placed under experimental scrutiny. Once Erdmann and Dodge (1898) had recognized that vision might be suspended during saccades, the question then became one of discovering the nature of this suspension. Two main suggestions arose during the early work on vision during saccades. First, that there might be a central anaesthesia that suppresses vision for the duration of the saccade; this notion was heralded by Holt (1903). Second, rather than a complete anaesthesia during saccades, it may be that vision is reduced during an eye movement; this position was argued by Dodge (1900, 1905).

Edwin Bissell Holt (1873–1946) was a student of William James before graduating with a PhD from Harvard in 1901. In the early part of his career Holt investigated visual perception during eye movements and, like Erdmann and Dodge (1898), suggested that vision was not clear during fast eye movements (Holt, 1903). Where Holt and Dodge disagreed was in their explanation of how and why clear vision did not occur during eye movements. Holt suggested that during fast eye movements vision was suppressed centrally and no perception of any sort occurred. Thus Holt was arguing for a central anaesthesia during saccades. Holt maintained that even in situations where there was an apparent perception during an eye movement (such as in Dodge's rotating disk experiments explained below) this was a false perception. Holt argued that in such situations the retinal image from within a saccade might stay dormant and then be perceived once the saccade was over and the eye was at rest once more (Holt, 1903).

Dodge was not convinced by the notion of a central anaesthesia during saccades. Rather he preferred the idea that vision was merely reduced rather than completely suppressed. As we have seen in previous chapters, Dodge was a gifted designer of experimental apparatus for testing his ideas about visual perception, and he used this ability to conduct an elegant series of experiments in 1900 that were designed to investigate vision during saccades. The starting point for Dodge's rejection of the notion of central anaesthesia, was the simple observation that one can perceive 'long streaks of light seen when the retina moves across the image of a bright point of light on a dark background' (Dodge, 1900, p. 458). This observation was followed up with an experiment in which:

A disk of black cardboard thirteen inches in diameter, in which a circle of one-eighth inch round holes, one-half inch apart, had been punched close to the periphery all around, was made to revolve at such a velocity that, while the light from the holes fused to a bright circle when the eye was at rest, when the eye moved in the direction of the disk's rotation from one fixation point, seen through the fused circle of light, to another one inch distant, three clear-cut round holes were seen much brighter than the band of light out of which out of which the seemed to emerge. (p. 458)

Dodge believed that this simple result was clearly incompatible with the suggestion of central anaesthesia during saccades; if vision was suspended during eye movements as the anaesthesia explanation suggested, then the spots of light should not be visible during the saccade. Satisfied that this experiment discredited the central anaesthesia explanation, Dodge went on to scrutinize the details of what could be seen during a saccade. Dodge devised an experiment whereby a visual stimulus was only exposed during the eye movement and remained hidden from view during the fixations before and after the saccade. This was achieved by making an eye movement across a slit in a screen, behind which visual stimuli could be placed at such a position that they were obscured at the start and end of the eye movement, but exposed over an extent of 10° during the saccade. Behind the screen, Dodge placed either white or coloured cards and found that: 'The first experiments with this apparatus were altogether negative. White cardboard filling the whole ten degrees of the field of exposure was wholly unseen. The result was the same when colored surfaces were substituted for the white' (Dodge, 1900, p. 460). This negative result was contrary to what Dodge had anticipated given his experiments with the rotating disc. One problem with the experiment that used a slit in the screen to expose stimuli only during saccades was that it required a saccade of approximately 80°. Dodge wondered whether the unnaturally large eye movement might be the source of his negative result and so modified the apparatus so that a movement of only around 50° was necessary. Once again, the result was negative; nothing was seen during the saccade. Not deterred by these negative results, Dodge wondered whether the failure to perceive stimuli during saccades might be because his stimuli were not sufficiently bright. Consequently, he decided to increase the illumination of the intra-saccadic stimulus:

These failures suggested an increase of the illumination of the field of exposure. A ground glass plate, illuminated from behind by a bright, sunlit landscape, was substituted for the white cardboard in the first form of apparatus. Under these conditions a long band of light was immediately evident at each movement of the eye. (Dodge, 1900, p. 461)

Thus, by increasing the illumination of the intra-saccadic stimuli, a stimulus that was only available during a saccade could be perceived. If coloured plates were used, the intra-saccadic perception of a smear of light was coloured appropriately, albeit rather dully. These experiments highlight an aspect of intra-saccadic vision that has become a much more modern concern. Namely, the possibility that the suppression of vision during saccades might not be an absolute absence of visual perception during saccades (as had been argued by Holt, 1903, and debated by Dodge, 1900, 1905), but rather that contrast sensitivity might be lowered during saccades (e.g. Diamond et al., 2000). This modern account of saccadic suppression argues that contrast sensitivity is reduced to such an extent that under natural conditions nothing will be perceived during a saccade, but that if contrast is very high, then vision can proceed. This explanation is entirely consistent with Dodge's results; although he did not explicitly discuss the possible implications of his observation that bright illumination of the intra-saccadic stimulus (and therefore high contrast with the black cardboard) was needed for perception during the saccade. Rather, Dodge proposed that the failure to perceive the fainter stimuli was due to attentional factors. He believed that given sufficient training the observer would be able to learn to attend to and perceive the fainter stimuli during saccades.

Dodge was chiefly concerned with discrediting the notion of a complete central anaesthesia and characterizing the nature of the percept during saccades. With regard to the character of the intra-saccadic percept, Dodge suggested that the light arriving at the retina during the saccade formed a fused smear. The evidence from this came mainly from variants of his experiments described above in which the intra-saccadic stimulus was not a uniform colour, but comprised a set of slits, each one degree in width and one degree apart. When each slit contained a different colour, the percept was of a smear of a single, fused colour, the hue of which depended upon the individual colours present in the slits (Dodge, 1900).

One problem arising from Dodge's work demonstrating intra-saccadic fused perception was that this was clearly unlike our normal, everyday experience of vision. In a follow up article in 1905, Dodge continued his debate with Holt and clarified his position regarding the possible reasons why we do not normally experience percepts during saccadic eye movements. Dodge maintained his preference for inhibition rather than complete anaesthesia, and further disagreed with Holt's suggestions regarding the source of the inhibition:

> With regard to the causes of the inhibitory processes my disagreement with the Harvard Studies is more radical. Mr. Holt conjectures that the eye-movement anaesthesia is the effect of 'muscle sensations of present movement streaming to consciousness to form the basis of the new post-motum localisation.' Without admitting the efficacy of such sensations of eye movements to produce a visual anaesthesia I must protest again that I do not find in myself sensations of eye movements 'streaming to consciousness'; and moreover, that a careful examination of a considerable number of persons during the last ten years makes it clear that in this respect I am not altogether abnormal. (Dodge, 1905, p. 194)

It is clear that Dodge disagreed with Holt's suggestion that processes rather like the afference or inflow, proposed by Sherrington and others to account for perceptual stability during pursuit eye movements, might account for perceptual suppression during saccadic eye movements. Rather, Dodge suggested that a combination of central and peripheral factors contributed to our failure to perceive the fused stimuli that he had previously demonstrated to be visible during saccades, and that the relative contribution of these factors varied according to the size of the eye movement. For small amplitude eye movements, Dodge suggested that our failure to perceive the intra-saccadic fused smear was due to peripheral (namely, retinal) factors:

> Chief in the first group is to be reckoned the after effects of stimulation. These alone would account for the nonperception of a fused visual field during short eye movements. An eye movement of 5° occupies about 30 σ, but the positive after image of a moderate stimulation may last 30 σ without perceptible diminution of intensity. A second and probably equally important peripheral factor consists in the inhibitive action of the new stimulation at each new point of regard. These two facts obviously work together to prevent perception of the faint fusion stimulus during short eye movements. (Dodge, 1905, p. 197)

The second factor suggested by Dodge in the above quotation again parallels much more modern suggestions that saccadic suppression might arise because the image on the retina from the post-saccadic fixation effectively masks the percept of the saccade that immediately preceded it; an explanation known as backward masking (see Breitmeyer and Ogmen, 2000). A variety of other possible masking effects that might account for saccadic suppression have also been suggested, but again these have been relatively modern developments in our consideration of eye movements and perception (e.g. Alpern, 1969; Bridgeman, 1971; Davidson et al., 1973; MacKay, 1970; L. Matin, 1972; E. Matin, 1974; Weisstein, 1972).

For larger amplitude saccades, Dodge suggested a more pivotal role for central inhibitory processes, but argued that these central processes were attentional in nature rather than being an anaesthesia:

> The fencing mask, the muscæ volitantes, and involuntary winking, are all illustrations to the point. The real objects of interest in the visual field are the present object of fixation and that peripheral object which is about to become, at the completion of an eye movement, the new object of fixation. Other parts of the field are of lesser attention value, otherwise they would be substituted for the object of fixation. During moments of clearest vision, then, the space about to be traversed by the line of regard during an eye movement of the first type is without especial interest to us; and it is reasonable to suppose that what is without especial interest during clear vision, when the eye is at rest, would arouse no new interest during the confused stimulation incident to eye movements of the first type. (Dodge, 1905, p. 198)

An attentional account of saccadic suppression did not prove popular in the years that followed and is completely absent from Volkmann's (1976) review of the subject, in which the possible explanations of saccadic suppression were discussed. Volkmann's review brought together much of the preceding research on saccadic suppression, becoming a key point of historical reference, and helped to define the direction for much of the eye movement research that followed. While becoming unpopular for almost a century, Dodge's possibility that attention might play a role in saccadic suppression has recently re-surfaced. Moore et al. (1998) recorded neuronal activity in area V4 in macaque monkeys and found evidence for the maintenance of visual representations during saccades. They proposed that attention might serve to maintain this representation during the saccade and thus suppress perception of the blurred retinal image during eye movements, and pointed out the parallels between their conclusions and those of Dodge in 1905.

It is interesting that the disagreement between Holt and Dodge over the reasons why we do not appear to perceive retinal input during saccades is echoed in modern research. We still do not fully understand the source of visual suppression during eye movements in spite of nearly a century of exploration of this issue. Current accounts include central suppression (e.g. Burr et al., 1994), backward masking (see Breitmeyer and Ogmen, 2000), and retinal shear (Castet and Masson, 2000; Castet et al., 2001).

6.3.1 Perceptual stability across fixations

The recognition that clear vision was interrupted during saccades has led to a wealth of research into the likely cause of saccadic suppression. However, it has also raised a parallel but subtly different issue that has become a particularly prominent area of research. Namely, how we can account for the smooth visual perception of the world around us that we all experience, given that vision is interrupted by brief periods of blindness at a frequency of about three times in every second. Furthermore, as our understanding of the saccade-and-fixate strategy of normal oculomotor behaviour became clearer at the end of the nineteenth and early twentieth centuries (see Chapter 4), so the problem grew more complex. If we are effectively blind (or at least unaware) during saccadic eye movements, yet the eye remains relatively stable during the fixation periods between these eye movements, the consequence must be that the input to the visual system supplied by the eye must be in the form of a series of relatively static snapshots of the world, arriving at about three or four per second. This is very unlike the smooth and continuous perception of the world that we experience. While explanations of saccadic suppression can account for why we do not perceive disruptions from saccades, they do not as readily allow us to explain the smooth continuity of our visual experience over successive fixations.

As our understanding of vision and eye movements developed, so it became clear that purely retinal accounts of the input to the visual system could not account for our visual experience. First, as retinal anatomy developed, it became evident that vision was only distinct in the centre of the visual field, and became increasingly degraded in the periphery (see Chapters 1 and 2). Second, saccades and fixations meant that vision was disrupted, producing a disjointed, staccato perceptual input. Thus accounts of vision began to appeal to notions of internal representation to explain our smooth and complete experience; distinct vision necessitated eye movements for a complete impression of the scene and saccades seemed to suggest the need to store this information and use it to construct a representation of the scene.

An intuitively appealing account of visual stability across fixations is to suggest that faithful copies of the images received at the eye might be stored in the brain and fused together, such that, over a number of fixations, we might be able to construct a relatively detailed and extensive representation of our surroundings. Such notions of an 'internal picture' in the brain were commonly found in the literature until the later part of the twentieth century (e.g. Marr, 1982), and the existence of a low-level integrative buffer that serves this purpose has specifically been suggested and investigated (e.g. McConkie and Rayner, 1976; Rayner, 1978).

The idea of a faithful internal copy of our visual environment is no longer accepted widely. Evidence against this notion has been available for some time (e.g. Bridgeman et al., 1975; Irwin, 1991, 1993; Irwin et al., 1983; McConkie and Zola, 1979; Pollatsek and Rayner, 1992; Rayner and Pollatsek, 1983; Rayner et al., 1980). The most compelling evidence against this notion, however, has come to light from a large literature on change detection (since Grimes, 1996). Observers often fail to detect even quite large changes to the position, colour or presence of an object in a complex scene, if that change occurs at the time of a saccade (e.g. Grimes, 1996; McConkie and Currie, 1996), blink (O'Regan et al., 2000), or brief artificial interruptions (Rensink et al., 1995, 1997, 2000).

Our surprising blindness to changes in complex scenes has led researchers to reject the notion of an integrative, richly detailed internal representation of our surroundings and has lead to a considerable body of literature devoted to attempting to characterize what the nature of our visual representation might be, or even if we construct one at all. Current opinion is divided into those who believe that we do construct a representation, but that it is not a point-by-point pictorial copy of the world (e.g. Hollingworth and Henderson, 2002; Tatler, Gilchrist et al., 2005), and those who believe that no internal representation is constructed (e.g. O'Regan and Noë, 2001). While this debate over the nature of visual representation appears an extremely modern concern, the ideas championed by both camps have much older origins.

6.3.2 Mental representation

The notion that we form an internal representation of what we see has a long history, and the debate as to its likely nature is almost as old. Aristotle held the view that we form in our minds an exact replica of the object that we view. To Aristotle, the object in the mind was not really a representation at all, but rather was a copy of the object itself. This might also have been founded on an aspect of perception: a reflected image of the object could be seen by another person. The concept of some copy of objects, carried through the air to the eye, was to have widespread and longlasting appeal, and it was referred to by many names. Indeed, by the end of the thirteenth century, Roger Bacon was able to list the terms image, species, idol, simulacrum, film, phantasm, form, intention, passion, impression, used by authors of works on vision (Lindberg, 1983), to which could be added effigies, figures, and membranes. There was an obvious source of observational support for such a theory: the image of an object could be seen reflected from the eye of an observer.

Aristotle believed that 'phantasms' from objects projected into the eyes and formed an internal replica of the object viewed. Aristotle's views on internal models of objects were to become highly influential upon later writings, due in no small part to the intuitive appeal of the idea that we have in our minds a replica of what we view. While Aristotle's writings suggest that he viewed the internal replica of the object as an exact copy, some limited degree of abstraction is compatible with his ideas. Aristotle articulated this in his *De Anima*:

> Let us now summarize our results about soul, and repeat that the soul is in a way all existing things; for existing things are either sensible or thinkable, and knowledge is in a way what is knowable, and sensation is in a way what is sensible: in what way we must inquire. Knowledge and sensation are divided to correspond with the realities, potential knowledge and sensation answering to potentialities, actual knowledge and sensation to actualities. Within the soul the faculties of knowledge and sensation are potentially these objects, the one what is knowable, the other what is sensible. They must be either the things themselves or their forms. The former alternative is of course impossible: it is not the stone which is present in the soul but its form. (Ross, 1927, p. 431*b*)

This is an important point and one that was returned to by Thomas Aquinas (1225–1274; Fig. 6.9, left) in the thirteenth century. Aquinas largely echoed the Aristotelian perspective, arguing

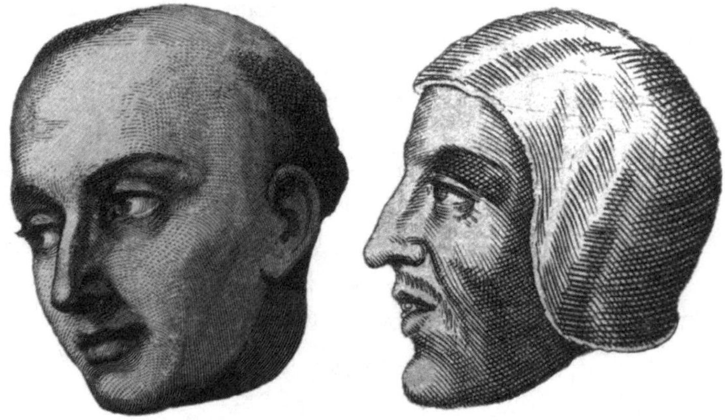

Figure 6.9
Left, Thomas Aquinas (1225–1274) after an engraving in Figuier (1866). Right, John Duns Scotus (c. 1265–1308) after a woodcut in Freher (1688).

in his *Summa Theologicæ* (1266–1273/1963–1970) and his *De Veritate* (1256–1259/1994) that 'intelligible species' from objects (equivalent to Aristotle's phantasms) formed internal replicas of viewed objects. While his viewpoint appears generally to be that the internal copy is a true likeness of the external object, he went to considerable lengths in his *Summa Theologicæ* to clarify his position that the internal model is a 'likeness' rather than being exactly the same as the external object:

> We must say, therefore, that species stand in relation to the intellect as *that by which* the intellect understands. To make the matter clear: although there are two kinds of activity—one that remains within the agent (e.g., seeing or understanding), and one that passes over into a thing outside (e.g., heating or cutting)—nevertheless each is produced in accord with a form. Now just as the form from which an activity extending to a thing outside proceeds is like the object of the activity (for instance, the heat of a heater is like that of the thing heated), so also, in a similar way, the form from which an activity remaining within an agent proceeds is a likeness of the object. Thus it is according to a likeness of a visible thing that the faculty of sight sees, and likewise a likeness of a thing understood, i.e., a species, is the form according to which the intellect understands. However, since the intellect reflects upon itself, by such a reflection it understands both its own understanding and the species by which it understands. Thus species are secondarily that which is understood. But what is understood first is the reality of which a particular species is a likeness. (Aquinas, 1266–1273/1963–1970, Vol. X, p. 61, original italics)

Clearly, the possibility of abstract representations was being entertained even in the thirteenth century. The debate as to the nature of visual representation was far from over. The Scottish philosopher and theologian John Duns Scotus (ca. 1265–1308; Fig. 6.9, right), built upon Aquinas' ideas of abstraction, taking them a step further by suggesting that the internal model of an object comprises both the form of the object represented and the act of representing it. Duns Scotus began to move away from the old notions that what was in the mind was a copy of the object itself, and instead appeal to what we now understand by the term representation. Duns Scotus' ideas increased the notion of abstraction from the object, but was still based upon the earlier ideas of Aquinas and Aristotle that the representation was a likeness of the object. While Duns Scotus redefined the question to being one of representation rather than internalization of objects, the debate as to the nature of the representation continued.

A bolder departure from the Aristotelian tradition was proposed by William of Ockham (1288–1348), who is thought to have been a pupil of Duns Scotus, in his *Summa Logicae* (ca. 1323/1974). Ockham pointed out that many different things can act as representations of an object and that these need not be image-like. It is from the writings of Ockham that notions of symbolic and language-based representations of objects begin to emerge. In spite of Ockham's suggestion that representation might be more abstract than previous writers had suggested, the notion of an image-like representation remained popular with other writers. William Crathorn (fl. 1330) adhered to the Aristotelian view of image-like veridical representations even more strictly than Aquinas. Crathorn believed that a representation must be the same as that which it represents; that is, a representation of a red object must itself be red: 'a soul seeing and intellectively cognizing color is truly colored, not by any color existing outside the soul but by its likeness, which is a true color. And the same has to be said of a soul's *intellectual* cognition, whenever a natural word of that color is formed within it' (Pasnau, 2002, p. 288, original italics). In spite of Crathorn's attempted return to strict notions of image-like representations, his ideas were not popular and the accounts of representations that at least appealed to some notion of abstraction from the actual object remained popular. A similar argument and opposition can be found in the twentieth century with the Gestalt concept of isomorphism and the objections to it (see Asch, 1995).

In the seventeenth century, our understanding of vision was transformed by the work of Kepler, Platter, and Scheiner (see Chapter 1). Kepler described how the eye operated as an optical instrument, focusing light onto the retina to form an image. This discovery necessitated a radical review of the old notions of how mental representations of objects might be formed and what their nature might be. Kepler's description of an inverted and reversed image on the retina clearly redefined the questions of visual experience. Kepler did not himself feel able to comment on how the brain might deal with turning the retinal image into what we experience: 'I leave it to natural philosophers to discuss the way in which this image or picture (*pictura*) is put together by the spiritual principles of vision' (Crombie, 1964, p. 147). As oculomotor anatomy improved, so the realization that vision was only clear in the centre of the field not only refined the questions of representation but also suggested that representation was a necessary part of understanding vision. Given poor peripheral resolution, a representation that was a faithful likeness of the visual world could not arise perceptually because there was no complete retinal image supplied by the eye. Thus a complete impression of a scene necessarily required that the eyes be moved around and that the information gathered be used to construct an internal representation of the scene. The seventeenth century revolution in optics and ocular anatomy, therefore, led to a resurrection and redefinition of the question of mental representation.

Thomas Hobbes (1588–1679; Fig. 6.10, left) is best known for his political philosophy, but he also discussed issues of sensation and perception (Hobbes, 1651/1996, 1656/1839–1845). Hobbes devoted a section of *Leviathan* to the senses: he discussed

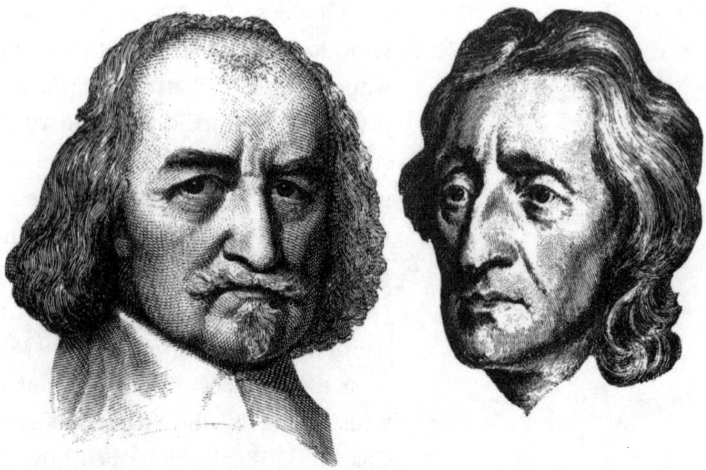

Figure 6.10
Left, Thomas Hobbes (1588–1679) after an engraving in Molesworth (1839). Right, John Locke (1632–1704) after an engraving in Birch (1743).

his ideas of sensation, imagination, and memory and made clear his belief in the importance of representations:

> Concerning the Thoughts of man, I will consider them first *singly*, and afterwards in *Trayne*, or dependence upon one another. *Singly*, they are every one a *Representation* or *Appearance*, of some quality, or other Accident of a body without us; which is commonly called an *Object*. Which object worketh on the Eyes, Eares, and other parts of mans body; and by diversity of working, produceth diversity of Appearances. The Originall of them all, is that which we call SENSE; (For there is no conception in a mans mind, which hath not at first, totally, or by parts, been begotten upon the organs of Sense). The rest are derived from that originall. (Hobbes, 1651/1996, p. 13, original italics and capitals)

Hobbes evidently regarded representations as central to our experience, yet his precise position on the issue of the nature of representation is somewhat unclear. In places he clearly alludes to the idea of abstracted forms of representation:

> For after the object is removed, or the eye shut, wee still retain an image of the thing seen, though more obscure than when we see it. And this is it, the Latines call *Imagination*, from the image made in seeing; and apply the same, though improperly, to all the other senses. But the Greeks call it *Fancy*, which signifies *appearance*, and is as proper to one sense, as to another. (Hobbes, 1651/1996, p. 15, original italics)

However, in other passages of *Leviathan* Hobbes' descriptions appear to imply a more image-like pictorial notion of representation. For example, Hobbes states that 'IMAGINATION, therefore, is nothing but *decaying sense*; and is found in men, and many other living Creatures, as well sleeping, as waking' (p. 15, original italics and capitals). The reference to imagination as being decaying sense seems to appeal to notions of an internal picture-like representation that decays over time, rather like later ideas of iconic memory (Sperling, 1960, 1967). Later in the same section, Hobbes is more explicit in stating this possibility:

> And any object being removed from our eyes, though the impression it made in us remain; yet other objects more present succeeding, and working on us, the Imagination of the past is obscured, and made weak; as the voyce of a man is in the noyse of the day. From whence it followeth that the longer the time is, after the sight or Sense of any object, the weaker is the Imagination. (Hobbes, 1651/1996, p. 16)

Contemporary with Hobbes, both René Descartes and John Locke (1632–1704; Fig. 6.10, right) discussed the nature of representation and both held the view that they were abstractions rather than image-like replicas. In his *Essay concerning human understanding*, Locke argued the case for linguistic and generalizable representations:

Whatever therefore be the secret abstract nature of *substance* in general, all *the ideas we have of particular distinct sorts of substances*, are nothing but several combinations of simple ideas, co-existing in such, though unknown, cause of their union, as makes the whole subsist of itself. 'Tis by such combinations of simple *ideas*, and nothing else, that we represent particular sorts of *substances* to ourselves; such are the ideas we have of their several species in our minds; and such only do we, by their specific names, signify to others, *e.g.*, *man*, *horse*, *sun*, *water*, *iron*; upon hearing which words, everyone, who understands the language, frames in his mind a combination of those several simple ideas, which he has usually observed, or fancied to exist together under that denomination. (Locke, 1690/1997, p. 270, original italics)

René Descartes' contribution to vision demonstrates the close relationship between the science of optics and visual anatomy and of mental representation that developed during this period. Descartes (1637, 1662, 1664) was a central figure in the development of our knowledge of optics (see Chapters 1 and 2) and also recognized the importance that this new understanding placed upon notions of mental representation. Descartes felt that these issues were necessarily related and were both of crucial importance to understanding vision as a whole.

The Scottish philosopher David Hume (1711–1776) considered the nature of representation in his *An enquiry concerning human understanding* (1748/1902):

Every one will readily allow, that there is a considerable difference between the perceptions of the mind, when a man feels the pain of excessive heat, or the pleasure of moderate warmth, and when he afterwards recalls to his memory this sensation, or anticipates it by his imagination. These faculties may mimic or copy the perceptions of the senses; but they never can entirely reach the force and vivacity of the original sentiment. The utmost we say of them, even when they operate with greatest vigour, is, that they represent their object in so lively a manner, that we could *almost* say we feel or see it: But, except the mind be disordered by disease or madness, they never can arrive at such a pitch of vivacity, as to render these perceptions altogether undistinguishable. (Hume, 1748/1902, p. 17, original italics)

This quotation suggests that Hume's conception of representation is somewhat of a return to the more image-like internal copy of earlier writers, albeit with an admission that the internal copy is of lesser vivacity than the sensation itself. Hume recognized the controversy that surrounded the debate of the nature of representation and the pitfalls of appealing to the intuitive notion of image-like copies of objects, rather than abstractions of them:

> This is a topic, therefore, in which the profounder and more philosophical sceptics will always triumph, when they endeavour to introduce an universal doubt into all subjects of human knowledge and enquiry. Do you follow the instincts and propensities of nature, may they say, in assenting to the veracity of sense? But these lead you to believe that the very perception or sensible image is the external object. Do you disclaim this principle, in order to embrace a more rational opinion, that the perceptions are only representations of something external? You here depart from your natural propensities and more obvious sentiments; and yet are not able to satisfy your reason, which can never find any convincing argument from experience to prove, that the perceptions are connected with any external objects. (Hume, 1748/1902, pp. 153–154)

Just as the revolution in optics and ocular anatomy in the seventeenth century redefined questions of visual representation and brought them back into prominence in visual science and psychology, so the nineteenth century revolution in our understanding of eye movements (see Chapter 4) also had a profound impact upon notions of representation. Once again, discoveries in the way that the eyes operate and the perceptual input that they supply to the visual system redefined the questions of representation. In many ways the need for representation was emphasized by the development of our understanding of saccades and fixations; as the gap widened between what was understood to be the perceptual input to the visual system and the cognitive experience that we have of vision, so the role of representation as a means to bridge that gap assumed increasing importance.

The debate about the nature of representation has resumed its significance in accounts of vision and visual experience in recent years. This is in consequence of the change detection studies described earlier; the question of the nature of visual representation has returned to prominence in psychological and philosophical research. It is in this most recent resurgence of interest in mental representation that the role of eye movements in the construction of representations has become particularly crucial. Increasingly, researchers are stressing the implausibility of image-like representations in vision and favouring descriptions of abstract representation (e.g. Rensink, 2000*a*,*b*). The question has once again turned to trying to discern what form this abstract representation might take and how it might be constructed and maintained (e.g. Hollingworth and Henderson, 2002; Tatler, Gilchrist et al., 2005). The advantage that we now have over the earlier writers is the knowledge of the oculomotor saccade-and-fixate strategy and the technology with which to explore these questions.

6.3.3 Is representation necessary?

While we have seen that there is a long tradition of attempts to explain vision by appealing to notions of representation, other researchers have preferred the possibility that perhaps we do not require an internal representation of our surroundings. This has become a very modern concern arising principally from the work of O'Regan and colleagues (O'Regan, 1992; O'Regan and Noë, 2001). In these accounts they suggest that vision need not require an internal representation, either image-like or abstract, because the best model of the world, is the world itself. That is, the world can effectively act as its own 'outside memory' (O'Regan, 1992). They explain that given the mobility of the eyes, if we require detailed information about any part of the scene the most efficient strategy is to direct the eyes towards that part of the scene, rather than to inspect some internally reconstructed representation of it. Clearly this notion has considerable merit and appeal and indeed is consistent with the well-established knowledge that in real-world tasks, we do tend to look at that which we require information about (Ballard et al., 1992; Ballard et al., 1995; Land and Hayhoe, 2001; Land et al., 1999). While the notion of the world acting as its own memory and not requiring internalization may appear an entirely modern development in the representation debate, it too has much older origins.

The most recent antecedent of such ideas is the work in perception of Gibson (1950, 1966, 1979). In these books Gibson stressed the importance of vision in guiding action, and also that vision cannot be divorced from the dimension of time. In particular he argued that natural perception depends on complex patterns of stimulation, involving active exploration of the environment by the perceiver. He drew attention to the lawfulness of the transformations that take place with eye and object motions and he suggested that we use them to determine both our posture and the motion of objects in the world. Gibson regarded perception as wholly independent of cognition, and determined entirely by a direct response to patterns of stimulation without any intervening process.

While he did not specifically discuss the issue of whether or not there may be a representation underlying visual perception, some of Raymond Dodge's comments do raise the possibility that he may also have regarded a representation as unnecessary. In his article in 1905 where he proposed his attentional account for saccadic suppression (see above), his statements could be interpreted as having implications for representations. When he states that: 'The real objects of interest in the visual field are the present object of fixation and that peripheral object which is about to become, at the completion of an eye movement, the new object of fixation. Other parts of the field are of lesser attention value, otherwise they would be substituted for the object of fixation'. (Dodge 1905, p. 198)

This argument could be interpreted in the same context as those later suggestions by Gibson and by O'Regan and Noë that vision does not require a representation; if an object is of interest to us we do not require a representation to scrutinize it, rather we simply require that we move our eyes to it.

While we have seen that there have been several twentieth century instances of writers entertaining the idea that representation may not be required, to a large extent these are modern re-incarnations of the ideas heralded by Berkeley (1709/1910):

> Now I do not find that I can perceive, imagine, or any wise frame in my Mind such an abstract *Idea*, as is here spoken of. A Line, or Surface which is neither Black, nor White, nor Blue, nor Yellow, &c. Nor Long, nor Short, nor Rough, nor Smooth, nor Square, nor Round, &c. is perfectly incomprehensible. This I am sure of as to my self, how far the Faculties of other Men may reach, they best can tell. (Berkeley, 1709/1910, p. 69, original italics)

Rather than appealing to notions of representation to explain visual experience, Berkeley proposed that geometrical factors regarding the direction of the eyes, and, importantly, the effect that moving the eyes has upon the image that they receive of an object were of central importance in generating our visual perception and experience:

> Nor do I see, how I can easily be mistaken in this Matter. I know evidently that Distance is not perceived of it self. That by consequence, it must be perceived by means of some other *Idea* which is immediately perceiv'd, and varies with the different Degrees of Distance. I know also that the Sensation arising from the Turn of the Eyes is of it self, immediately perceiv'd, and various Degrees thereof are connected with different Distances; which never fail to accompany them into my Mind, when I view an *Object* distinctly with both Eyes, whose Distance is so small that in respect of it, the Interval

between the Eyes has any considerable Magnitude. (Berkeley, 1709/1910, p. 17, original italics)

That eye movements might be of fundamental importance for generating perceptions was echoed by Brücke (1841) and Brewster (1844, 1856) who argued for the role of changes in convergence and accommodation in their explanations of binocular vision and space perception (see Section 2.2). These suggestions that the perception of an object might arise from the act of moving the eyes when viewing it are remarkably similar to the suggestions made by O'Regan and Noë (2001) in their account of visual experience. O'Regan and Noë suggest that visual perception arises as a result of the changes that occur in the projection of an object on the retina as a result of moving the eyes when viewing the object. They refer to this idea as sensorimotor contingencies, whereby three-dimensional object perceptions can be generated simply from the act of moving the eyes over an object. Again we find that an apparently modern notion is in reality grounded in a much longer history.

6.4 Stability and fixations

The stability we have discussed so far concerns that of perception despite eye movements that pursue objects or make saccadic movements over a scene. In this section we will examine another aspect of stability—that of the eye itself when attempts are made to maintain fixation. This has been investigated by imposing artificial stability on the image presented to the retina. Such studies have brought to light a fascinating array of minute involuntary eye movements, and they have shown how vital they are to vision. Of course, without the artificial devices the eyes do indeed move during fixation, so that the image is moving over the retina. The maintenance of perceptual stability during the changes is yet another remarkable achievement of vision.

The fact that the eyes are rarely stationary was evident from Robert Darwin's (1786) observations of coloured silk (Section 4.2.1) and from the demonstration of your own afterimage motion with Fig. 1.8. Since the dominant metaphor in vision since the time of Kepler has been the equation of eye and camera, a constantly moving eye seemed to pose problems for vision. With the invention and development of photography the demands of a stable and stationary camera became paramount. If the highest visual acuity is restricted to a small region around the fovea then it was possible that keeping this still would enhance acuity. It was precisely this problem that led to some of the earliest work on compensating for involuntary eye movements in the 1950s. What was considered to be surprising was that vision faded rapidly with a stable image on the retina.

This should not have been a surprise, as attempts to maintain steady fixation and a stable image on the retina had been made many years earlier. However, the perceptual fading was considered to be restricted to the peripheral retina, despite clear descriptions of central fading. Ignaz Paul Vitalis Troxler (1780–1866; Fig. 6.11, left) described how peripheral targets fade and disappear, and it is now known as the Troxler effect. Troxler (1804) initially placed three small white figures in a line on a blue wall and noted that with fixation on one of them the others would suddenly disappear. He then elaborated upon this procedure: he arranged a sequence of colour patches on a wall so that they extended into the periphery of vision. When he fixated on one, after some time the most peripheral ones disappeared, followed by those closer to the fixation point. In all cases, the lost patterns were replaced by the blue wall, which was the background: 'I stuck a long row of all types of brightly coloured stripes and patches on a light blue surface, and always arranged them at a particular distance and direction from my eyes and the row disappeared to be replaced by the blue surface' (Troxler, 1804, p. 7). Troxler's

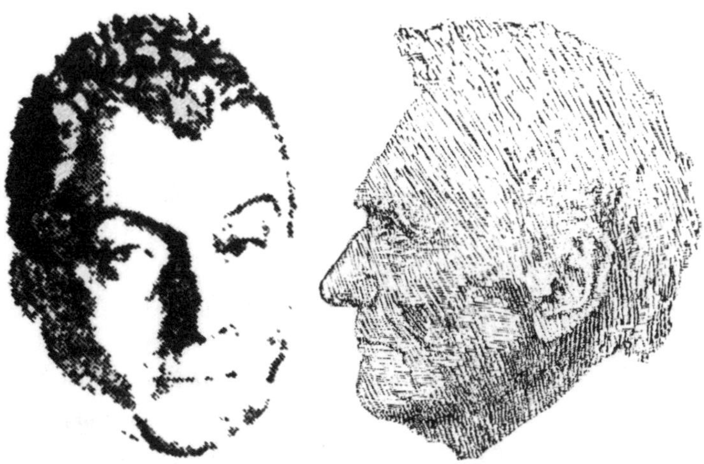

Figure 6.11
Left, Ignaz Paul Vitalis Troxler (1780–1866) after an illustration in Attinger et al. (1932). Right, Jan Evangelista Purkinje (1787–1869) after a frontispiece illustration in Purkinje (1918).

effect has become associated almost exclusively with the disappearances of peripheral targets, but it is noteworthy that Troxler himself reported that the central fixation target disappeared after prolonged observation.

The last aspect was actually amplifying a point made a decade earlier by Erasmus Darwin; he described the perceptual fading of a centrally fixated pattern: 'On looking long on an area of scarlet silk of about an inch in diameter laid on white paper . . . the scarlet colour becomes fainter, till at length it entirely vanishes, though the eye is kept uniformly and steadily upon it' (Darwin, 1794, p. 19). Brewster (1818), on the other hand, maintained that fixated objects never disappeared, whereas peripheral ones did, even when viewed binocularly:

> When the eye is steadily fixed upon any object, this object will never cease to become visible; but if the eye is steadily directed to another object in its vicinity while it sees the first object indirectly, the first object will, after a certain time, entirely disappear, whether it is seen with one or both eyes, whatever be its form or colour, or its position with respect to the axis of vision. When the object is such as to produce its accidental colour before it vanishes, the accidental colour disappears, also, along with the object. (Brewster, 1818, p. 151)

The effect of peripheral fading was confirmed by Purkinje (1823*b*; Fig. 6.11, right): the patterns were replaced by cloudy streaks.

> I distributed several pieces of paper evenly on a dark ground, removed any lighting from the side of the eye, and fixated on the central piece. After a short time the pieces of paper started to disappear. I waited until the effect reached its maximum, blew the papers away, and saw the well-known cloudy streaks appear in motion, wander around and disappear in their usual way. This is related to the disappearance and reappearance of letters seen when one becomes sleepy while reading, because that is the best time to experience the cloudy circles. (Purkinje, 1823*a*, p. 78)

How he was able to conduct the experiment described is puzzling, since the act of blowing the pieces of paper away would have resulted in some eye or head movement, and such movements are known to restore faded images. Purkinje (1823*a*) described another aspect of careful fixation that was subsequently linked to visual acuity—the distortions that are attendant on viewing high spatial frequency gratings: 'During intense viewing of the parallel lines of an engraving one observes an oscillation of the lines which on closer inspection involves some being closer together and others farther apart, so that the lines appear in the form of waves' (p. 122). Helmholtz (1867*a*) interpreted this waviness to the lines falling over the elements of the retinal mosaic (see Wade, 2004*b*).

6.4.1 Stabilized retinal images

The demonstration of ocular instability during fixation appeared to create a problem for visual resolution if the eye–camera analogy was adopted. However, a possible advantage of such instabilities was speculated upon at an early stage. In his essay on distinct vision Jurin (1738) determined that measures of visual resolution differed with the stimuli employed. For example, a white line flanked by large black squares ceased to be resolved when a black line of the same dimensions was still visible. He suggested that this could be because of the 'instability of the eye'. He gave an even more telling example:

> For instance, The hour I. upon a dial-plate may be seen at such a distance, as the hours II, III, IIII. are not to be distinguished at, especially if the observer be in motion, as in a coach or on horseback, or even in a boat upon the water. This may easily be experienced in looking at a dial where the intervals between the black or gilt strokes are equal to the breadth of those strokes; and much more easily where the intervals are of a less breadth, which is a defect in large dials that are to be seen at a great distance. For in these, the intervals ought to be considerably broader than the strokes. Likewise, *AB*, is a compound object consisting of three parts, *viz*. the two black lines and the white line lying between them: But *CD* is a single object consisting of one black line only on a white ground: And *IK* is to be considered as a single object consisting of one white line only upon a black ground. Now in viewing either of these single objects, if the eye be imperceptibly moved, all the effect from that motion will be only, that the object will be painted upon a different part of the *retina*; but wherever it be painted, there will be but one picture, single and unconfounded with any other. But in viewing a compound object *AB*, if the eye be supposed to fluctuate ever so little, the image of one or other of the black lines will be shifted on to that part of the *retina*, which was before possessed by the white line; and this must occasion such dazzle in the eye, that the white line cannot be distinctly perceived and distinguished from the black lines, which by their continual fluctuation will alternately occupy the space of the white line, whence must arise an appearance of one broad dark line without any manifest separation. (Jurin, 1738, p. 151, original italics)

Jurin was not able to measure the instability of the eye but he did point to the aspect of vision to which such measurements would be directed—visual acuity. The instability of fixation could readily be demonstrated in the nineteenth century but the detailed characteristics of the eye movements required technological advances that were not then available. The photographic recording techniques developed by Dodge and others were not precise enough to resolve such small eye movements. From the early 1950s optical techniques were employed to measure such small eye movements and also to present stimuli that were optically stabilized on the retina; that is, they moved with movements of the eyes. Three research groups were very active in this initial phase, Ditchburn and Ginsborg at Reading University, and Riggs and Ratliff at Brown University, as was Barlow at Cambridge.

Ratliff and Riggs (1950) employed an optical lever system and photography to record the involuntary motions of the eye during fixation. They found small rapid motions of about 17.5 s of arc at 30–70 Hz, slow motions of irregular frequency and extent, slow drifts and rapid jerks. Barlow (1952) placed a droplet of mercury on the cornea and photographed the eye during motion and fixation; the instabilities during fixation were small but measurable. He confirmed his photographic measurements by comparing them with afterimages. At about the same time, Ratliff (1952) specifically investigated the effects of the instabilities on visual acuity. His conclusions were quite contrary to the speculations advanced by Jurin:

> Involuntary drifts of the visual axis during the presentation of the test object are clearly detrimental to monocular acuity; Relatively large amounts of the minute rapid tremor during presentation of the test object are a hindrance to monocular acuity. These findings are compatible with the assumption that acuity, as measured by a typical grating test object, depends upon simultaneous differential responses of adjacent receptors. They are not in agreement with the assumption that the small involuntary eye movements contribute to visual acuity by providing temporal variations in the stimulation of each receptor as it is exposed to various parts of the retinal image. (Ratliff, 1952, p. 171)

Two of the initial systems employed to stabilize images on the retina are shown in Fig. 6.12. Both used contact lenses on the eye with small mirrors attached to them from which images could be reflected. These devices were developments of the contact lens eye trackers described in Section 1.3.2.

Broadly similar results were reported by both groups. Ditchburn and Ginsborg (1952) used a disc subtending 1° separated into halves vertically. Luminance differences between the two parts were visible initially but disappeared after two or three seconds;

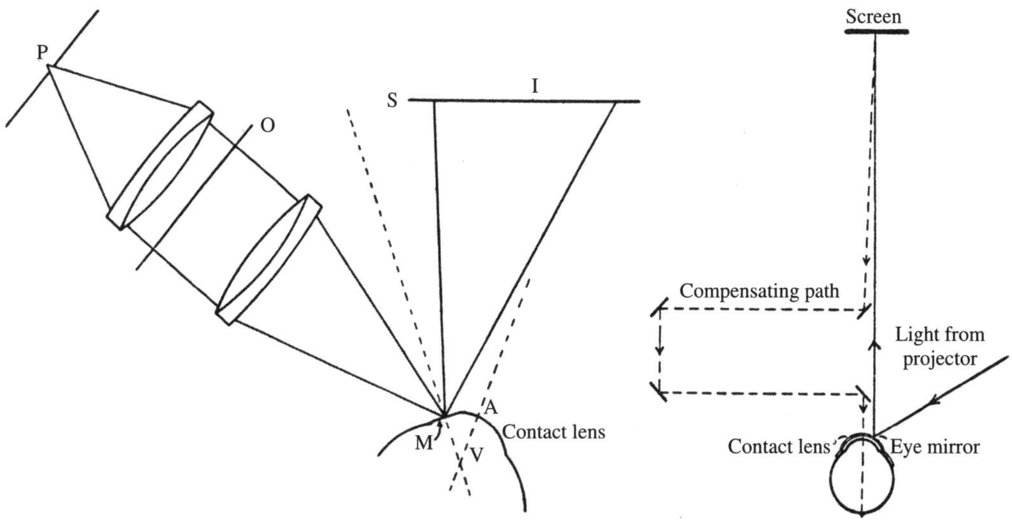

Figure 6.12
Left, the optical system employed by Ditchburn and Ginsborg (1952) for stabilizing an image on the retina; right, that used by Riggs et al. (1953).

the diffuse disc remained visible with occasional reappearances of the bipartite disc. Riggs et al. (1953) conducted more systematic experiments with line stimuli in a circular annulus; they found that the line faded and then disappeared all together. They also examined the effects of the involuntary eye movements on visual acuity. With very brief presentations (less than 0.1 s) acuity was superior with a stabilized image. Their succinct conclusion was 'that eye movements are bad for acuity but good for overcoming the loss of vision due to uniform stimulation of the retinal receptors' (Riggs et al., 1953, p. 501). Yarbus developed a fuller-fitting contact lens which retained its position by suction (see Fig. 1.10); the studies were published in Russian from the mid-1950s, and are summarized in Yarbus (1967). With his optical system he found that 'in any test field, unchanging and stationary with respect to the retina, all visible differences disappear after 1–3 sec, and do not reappear in these conditions' (Yarbus, 1967, p. 59).

The source of the differences between the various studies was examined by Barlow (1963). He used a full-fitting contact lens and a suction cap after the manner of Yarbus in order to compare their possible slippage; an afterimage was used as a perfectly stabilized target. The suction cap was more stable than the full-fitting contact lens, but neither was free from some slippage.

His conclusion was that 'Good-quality images stabilized as well as possible . . . "blur" and lose contrast rapidly: detail and texture cease to be visible, and do not reappear' (Barlow, 1963, p. 50).

Higgins and Stultz (1953) examined the minute involuntary tremor motions of the eye by photographing a blood vessel in the sclera (see Section 1.3.3): the tremors occurred with a frequency of 50 Hz and an average amplitude of 1.2 min of arc. Rapid technical advances were made thereafter (see Ditchburn, 1973), and attention was directed to the pattern characteristics of disappearances (see Pritchard, 1961). They resulted in a more accurate understanding of the involuntary eye movements, which have three components: high-frequency tremor, slow drifts, and microsaccades (see Fig. 6.13).

6.4.2 Entoptic phenomena

Barlow also drew attention to other naturally occurring stabilized images that have not received so much attention. One of these is called the Purkinje tree; it is the pattern of retinal blood vessels that lie over the receptors, and it can be rendered visible by shining light into the eye from the side. The phenomenon was described before Purkinje, and also appropriately interpreted before his account in 1823; Purkinje not only described them but also represented them graphically (Purkinje, 1823*a*; Wade and Brožek, 2001). Pecquet (1668) described the structure of the vessels in the context of Mariotte's (1668) contention that the retina

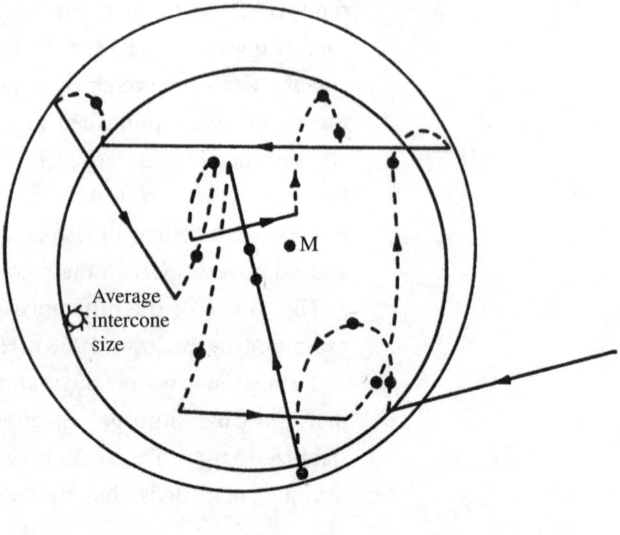

Figure 6.13
Involuntary eye movements during fixation. The high-frequency tremor is superimposed on the slow drifts (dashed lines), with intermittent microsaccades (after Ditchburn, 1973).

was not the receptive surface for vision. Pecquet's anatomical observations were detailed, but they seem to have been shrouded by the controversy over the blind spot, and not related to their observation. Bell's (1803) observations were more pertinent since he appreciated that the visible ramifications were shadows on the retina cast by the vessels. An even more precise description was provided by Wheatstone in his review of Purkinje's book (written over the initials C. W.):

> This is an easy experiment to repeat, and is certainly a singularly beautiful one; the blood-vessels of the retina, with all their ramifications, are distinctly seen projected, as it were, on a plane without the eye, and greatly magnified. I have found the experiment to work more perfectly when, the eye being stedfastly directed forwards, the light is made to move right and left below the eye, or upwards and downwards at the side of the eye; for when the flame is in the field of view the image is indistinct: the eyelids of the unemployed eye should not be closed, but the light should be obstructed by the hand or any other covering. It is indispensable that the light be in motion, for directly it becomes stationary the image breaks into fragments and disappears: during the motion of the light the image also moves, and in a contrary direction to that of the light... One of the most remarkable circumstances of this phenomenon is that the point corresponding to the foramen centrale, a crescent-image is occasionally observed... That the variable mark just mentioned is in the centre of distinct vision I ascertained by the following experiment: I impressed on my eye the spectrum [after-image] of a coloured wafer, by looking intently at a black dot at its centre; on causing then the vascular image to appear, I saw the centre of the spectrum coincide with that of the mark... The mark in the middle of the field of vision is most probably a shadow, occasioned by a slight convexity or concavity of the retina at that point... The absence of vessels at the centre of the retina will probably account for the greater distinctness with which small objects are there seen, and also for the difference of colour observed by anatomists in that part of the nervous expansion. (C. W., 1830, pp. 111–112)

Thus, Wheatstone directed a narrow, moving beam of light into the corner of the eye and noted that the shadows moved in the opposite direction to the light source; if the motion stopped the ramifications fragmented and disappeared. Of greater anatomical significance was the crescent-shaped shadow cast by the foramen centrale (fovea). He demonstrated that this region did correspond to the centre of the visual axis by generating a foveal afterimage and then locating it with respect to the crescent shadow. Thus he was using the afterimage as a stabilized retinal image in order to define the relative location of other retinal structures. He suggested a slightly different procedure for observing the finer vessels: a card with a large pinhole was moved by the side of the eye, so that diffuse light incident on its back surface could enter the eye. He could not see any vessels around the fovea, and his reference to the 'differences of colour observed by anatomists' was an allusion to Soemmerring's yellow spot. Later in the nineteenth century the Purkinje tree was used by Heinrich Müller (1855) to locate the various structures in the retina and to provide evidence of the fibres connecting the receptors with the ganglion cells. Ratliff (1971), in reviewing the impact of Purkinje's approach to subjective vision in general and to this phenomenon in particular, remarked that Purkinje's observations of the retinal blood vessels 'altered the character of the entire field of the study of mental phenomena' (p. 91). Modern studies of the visibility of retinal blood vessels can be found in Sharpe (1972) and Drysdale (1975*a*).

Entoptic phenomena, like the Purkinje tree, provided the basis for some of the earliest systematic studies of stabilized images. Brewster also pursued the branches of Purkinje's tree, but not with the sharpness of Wheatstone's intellect. Following a paper delivered to the British Association in 1832 by Brewster, Wheatstone (1832) described the best method of viewing the retinal blood vessels and then made the astute (italicized) generalizations:

> The experiment succeeds best in a dark room, when, one eye being excluded from the light, the flame of a candle is placed by the side of the unshaded eye, but so as not to occupy any of the central part of the field of view. So long as the flame of the candle remains stationary, nothing further occurs than a diminution of the sensibility of the retina to light; but after the flame has been moved upwards and downwards, through a small space, for a length of time, varying with the susceptibility of the individual on whom the experiment is tried, the phænomenon presents itself. The blood-vessels of the retina, with all their ramifications, exactly as represented in the engravings of Sœmmerring, are distinctly seen, apparently projected on a plane before the eye, and greatly magnified. The image continues only while the flame is in motion; directly, or soon after, the flame becomes stationary, it dissolves into fragments and disappears ... There was no difficulty in accounting for the image; it evidently was a shadow resulting from the obstruction of light by the blood-vessels spread over the retina; the real difficulty was to explain why this shadow is not always visible. To account for this Mr. W. adduced several facts, which tended to prove *that an object, either more or less luminous than the ground on which it is placed, when continuously presented to the same point of the retina, becomes invisible; and the rapidity of its disappearance is greater as the difference of luminous intensity between the object and the ground is less; but by continually shifting the place of the object on the retina, or by making it act intermittently on the same point, the object may be rendered permanently visible.* (Wheatstone, 1832, p. 550, original italics)

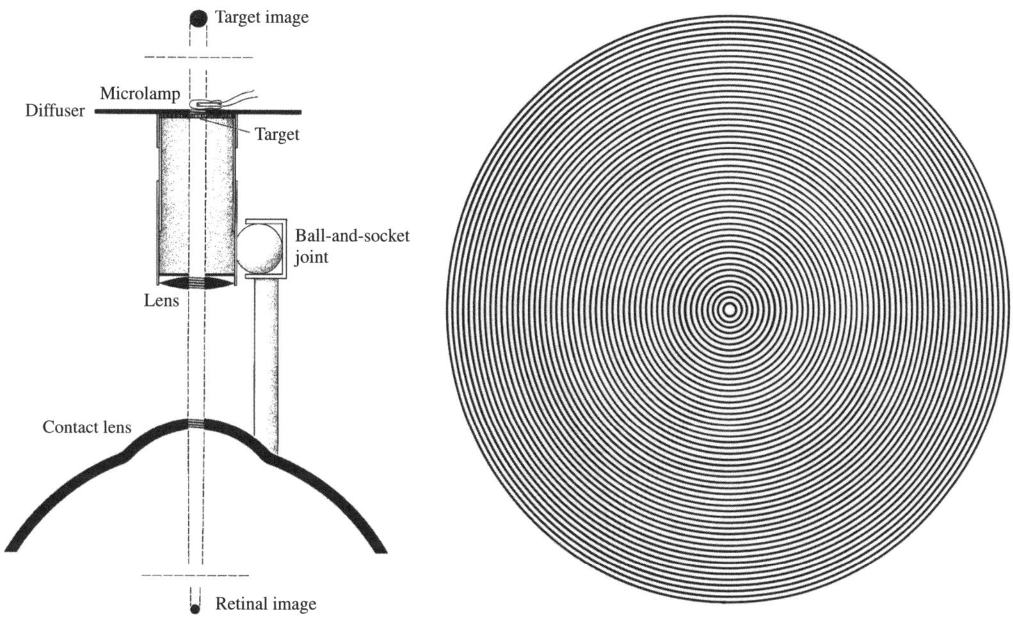

Figure 6.14
Left, the optical system employed for presenting complex patterns to the eye (after Pritchard, 1961). Right, a pattern of concentric circles that generates radiating spokes with unstabilized viewing. This particular pattern also contains a portrait of Purkinje, who first described the distortions (from Wade, 1995).

Another factor that distinguishes optically stabilized images from afterimages is that structures within the eye (like the lens) can modulate the image on the retina. This has proved particularly pertinent in studies of certain geometrical patterns, like concentric circles (see Fig. 6.14, right); when optically stabilized with an eye stalk device of the type developed by Pritchard (1958; Fig. 6.14, left) the radiations were still reported, but when viewed as an afterimage the pattern was visually stable (Evans and Marsden, 1966). The radiating spokes have been interpreted as reflecting transient changes in the axis of astigmatism due to variations in tension around the circumference of the lens (Millodot, 1968; Wade, 1982); these would not be influenced by optical image stabilization unless the lens was immobilized. In all probability, they could have amplified the motion over the retina due to transient astigmatism during optical stabilization because of the high degree of accommodation required.

Despite the differences in the degrees of image stabilization with afterimages, contact lens devices and steady fixation, these procedures have been found to yield similar patterns of disappearances when geometrical figures are viewed (MacKinnon et al., 1969; Wade, 1977, 1978). For example, the sides of an outline square tend to disappear as units under all conditions, although such effects are not free from response biases (see Swanston and Wade, 1981). Attention was subsequently directed to the factors involved in the patterns of fragmentation, rather than in the details of eye movements over such figures.

7

Summary and conclusions

7.1 Introduction

In an historical context, investigations of eye movements pose a paradox. On the one hand, they are a fundamental feature of our exploration of the world. We are aware that our own eyes move and we can readily observe movements in the eyes of those we observe. Indeed, eye movements are potent cues in social intercourse—we might see 'eye to eye' with someone, we might determine honesty when we 'look someone straight in the eye' or we might denigrate someone because they have a 'shifty look'. Moreover, we are exceedingly sensitive to binocular misalignments in the eyes of those who have squints. It is the binocular features of eye movements that were amongst the first aspects that were subject to scrutiny. In large part this was because a consequence of squinting is the disruption of binocular single vision, and this has been an overarching issue in the study of vision. On the other hand, throughout the long descriptive history of studies of eye movements a vital characteristic of them remained hidden from view, both in ourselves and in our observations of others. The rapid discontinuous nature of eye movements is a relatively recent discovery, as are the small involuntary movements that accompany fixation. For most of recorded history, the eyes were thought to glide over scenes to alight on objects of interest, which they would fix with unmoved accuracy.

In this book we have tried to indicate how changes in the understanding of eye movements came about. Some problems, like accommodation, became obvious as soon as the nature of light and the structure of the eye had been elucidated in the early seventeenth century. Interest in this aspect of internal eye movements was fostered by the analogy of the eye with a camera containing a lens of fixed curvature. On the one hand, the changes in the range of accommodation with ageing were well known and corrections were available for them from the late thirteenth century; individual differences in the range of accommodation, particularly short-sightedness, were commonplace. On the other hand, the manner in which a camera could focus on objects at nearer distances was a matter of common practice—either the length of the camera could be changed so that the lens moved away from the screen or the lens itself could be changed to another of greater curvature. These analogies informed theories of accommodation, and the theories vied with one another for over two centuries. When the elastic properties of lens were appreciated and the manner in which tension around it modulates its curvature was described by Cramer (1853) and Helmholtz (1855), interest shifted to its physiology rather than its psychology. That is, the mechanisms involved in accommodation assumed a greater significance than the functions that it served. Similar shifts in emphasis have occurred for movements of the pupil.

Experimental investigations of external eye movements lagged behind those of the internal movements. Occasional astute observations regarding their functions were made, as was the case for Porterfield (1737), but methods of lending substance to such speculations were wanting. It is to the development of novel methods that we now turn our eyes.

7.2 Emergence of methods for measuring eye movements

Another paradox in the study of eye movements is that initial knowledge about them derived from generating stimuli that did not move with respect to the eye when the eye moved. The first of these was the afterimage which, since the late eighteenth century, has been applied to determining the ways the eyes moved. More complex photographic recording devices appeared a century later, and the assistance of computers was incorporated three quarters of a century later still. Nonetheless, the insights derived from the skilful use of afterimages have tended to be overlooked in the histories of eye movements. One of the reasons that less attention has been paid to studies using afterimages is that they became tainted with other 'subjective' measures of eye movements as opposed to the 'objective' recording methods of the twentieth century. A second factor was that the early studies were concerned with vertigo, which resulted in involuntary movements of the eyes. Moreover, histories of vertigo have been similarly blind to the early studies of it employing afterimages.

These points apply particularly to the experiments conducted by Wells (1792), both in the context of voluntary and involuntary eye movements (see Wade, 2000*a*). In the case of voluntary eye movements, Wells demonstrated that afterimages appeared to move with active eye movements whereas they appeared stationary when the eye was moved passively (by finger pressure); this procedure became one of the critical tests of afference versus efference, of inflow versus outflow. Thus, the essential aspects of visual stability during eye movements were examined using afterimages, and the procedure was repeated throughout the nineteenth century. There was nothing novel about afterimages themselves at that time. Wells produced them by the time-honoured technique of viewing a bright stimulus (like a candle flame) for many seconds; the afterimage remained visible for long enough for him to examine its apparent movement under a range of conditions. One of these was vertigo generated by rotating the body around a vertical axis.

Porterfield (1759*b*) had argued that the visual motion that occurs when body rotation ceases was not a consequence of eye movements. His evidence was based on a truly subjective technique—the feeling that his eyes were not moving in the sockets following rotation. Porterfield was quite right, as Wells (1792) confirmed. That is, the eyes did not feel as though they were moving. However, Wells then adopted the simple expedient of observing the eyes of someone who stopped after revolving the body and noted that the eyes rotated slowly in one direction and rapidly in the other. This converging operation supported his conclusions based on afterimage motion. Moreover, Wells did not simply observe afterimages, but he compared them with real images visible simultaneously. When he directed the afterimage (following body rotation) to coincide with a point placed on a wall, the point and the afterimage moved slowly apart and then were suddenly superimposed, only for this sequence to be repeated for some cycles. This provided a means of measuring nystagmus, and Wells was able to relate the direction of the slow and fast phases to the orientation of the head during rotation.

Vertigo was also examined by Purkinje (1820), but he did not investigate eye movements with the rigour that had been adopted by Wells. Nonetheless, Purkinje (1820, 1825) did describe optokinetic nystagmus but it was not in the context of vertigo. He observed moving patterns for some time and then noted the motion aftereffects (in the opposite direction) that ensued. When observing a cavalry parade for a considerable time he realized that his eyes followed a particular rider and then moved rapidly in the opposite direction to pursue another. When he looked away from the cavalry parade he noticed that stationary objects appeared to move in the opposite direction to the parade. These he attributed to the continuing cyclical movements of the eyes. A similar observation was made following viewing descending water in a waterfall (Addams, 1834). Although optokinetic nystagmus was clearly described it was not measured with the skill that Wells had applied to eye movements in vertigo.

The major advance that Wells introduced to the measurement of eye movements was not just the use of afterimages as stabilized retinal images. Rather, it was the comparison of afterimages with real images. Wells applied this to determine the characteristics of eye movements. It could also be adopted to examine eye orientation by comparing the orientation of an afterimage formed in the primary position of the eye with vertical lines located in secondary and tertiary positions. This was the procedure introduced by Ruete (1845) and adopted by Helmholtz (1867*a*) and Hering (1879*a*). Eye rotations in tertiary positions are small relative to the large displacements that accompany vertigo, and it was the latter that led to the broader understanding of eye movements towards the end of the nineteenth century.

Wells' work was forgotten, but the techniques he pioneered were rediscovered by those scientists puzzling over the mechanisms of vestibular function. Mach (1873, 1875), Breuer (1874), and Crum Brown (1874, 1895*b*) all employed afterimages to measure the movements of the eyes after body rotation. They were able to link visual vertigo with their hydrodynamic theory of semicircular canal activity. Crum Bown forged the link between eye movements during vertigo and normal scanning of scenes; again afterimages were the tool used to demonstrate how scanning proceeds via a sequence of rapid movements interspersed with brief stationary pauses. Afterimages had been enlisted to attempt to examine eye movements during reading by Javal (1878*c*) but the contrast between the printed letters and paper made the afterimage difficult to discern. Novel methods were required and he was instrumental in trying some, but with little success. Javal's colleague, Lamare (1892), developed an indirect method that was more successful and yielded interesting and unexpected results. Lamare's technique was to use a tube attached to the eyelid or conjunctiva, from which sounds could be heard by the observer whenever the eyes moved. Using this technique, Lamare observed that, contrary to expectation and introspection, eye movements during reading were discontinuous. A very similar acoustic technique had been employed by Hering (1879*b*) to observe eye movements. However, Hering's technique had the added advantage of comparing the sounds thought to arise from eye movements to the movement of afterimages. Thus, Hering was able to confirm that the sounds coincided with movements of the afterimage and were therefore likely to be associated with eye movements.

As the nineteenth century ended and the twentieth began there was a proliferation of eye tracking technologies. Huey (1898, 1900) and Delabarre (1898) developed an eye tracker that used a lever attached to an eye-cup to record movements of the eyes on the surface of a smoked drum. Lever devices were limited by their mechanics; they applied additional force to the eye and their inertia resulted in considerable overshoots in the eye movement traces recorded. Alternative devices were developed rapidly in which direct attachment between eye and recording surface was not required. Orschansky (1899) attempted to record light reflected from a mirror attached to the surface of an eye-cup and variants of this principle were used throughout the twentieth century. An alternative to recorded light reflected from an eye-cup, or other attachment on the surface of the eye, was to record light reflected directly from the surface of the eye itself. The key figure in the development of such devices was Dodge (Dodge, 1903, 1904; Dodge and Cline, 1901). Photographic devices that required no attachment on the eye were more comfortable for the participants and many of the modern eye trackers are based on this principle.

The objective eye trackers developed in the late nineteenth and early twentieth centuries allowed crucial new insights into the true nature of eye movements (see Venezky, 1977). Researchers were unanimously surprised by what they found; eye movements were not as smooth and continuous as they subjectively appeared. With these new devices for measuring eye movements so began a proliferation of interest in the nature of eye movements. The technological advancements allowed new questions to be addressed and indeed identified new and unexpected questions in the psychology and physiology of eye movements and their relation to cognition and visual experience. Eye tracking technology continues to evolve, and with it so do the range of questions that we can address.

7.3 Eye movement and eye position

Wells' technique for studying eye movements was to stabilize an image on the retina and then to compare its apparent motion and position with that of a real image. By this means he was able to establish the rudiments of eye movements like the fast and slow phases of nystagmus and saccadic suppression (although he did not use these terms). His afterimage method (when rediscovered independently by Ruete) proved to be the standard technique adopted in the nineteenth century. However, it was not enlisted to examine eye movements but to measure eye position. This was epitomized in Helmholtz's (1867*a*) lengthy treatment of eye movements in volume 3 of his *Handbuch*. His coverage of eye movements, like those in vertigo, was not only cursory, but it was not even in the section entitled 'Movements of the eyes'. For Helmholtz and his contemporaries, eye movements were synonymous with eye position following an eye movement, that is, with eye orientation in tertiary positions of the eye or with differing degrees of convergence.

It could be argued that contemporary concern with eye movements shows a similar preoccupation with eye position. The saccade-and-fixate strategy that is subject to such detailed scrutiny in tasks like reading is much more concerned with the characteristics of fixation that with those of saccades (other than noting their size and direction). However, the very stability of eye position during fixation has been shown to be less than precise. The first indications of this instability derived from the movements of afterimages with attempts at fixation. Robert Darwin (1786) commented on this, and his observations were given greater substance when contact lens devices provided more precise measures of positional deviation. Several research groups in the early 1950s were able to chart the tremor, drift, and microsaccades that accompany attempts to maintain fixation. When doubts about the stability of the contact lenses themselves were voiced by Barlow (1963), it was the afterimage that provided the index of perfect stabilization. Moreover, patterned afterimages were employed thereafter to study the perceptual fragmentation that occurs when geometrical figures are stabilized on the retina.

7.3.1 Saccadic and pursuit eye movements

Where researchers did consider eye movements, it was, for much of history, pursuit movements that they dwelt upon; rapid, discontinuous saccadic eye movements were largely neglected until the end of the nineteenth century. The reasons for this focus upon pursuit, yet neglect of saccadic movement might have arisen because the former is available to our awareness and introspection, whereas the latter is not. As Dodge pointed out, introspection does not reveal the true nature of saccadic eye movements: 'If the observer takes the precaution to have some one watch his eyes, as recommended, he will find that what in self-observation passes for a slow movement of the eyes is in reality broken by one or more clearly defined full stops' (Dodge, 1900, p. 457). In contrast, it was easy to introspect upon the nature of pursuit eye movements. Moving objects often elicit eye movements in their pursuit, and over two thousand years ago Euclid discussed this in the context of an array of objects moving at different speeds: *If, when several objects move at unequal speed, the eye also moves in the same direction, some objects, moving with the same speed as the eye, will seem to stand still, others, moving more slowly, will seem to move in the opposite direction, and others, moving more quickly, will seem to move ahead.* (Burton, 1945, p. 371, original italics)

Why is it that we are aware that our eyes can pursue a moving target, yet we are unaware of saccades, which form the vast majority of the eye movements that we make in daily life? One reason is that clear vision continues throughout pursuit, but is suspended during saccades. It is possible to observe one's own eyes during pursuit; for example, one can look at one's own eyes in the mirror and then turn the head from side to side and observe the movements of the eyes in the socket. In contrast, we cannot normally observe our own saccades:

> when the head was held perfectly still we could never catch our own eye moving in a mirror. One may watch one's eyes as closely as possible, even with the aid of a concave reflector, whether one looks from one eye to the other, or from some more distant object to one's own eyes, the eyes may be seen now in one position and now in another, but never in motion. (Dodge, 1900, p. 456)

It is only recently that a technique has been described that allows observers to see their own saccades (Tatler and Trościanko, 2002). This technique exploits the Pulfrich pendulum phenomenon (Morgan and Thompson, 1974; Pulfrich, 1922). Pulfrich found that if a dark filter was placed in front of one eye, then, after a short time, a swinging pendulum would appear to move in an elliptical orbit. This is because the filter causes slight dark adaptation in the filtered eye, and this dark adaptation results in slight delays in the retinal and cortical signalling pathway. Because the unfiltered eye remains light adapted, there arises a temporal asynchrony between the signals from the two eyes. Tatler and Trościanko (2002) showed that the same principle can be used to reveal saccades, in conjunction with Erdmann and Dodge's (1898) simple self-observation technique using a mirror. If observers look at their own eyes in the mirror, but place a neutral density filter in front of one eye, then after sufficient time to dark adapt the filtered eye, they are able to catch a glimpse of their own saccades if they look from one eye to the other. This simple demonstration not only provides, as far as we know, the first glimpse of our eyes during saccades, but also has implications for the likely mechanisms of saccadic suppression. For the technique to be possible, suppression cannot be entirely due to retinal factors, such as mechanical shearing forces on the photoreceptors during movement (e.g. Castet and Masson, 2000; Castet, et al., 2001). Clearly, central factors must also be involved. It is interesting to note that even today techniques based upon careful self-observation and upon simple techniques employed over a century previously can offer useful insights into modern debates about eye movements.

While, for some time, saccadic eye movements were overlooked theoretically because they are overlooked perceptually, once they had been recognized, there followed a rapid proliferation of studies investigating them. Rapid rotations of the eye had been observed in nystagmus by Wells in 1792, but it was not until the late nineteenth century that it was realized that these movements were a general class of eye movement that occurred in many viewing situations. Javal is popularly accredited with being the first to describe saccades in reading, yet his description was in the form of a brief footnote highlighting the work of his colleague Lamare (Javal, 1879*e*). It is to Lamare (1892) and Hering (1879*b*) that much of the credit for this initial discovery should be accorded. Why, then, has their contribution been so overlooked? In the case of Lamare, it would appear that Javal's description of his work has overshadowed Lamare's actual report of it; perhaps due in part to Huey's (1908) influential text book, and, later to Woodworth's (1938), in both of which the work is accredited to Javal. In the case of Hering (1879*b*), the reasons are less clear. Perhaps his small article in which he described his technique for recording eye movements and made his crucial observations about their discontinuity, was overshadowed by the large chapter that he also published the same year in Hermann's *Handbuch der Physiologie* (Hering 1879*a*).

In the years that followed the descriptions offered by Javal, Hering, and Lamare, interest in saccades accelerated rapidly. Key early researchers in the field included the likes of Crum Brown, Dodge, Huey, Delabarre, Stratton, Judd, and Buswell. The discrepancies between the nature of eye movements (and therefore the retinal input for vision) and our subjective experience of vision became increasingly apparent and the work highlighted numerous new questions and directions in eye movement research. This critical period of research and thought revolutionized our understanding of vision and defined the direction of eye movement research to this day.

7.4 Normal and abnormal eye movements

Throughout this book we have focused on the normative aspects of eye movements on the basis that an adequate understanding of abnormalities is dependent upon establishing a normal baseline. Nonetheless, certain abnormalities have been described because their study was initiated so early and because they were evident from their perceptual consequences; the principal such condition has been strabismus. Deviations of one eye from the other have been remarked upon since antiquity and operations have been carried out to correct the misalignment since then and masks have been applied to assist the process. Concern with strabismus also reflected the central position that binocular eye movements have assumed: normal vision is binocular and the consequent perception is singular despite the two views of the world. These states can be disrupted by strabismus, and equivalent diplopia can be induced in those with normal vision by passively displacing one eye while keeping both open.

Several of the significant figures mentioned in the previous chapters who have advanced our understanding of eye movements also examined strabismus. For example Porterfield (1737) listed six possible causes of the condition, and Wells (1792) examined its theoretical implications regarding binocular visual direction, as did Helmholtz (1867*a*). Javal was led to the study of ophthalmology because both his father and sister had squints. Indeed, Javal is better known in ophthalmology for his work on squint than that on eye movements and reading. Duke-Elder remarked that Javal: 'will always remain one of the great figures in French and world ophthalmology, and, by recognizing the central anomaly in the development of squint and introducing the partnership of functional education and operative aid in its treatment, he revolutionized and set on a firm basis our knowledge of this subject'. (Duke-Elder, 1949, p. 3811)

Strabismus can now be detected using a variety of tests and it is dissected into many subcategories depending upon the muscle systems involved or the neural systems that are functioning abnormally (see Noorden, 1996). The range of categories is such that committees sit to set suitable systems of classification.

The same can be said of the other aspects of eye movements that have been described in previous chapters. For example, we have indicated how the discovery of nystagmus following body rotation resulted in the first evidence that eye movements can be discontinuous, with slow rotations in one direction and then rapid returns. The demonstration of such discontinuities was a great achievement, and subtle distinctions about the waveforms of the phases is a more modern preoccupation. When Crum Brown illustrated the saw-tooth curves of nystagmus during and after body rotation (see Fig. 4.11, right) there was little thought about different patterns of slow phase movements which are now known to exist. Moreover, the distinction between pendular and jerky nystagmus was not then recognized. Abnormal patterns of nystagmus can now be related to a variety of neural sources (Leigh and Zee, 1999). Despite this trend to increasing specialization, Carpenter's (1991) survey of normal and abnormal eye movements effectively divides them into two categories—gaze-holding and gaze-shifting. The examination of the historical origins of all abnormal eye movements is beyond the scope of this book, but would certainly be worthy of more detailed scrutiny.

7.5 Sleep and wakefulness

This book has not only concentrated on normal eye movements but also those that occur during wakefulness. Experiments have typically required observers to maintain fixation or to perform particular tasks (like reading), which result in eye movements. Despite the fact that sleep was surveyed by one of the prominent figures in eye movement research (Purkinje, 1846), the discovery of patterns of eye movements during different stages of sleep is relatively recent. Aserinsky and Kleitman (1953) reported that the eyes moved rapidly at certain periods during sleep. This could be observed directly by the movements of the eyes beneath the eyelids, but it could be recorded more precisely by electro-oculography and there were also correlated changes in the electro-encephalogram. The related discovery that dreams were more likely to be reported when people were awoken during rapid eye movement (REM) sleep led to an explosion of research (see Jouvet, 2001). However, the interests were not directed to the eye movements themselves but rather to their application as an index of dreaming. One change that is relevant to our considerations is that the proportion of sleep during which REM occurs is much higher in babies. It is to the developmental dimension that we now turn.

7.6 Developmental trends

An aspect of infant eye movements that was of early concern was binocular alignment. As Bartisch (1583) noted, treatment for strabismus should be introduced as soon after detection of the deviation as possible, and the chances of realignment are far higher for children than for adults. This developmental factor was of theoretical importance too. If muscular action was to inform vision of the spatial dimension of distance, as Berkeley (1709) argued, then any disruption in normal coordination between the eye muscles would have consequences for spatial vision. It is this aspect that led Hartley (1749) and Darwin (1778) to ruminate over strabismus. Hartley described a range of phenomena that was taken to support the close integration between sensation and action and they tended to be in the areas of the development of binocular single vision. For example, he remarked that 'new born Children move their Eyes in a congruous Manner; that the Motions are chiefly to the Right and Left, scarce upwards and downwards at all' (p. 216), but then speculated on the causes of squinting:

> The Circumstances which occasion Squinting in young Children, agree well with the Theory proposed here. Thus, if a Child be laid so into his Cradle, as that one Eye shall be covered, the external Influences of Light cannot operate upon it. And if this be often repeated, especially while the Association which confirms the Congruity of the Motions is weak, the Eye which is covered will obey the Influences which descend from the Brain, and turn upwards and inwards for the most part. What turns the Scale in favour of this Position, remains to be inquired. . . . The persons who squint, preserving the Sight of the squinting Eye, are obliged to move their Eyes in a congruous manner. (Hartley, 1749, pp. 218–221)

If the onset of strabismus occurs in adulthood then double vision results, but 'this ceases, and he gains the Power of seeing single again, provided the Distortion remains fixed to a certain Degree. For the Association between Points of the two *Retina's*, which corresponded formerly, grows weaker by degrees; a new one also between Points that now correspond, takes place, and grows stronger perpetually' (pp. 205–206, original italics).

In similar vein, Erasmus Darwin (1778) treated a five year-old boy with alternating dominance by constructing an artificial nose with a single hole through which the boy should look. Darwin considered that the treatment 'will, I believe, by resolute perseverance, entirely correct this unsightly deformity' (1778, p. 96). He did not, however, comment later whether his belief was justified. Squinting was not only a medical condition that warranted treatment but it provided a naturally occurring example of retinal noncorrespondence to which theories could be addressed.

It pointed to the importance of early experience and training, and it emphasized the integration of the senses. These ideas were not integrated into the emerging discipline of psychology, however.

In the late nineteenth century it was not thought that a great deal could be learned from studying vision in infants. This was famously expressed by William James whose views are often repeated because they were so wrong. His conclusion was based on the observation of their seemingly random and chaotic movements of the limbs and the eyes. More detailed study indicated that some aspects of behaviour were systematic and they could be used to determine what attracts the interests of infants. Many novel methods were devised to study infant vision in the 1960s. For example, it was noted that infants spent different amounts of time fixating on visual patterns and so infant perceptual discrimination was inferred from the patterns of preferential fixation. Recordings of eye movements in infants only a few days old showed that they were concentrated on contours or corners of simple patterns.

Contour extraction was also considered to be one of the first tasks tackled by the visual systems of newborns, and many novel methods were devised to study them. Fantz (1961) inferred infant perceptual discrimination from the patterns of differential fixation. He even suggested that there was an innate preference for viewing human faces, although the outline figures he used as stimuli had very little ecological validity, but his suggestions have generally been confirmed (see Johnson et al., 1991). Salapatek and Kessen (1966) recorded eye movements of infants only a few days old and found that they were concentrated on contours or corners. Subsequent research has shown that infants develop adult-like patterns of eye movements at an early age (see Atkinson, 2000; Hainline, 1993, 1998). For example, the dynamics of saccades are evident soon after birth and opto-kinetic nystagmus is present at birth; smooth pursuit takes a little longer to develop and vergence eye movements longer still.

7.7 Perceptual and cognitive processes

One of the main themes throughout this book has been that studies of eye movements have been stimulated by visual phenomena. The principal one has been the knowledge that visual acuity falls off rapidly with eccentric retinal stimulation. Writers on optics from Euclid onwards have commented on this, and it is a phenomenon that is independent of the theory of light that is adopted. It applied if light was thought to be emitted from the eye or if light was received by it. However, it was not until the seventeenth and eighteenth centuries that embryonic studies of eye movements were entertained. Porterfield (1737, 1759*b*), in particular, emphasized the necessity of moving the eyes over a scene in order to be aware of its contents; moreover the eye movements were rapid. His words are worth repeating:

> [In] viewing any large Body, we are ready to imagine that we see at the same Time all its Parts equally distinct and clear: But this is a vulgar Error, and we are led into it from the quick and almost continual Motion of the Eye, whereby it is successively directed towards all the Parts of the Object in an Instant of Time. (Porterfield, 1737, p. 186)

Porterfield was able to appeal to the 'quick and almost continual Motion of the Eye' but he was not able to measure it. In fact, the method that he employed when interpreting the visual motion that follows body rotation was the muscular feeling in his orbits. It was Wells' distrust of such subjective indices of eye movements that resulted in his adoption of afterimages as a measure. By this means he was able to chart the phases of nystagmus. Thus, the phenomenon of visual vertigo was another perceptual goad to the investigation of eye movements.

Another visual phenomenon, the motion aftereffect, was the stimulus for describing opto-kinetic nystagmus. Purkinje (1820) applied it in accounting for the visual motion that is subsequently seen when viewing stationary objects. The lure of eye movements as interpretations of visual motion illusions was more widely adopted in the nineteenth century, particularly by Helmholtz (1867*a*). The interpretation was applied to a range of motion illusions, but it could only be sustained for visual vertigo. In general, eye movement theories were rejected on the basis of psychophysical experiments rather than by measurements of eye movements themselves.

Nonetheless, Porterfield's 'vulgar Error' was retained in precisely the areas he had railed against—surveying scenes and reading. Until almost the end of the nineteenth century, the eyes were believed to glide over scenes rather than move jerkily across them. The obvious characteristic of smooth pursuit eye movements could well have favoured this view. Javal (1878*c*) initially considered that the eyes glided along lines of text until he was convinced otherwise by his co-worker Lamare (1892). When Dodge (1900) applied his technical skills to recording eye movements during reading, the discontinuous pattern of eye movements was established firmly. Thereafter, the study of eye movements was concentrated on the task of reading. It could be said that from that time the impetus for eye movement studies stemmed from cognitive rather than perceptual concerns. With the increased understanding of saccade and fixate behaviour, it became clear that perceptual accounts, based primarily on the eye and its movements, were inadequate as accounts of visual experience. In order to address the question of visual experience the emphasis had to be shifted towards the cognitive; it was now necessary to consider how cognitive processes gave rise to visual experience. Eye movements still retained their central position in vision research as they offered objective tools for scrutinizing vision and understanding how the perceptual input might relate to the cognitive experience. Indeed it is for this reason that emphasis has shifted back from being centred upon eye movements themselves, to the earlier interest in the fixations that occur between them. The re-defining of the central issues in eye movement research arose alongside the understanding that clear vision was confined to fixations and was disrupted during saccades. Thus, to understand the relationship between perceptual input and visual cognition, it is to the fixations that we must look.

While much research considered eye movements in reading, some did continue to examine a wider range of stimuli. Stratton and Judd were the first to record eye movements while observers viewed patterns, line illusions, and simple forms (Judd, 1905*a*,*b*; Judd et al., 1905; Stratton, 1902, 1906). Buswell's (1935) seminal work on eye movements during picture viewing is often overlooked, yet it can be seen to raise and consider many of the issues that defined twentieth century eye movement research.

One of the earliest areas of research to be generated by the discovery of the saccade-and-fixate strategy and the proliferation of eye movement research at the start of the twentieth century, was the question of how our smooth and complete visual experience might arise from the discontinuous input supplied by the eye. Dodge and Holt debated the mechanisms that might underlie the suspension of vision during saccades (Dodge, 1900, 1905; Holt, 1903); this question remained throughout the twentieth century and was the topic of much research and interest. The possible nature of visual representation re-emerged as a crucial topic in eye movement research; an internal representation might serve to explain how the disjointed input from the eyes might be transformed into our smooth visual experience. Researchers in the twentieth century revisited traditional notions of visual representation, but were now armed with a greater understanding of the input supplied by the eyes.

The latter part of the twentieth century saw increasing interest in what might underlie the targeting of eye movements; are the eyes primarily reactive to external stimuli, or proactive in response to internal goals? Yarbus (1967) is typically regarded as the first to consider this relationship systematically. Yarbus showed an observer the same picture several times, but each time they were given different instructions prior to viewing it (including instructions such as to estimate the material worth of the people, to estimate their ages, or to remember the positions of objects). He found that the pattern of eye movements made by the observer was very different depending upon the instructions given. This was an elegant example of the fact that eye movement targeting can be influenced by our internal goals. It is rarely noted, however, that Buswell (1935) had also considered this question. Buswell found differences in the eye movements according to the instructions given to observers before viewing. While it was not investigated systematically, earlier researchers also found that eye movements did not relate as closely to the stimulus as would be expected if they were directed by it (e.g. Cameron and Steele, 1905; Judd, 1905*a*,*b*; Judd and Courten, 1905; Stratton, 1902, 1906).

In the last few decades, technologies that allowed eye movements to be recorded under more naturalistic, real world settings emerged. This provided a new tool for investigating the role of eye movements in everyday vision, and provided new insights into the operations of the eyes and vision. Real world studies have highlighted the intricate relationship between vision and action (see Findlay and Gilchrist, 2003).

Developments in computer technology in the twentieth century did not only widen the scope and improve the precision of eye trackers, but also provided researchers with new tools for analysing eye movements. There has been a proliferation of computational modelling approaches in eye movement research; for example, computational modelling techniques were used to study the image statistics selected at fixation and therefore gain new insights into the factors that might guide eye movements (see Parkhurst et al., 2002; Tatler, Baddeley et al., 2005).

Even after over a century of research since the discovery of saccades in normal viewing, the same questions that were identified by Dodge, Stratton, Judd, and Buswell define contemporary research. We still cannot answer the question of the link between the retinal input and our cognitive experience of vision. Over the years, the emphasis of particular aspects of this question has evolved. In the middle of the twentieth century, emphasis was placed upon explaining the processes involved in saccadic suppression. Later in the twentieth century emphasis moved towards real world experimentation and computational modelling and this has provided us with new tools to investigate questions set out for us by those who initially characterized saccades. As Lamare stated at the end of his important paper describing saccadic eye movements in reading: 'Although the results of this work are incomplete and do not support any theory, they may be useful to those who wish to pursue this interesting work' (Lamare, 1892, p. 361). Today, we continue to 'pursue this interesting work' and the prominence that it still assumes in vision research is clearly evident from the huge volume of modern literature devoted to the study of eye movements and their relationship with visual cognition.

7.8 Moving tablets—literature on eye movements

Books specifically devoted to eye movements are a relatively recent enterprise, but the wider literature on vision and ophthalmology contains many references to this topic. Indeed, the first book addressed specifically to ophthalmology (Bartisch, 1583) has been cited many times in the previous chapters. Nonetheless, histories of ophthalmology tend to stress the neglect of eye movements and their disorders in the period prior to the nineteenth century (e.g. Albert and Edwards, 1996; Duke-Elder, 1932).

There are now many tablets covering a range of eye movements the origins of which we have examined. Many of the books are edited and often contain proceedings of conferences. The fact that there are regular meetings to discuss eye movement research speaks to the vitality of the endeavour. For example, the European Conference on Eye Movements meets biennially, and its proceedings have often appeared as books (Becker et al., 1999; D'Ydewalle and van Rensbergen, 1993, 1994; Gale and Johnson, 1984; Groner et al., 1983; Findlay et al., 1995; Hyönä, Munoz et al., 2002; Hyönä, Radach et al., 2002; Luer and Lass, 1987; Luer et al., 1988; O'Regan and Levy-Schoen, 1987; Schmid and Zambarbieri, 1991). Other edited books include Chekaluk and Llewellyn (1992), Groner et al. (1990), Monty and Senders (1976), Senders et al. (1978), Radach et al. (2002, 2004), Rayner (1983, 1992), and Underwood (1998, 2005). The individual chapters in all these books provide elegant examples of the sophistication now applied to measuring eye movements and interpreting the results obtained. Handbooks are also a valuable resource as they provide a broader survey of the field (e.g. Hallett, 1986). Tablets penned by one or two hands are less common than they used to be when Yarbus (1967) and Ditchburn (1973) placed their own studies in a broader context. Welcome exceptions to this are the two editions of Carpenter's (1977, 1988) book, and Findlay and Gilchrist's (2003) integration of eye movements and vision within the context of particular theoretical ideas. Ebenholtz (2001) has related oculomotor activity to the processes of perception that underlie it. He has also provided an overview of the extensive research he and his colleagues have conducted on eye movements in the context of accommodation, convergence, motion sickness, perceptual constancy, visual direction, and orientation.

Whereas Erasmus Darwin was prepared to 'reduce the facts belonging to ANIMAL LIFE into classes, orders, genera, and species; and by comparing them with each other, to unravel the theory of diseases' (1794, p. 1, original capitals), there seems now to be a reluctance to launch a similar expedition into the restricted terrain of eye movements.

7.9 Conclusion

The title of this book is taken from a line in Erasmus Darwin's poem *The temple of nature*, and the verse in which it occurred was given at the close of Chapter 1. Accordingly, it seems fitting to turn again to the poem to conclude our survey of the seen. The verse, also from Canto 3 (lines 131–144), is referred to by Darwin as 'Vision is the Language of Touch', and it provides an apposite ending to a book that has sought to unite vision with eye movements:

> Slow could the tangent organ wander o'er
> The rock-built mountain and the winding shore;
> No apt ideas could the pigmy mite,
> Or embryon emmet, to the touch excite.
> But as each mass the solar ray reflects,
> The eye's clear glass the transient beams collects;
> Bends to their focal point the rays that swerve,
> And paints the living image on the nerve.
> So in some village-barn, or festive hall,
> The spheric lens illumes the whiten'd wall;
> O'er the bright field successive figures fleet,
> And motley shadows dance along the sheet.—
> Symbol of solid forms is colour'd light,
> And the mute language of the touch is sight.

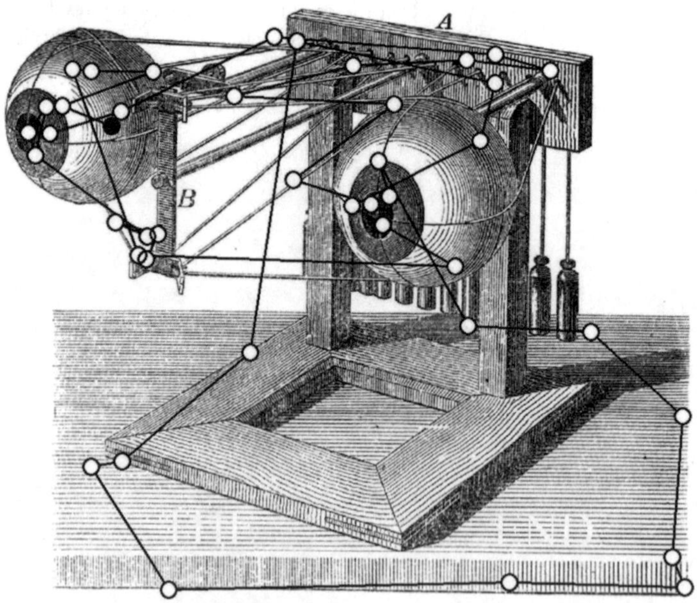
A
B
END

REFERENCES

Adams, H. F. (1912). The autokinetic sensations. *Psychological Review Monograph Supplement*, **14**, 1–45.

Addams, R. (1834). An account of a peculiar optical phænomenon seen after having looked at a moving body. *London and Edinburgh Philosophical Magazine and Journal of Science*, **5**, 373–374.

Adjouadi, M., Seslin, A., Ayala, M., and Cabrerizo, M. (2004). Remote eye gaze tracking system as a computer interface for persons with severe motor disability. In D. Burger, J. Klaus, K. Miesenberger, and W. Zagler (Eds.), *Computers helping people with special needs: 9th International Conference* (pp. 761–769). Berlin: Springer-Verlag.

Adler, F. H. and Fliegelman, M. (1934). Influence of fixation on visual acuity. *Archives of Ophthalmology*, **12**, 475–483.

Ægineta, P. (1844). *The seven books of Paulus Ægineta*. Vol. 1. (Trans. F. Adams) London: The Sydenham Society.

Aguilonius, F. (1613). *Opticorum libri sex. Philosophis juxta ac mathematicis utiles*. Moretus: Antwerp.

Ahrens, A. (1891). *Die Bewegung der Augen beim Schreiben*. Rostock: University of Rostock.

Aitken, J. (1878). On a new variety of ocular spectrum. *Proceedings of the Royal Society of Edinburgh*, **10**, 40–44.

Albert, D. M. and Edwards, D. D. (1996). *The history of ophthalmology*. Cambridge, MA: Blackwell Science.

Alhazen (1572). *Opticae Thesaurus*. F. Risner, (Ed.) Basel: Gallia.

Alpern, M. (1969). *Types of eye movement* In H. Davson (Ed.), *The eye*. Vol. 3. (pp. 65–163) New York: Academic Press.

Aquinas, T. (1256–1259/1994). Truth. (Trans. R. Mulligan, J. McGlynn, and R. Schmidt) Indianapolis, IN: Hackett.

Aquinas, T. (1266–1273/1963–1970). *Summa Theologicæ, Prima Pars*. Vols 1–15. (Trans. the Fathers of the English Dominican Province) Cambridge: Blackfriars.

Ariotti, P. E. (1973). A little known early seventeenth century treatise on vision: Benedetto Castelli's Discorso sopra la Vista. *Annals of Science*, **30**, 1–30.

Asch, M. G. (1995). *Gestalt psychology in German culture, 1890–1967. Holism and the quest for objectivity*. Cambridge: Cambridge University Press.

Aserinsky, E. and Kleitman, N. (1953). Regularly occurring periods of eye motility, and concomitant phenomena, during sleep. *Science*, **118**, 273–274.

Atkinson, J. (2000). *The developing visual brain*. Oxford: Oxford University Press.

Attinger, A., Godet, M., and Türler, H. (1932). *Dictionnaire Historique & Biographique de laSuisse*. Vol. 6. Neuchatel: Administration du Dictionnaire Historique et Biographique de la Suisse.

Aubert, H. (1865). *Physiologie der Netzhaut*. Breslau: Morgenstern.

Aubert, H. (1887). Die Bewegungsempfindungen. *Archiv für die gesammte Physiolologie des Menschen und der Tiere*, **40**, 459–480.

Augé, C. (Ed.) (1898). *Nouveau Larousse Illustré*. Paris: Libraire Larousse.

Ballard, D. H., Hayhoe, M. M., Li, F., Whitehead, S. D., Frisby, J. P., Taylor, J. G., and Fisher, R. B. (1992). Hand eye coordination during sequential tasks. *Philosophical Transactions of the Royal Society of London Series B-Biological Sciences*, **337**, 331–339.

Ballard, D. H., Hayhoe, M. M., and Pelz, J. B. (1995). Memory representations in natural tasks. *Journal of Cognitive Neuroscience*, **7**, 66–80.

Baloh, R. W. and Honrubia, V. (1990). *Clinical neurophysiology of the vestibular system*. (2nd edn.) Philadelphia, PA: Davis.

Bárány, R. (1906). Untersuchungen über den vom Vestibularapparat des Ohres reflektorisch ausgelösten rhythmischen Nystagmus und seine Begleiterscheinungen. *Monatsschrift für Ohrenheilkunde*, **40**, 193–297.

Bárány, R. (1913*a*). Der Schwindel und seine Beziehungen zum Bogengangapparat des inneren Ohres. Bogengangapparat und Kleinhirn. (Historische Darstellung. Eigene Untersuchungen.) *Naturwissenschaften*, **1**, 396–401.

Bárány, R. (1913*b*). Der Schwindel und seine Beziehungen zum Bogengangapparat des inneren Ohres. Bogengangapparat und Kleinhirn. (Historische Darstellung. Eigene Untersuchungen.) *Naturwissenschaften*, **1**, 425–428.

Barlow, H. B. (1952). Eye movements during fixation. *Journal of Physiology*, **116**, 290–306.

Barlow, H. B. (1963). Slippage of contact lenses and other artefacts in relation to fading and regeneration of supposedly stable retinal images. *Quarterly Journal of Experimental Psychology*, **15**, 36–51.

Barlow, H. B. and Hill, R. (1963). Evidence for a physiological explanation of the waterfall illusion and figural aftereffects. *Nature*, **200**, 1345–1347.

Bartisch, G. (1583). *ΟΦΘΑΛΜΟΔΟΥΛΕΙΑ. Das ist, Augendienst*. Dresden: Stockel.

Basler, A. (1910). Über das Sehen von Bewegungen. V. Mitteilung. Untersuchungen über die simultane Scheinbewegung. *Archiv für die gesammte Physiolologie des Menschen und der Tiere*, **132**, 131–142.

Baumann, C. (2002). *Der Physiologe Ewald Hering* (1834–1918). Frankfurt: Hänsel-Hohenhausen.

Becker, W., Deubel, H., and Mergner, T. (Eds.) (1999). *Current oculomotor research: physiological and psychological*. New York: Kulwer.

Bell, C. (1803). *The anatomy of the human body*. Vol. 3. London: Longman, Rees, Cadell and Davies. (Reprinted in N. J. Wade (2000). (Ed.) *The emergence of neuroscience in the nineteenth century*. Vol. 1. London: Routledge/Thoemmes Press.)

Bell, C. (1823). On the motions of the eye, in illustration of the uses of the muscles and of the orbit. *Philosophical Transactions of the Royal Society*, **113**, 166–186.

Bell, G. J. (Ed.) (1870). *Letters of Sir Charles Bell, selected from his correspondence with his brother George Joseph Bell*. London: John Murray.

Berkeley, G. (1709). *An essay towards a new theory of vision*. Dublin: Pepyat.

Berkeley, G. (1910). An essay towards a new theory of vision. In E. Rhys (Ed.) *A new theory of vision and other select philosophical writings by George Berkeley, bishop of Cloyne*. (pp. 1–86) London: J. M. Dent and Sons.

Berry, W. (1922). The flight of colors in the after-image of a bright light. *Psychological Bulletin*, **19**, 307–337.

Birch, T. (1743). *The heads of illustrious persons of Great Britain*. Vol. 1. London: Knapton.

Boissier de Sauvages, F. (1772a). *Nosologie méthodique, ou distribution des maladies en classes, en genres et en especes, suivant l'esprit de Sydenham, & la méthode des botanistes*. Vol. 4. Lyon: Bruyset.

Boissier de Sauvages, F. (1772b). *Nosologie méthodique, ou distribution des maladies en classes, en genres et en especes, suivant l'esprit de Sydenham, & la méthode des botanistes*. Vol. 7. Lyon: Bruyset.

Boring, E. G. (1942). *Sensation and perception in the history of experimental psychology*. New York: Appleton-Century.

Bourdon, B. (1898). La perception monoculaire de la profondeur. *Revue Philosophique*, **46**, 124–145.

Bourdon, B. (1902). *La perception visuelle de l'espace*. Paris: Librairie Schleincher Frères.

Bowditch, H. P. and Hall, G. S. (1881). Optical illusions of motion. *Journal of Physiology*, **3**, 297–307.

Boyle, R. (1663). *Experiments and considerations touching colours*. London: Herringman. (See also Boyle, R. (1996). *The works*. Vol. 1. T. Birch, (Ed). Hildesheim: Olms.)

Brandt, T. (1991). Man in motion. Historical and clinical aspects of vestibular function. A review. *Brain*, **114**, 2159–2174.

Brandt, T., Dietrich, M., and Strupp, M. (2004). *Vertigo and dizziness: common complaints*. New York: Springer.

Breitmeyer, B. G. and Ogman, H. (2000). Recent models and findings in visual backward masking: a comparison, review and update. *Perception and Psychophysics*, **62**, 1572–1595.

Breuer, J. (1874). Über die Function der Bogengänge des Ohrlabyrinthes. *Wiener medizinisches Jahrbuch*, **4**, 72–124.

Breuer, J. (1875). Beiträge zur Lehre vom statischen Sinne. *Wiener Medizinisches Jahrbuch*, **5**, 87–156.

Brewster, D. (1818). On a singular affection of the eye in the healthy state, in consequence of which it loses the power of seeing objects within the sphere of distinct vision. *Annals of Philosophy*, **11**, 151.

Brewster, D. (1826). Farther observations on the supposed optical and physiological discoveries of Mr. Charles Bell. *Edinburgh Journal of Science*, **5**, 259–268.

Brewster, D. (1832). On the undulations excited in the retina by the action of luminous points and lines. *Report of the British Association for the Advancement of Science. Transactions of the Sections*. Oxford Meeting. (pp. 548–551).

Brewster, D. (1844). On the knowledge of distance given by binocular vision. *Transactions of the Royal Society of Edinburgh*, **15**, 663–674.

Brewster, D. (1856). *The stereoscope. Its history, theory, and construction*. London: Murray.

Bridgeman, B. (1971). Metacontrast and lateral inhibition. *Psychological Review*, **78**, 528–539.

Bridgeman, B., Hendry, D., and Stark, L. (1975). Failure to detect displacement of the visual world during saccadic eye movements. *Vision Research*, **15**, 719–722.

Brindley, G. S. and Merton, P. A. (1960). The absence of position sense in the human eye. *Journal of Physiology*, **153**, 127–130.

Brown, T. (1798). *Observations on the Zoonomia of Erasmus Darwin, M.D.* Edinburgh: Mundell.

Brücke, E. (1841). Über die stereoskopischen Erscheinungen und Wheatstone's Angriff auf die Lehre von den identischen Stellen der Netzhäute. *Archiv für Anatomie und Physiologie*, 459–476.

Bryan, C. P. (1930). *The Papyrus Ebers*. London: Geoffrey Bles.

Buffon, Comte de (1743). Dissertation sur les couleurs accidentalles. *Mémoires de Mathématique et de Physique de l'Académie Royale des Sciences*. 147–158.

Burr, D. C., Morrone, M. C., and Ross, J. (1994). Selective suppression of the magnocellular visual pathway during saccadic eye-movements. *Nature*, **371**, 511–513.

Burton, H. E. (1945). The optics of Euclid. *Journal of the Optical Society of America*, **35**, 357–372.

Buswell, G. T. (1920). An experimental study of the eye-voice span in reading. *University of Chicago supplementary educational monographs no. 17*. Chicago, IL: University of Chicago Press.

Buswell, G. T. (1922). Fundamental reading habits: a study of their development. *University of Chicago supplementary educational monographs no. 21*. Chicago, IL: University of Chicago Press.

Buswell, G. T. (1926). *Diagnostic studies in arithmetic*. Chicago, IL: University of Chicago Press.

Buswell, G. T. (1935). *How people look at pictures: a study of the psychology of perception in art*. Chicago, IL: University of Chicago Press.

Buswell, G. T. (1937). *How adults read*. Chicago, IL: University of Chicago Press.

C. W. (1830). Contributions to the physiology of vision. *Journal of the Royal Institution*, **1**, 101–117. (Charles Wheatstone).

Cameron, E. H. and Steele, W. M. (1905). The Poggendorff illusion. *Psychological Monographs*, **7**, 83–111.

Canosa, R. L., Pelz, J. B., Mennie, N. R., and Peak, J. (2003). High-level aspects of oculomotor control during viewing of natural-task images. In B. E. Rogowitz and T. N. Pappas (Eds.), *Proceedings IS&T/SPIE 15th Annual Symposium on Electronic Imaging: Human Vision and Electronic Imaging VIII*. Vol. 5007. pp. 240–251.

Cantor, G. (1977). Berkeley, Reid, and the mathematization of mid-eighteenth-century optics. *Journal of the History of Ideas*, **38**, 429–448.

Carmichael, L. (1926). Sir Charles Bell: a contribution to the history of physiological psychology. *Psychological Review*, **33**, 188–217.

Carpenter, R. H. S. (1977). *Movements of the eyes*. London: Pion.

Carpenter, R. H. S. (1988). *Movements of the eyes*. (2nd edn.) London: Pion.

Carpenter, R. H. S. (Ed.) (1991). *Vision and visual dysfunction. Vol. 8. Eye movements*. London: Macmillan.

Carpenter, R. H. S. (2001). Express saccades: is bimodality a result of the order of stimulus presentation? *Vision Research*, **41**, 1145–1151.

Carr, H. A. (1910). The autokinetic sensation. *Psychological* Review, **17**, 42–75.

Caspar, M. (Ed.) (1938). *Johannes Kepler Gesammelte werke*. Vol. 1. Munich: Beck.

Castet, E. and Masson, G. S. (2000). Motion perception during saccadic eye movements. *Nature Neuroscience*, **3**, 177–183.

Castet, E., Jeanjean, S., and Masson, G. S. (2001). 'Saccadic suppression'—no need for an active extra-retinal mechanism. *Trends in Neurosciences*, **24**, 316–317.

Cattell, J. M. (1900*a*). On relations of time and space in vision. *Psychological Review*, **7**, 325–343.

Cattell, J. M. (1900*b*). Vision with the moving eye. *Psychological Review*, **7**, 507–508.

Charpentier, A. (1886). Sur une illusion visuelle. *Comptes Rendus*, **102**, 1155.

Chaudhuri, A. (1991). Eye movements and the motion aftereffect: alternatives to the induced motion hypothesis. *Vision Research*, **31**, 1639–1645.

Chekaluk, E. and Llewellyn, K. R. (Eds.) (1992). *The role of eye movements in perceptual processes*. Amsterdam: North-Holland.

Collewijn, H., Erkelens, C. J., and Steinman, R. M. (1997). Trajectories of the human binocular fixation point during conjugate and non-conjugate gaze-shifts. *Vision Research*, **37**, 1049–1069.

Comrie, J. D. (1932). *History of Scottish medicine*. Vol. 2. London: Baillière, Tindall and Cox.

Cornsweet, T. N. and Crane, H. D. (1973). Accurate two-dimensional eye tracker using first and fourth Purkinje images. *Journal of the Optical Society of America*, **63**, 921.

Cox, J. M. (1804). *Practical observations on insanity*. London: Baldwin and Murray.

Cramer, A. (1853). *Het accommodatie-vermogen, physiologisch toegelicht*. Haarlem: Loosjes.

Crombie, A. C. (1964). Kepler: De Modo Visionis. In Mélange Alexandre Koyré I. (Ed.), *L'Aventure de la Science*. (pp. 135–172). Paris: Hermann.

Crum Brown, A. (1874). Preliminary note on the sense of rotation and the function of the semicircular canals of the internal ear. *Proceedings of the Royal Society of Edinburgh*, **8**, 255–257.

Crum Brown, A. (1875). On the sense of rotation and the anatomy and physiology of the semicircular canals of the internal ear. *Journal of Anatomy and Physiology*, **8**, 327–331.

Crum Brown, A. (1878). Cyon's researches on the ear. Part II: *Nature*, **18**, 657–659.

Crum Brown, A. (1895*a*). The relation between the movements of the eyes and the movements of the head. *Nature*, **52**, 184–188.

Crum Brown, A. (1895*b*). *The relation between the movements of the eyes and the movements of the head*. London: Henry Frowde.

Currie, C. B., McConkie, G. W., Carlson-Radvansky, L. A., and Irwin, D. E. (2000). The role of the saccade target object in the perception of a visually stable world. *Perception and Psychophysics*, **62**, 673–683.

Darwin, C. (1887). *The life of Erasmus Darwin*. (2nd edn.) London: Murray.

Darwin, E. (1778). A new case in squinting. *Philosophical Transactions of the Royal Society*, **68**, 86–96.

Darwin, E. (1789). *The botanic garden; a poem, in two parts*. Lichfield: Jackson.

Darwin, E. (1791). *The botanic garden; a poem, in two parts*. London: Johnson.

Darwin, E. (1794). *Zoonomia; or, the Laws of Organic Life*. Vol. 1. London: Johnson.

Darwin, E. (1795). *Zoonomia, oder, Gesetze des organischen Lebens*. (Trans. J. D. von Brandis) Hannover: Hahn.

Darwin, E. (1796). *Zoonomia; or, the Laws of Organic Life*. Vol. 1. (2nd edn.) London: Johnson.

Darwin, E. (1801*a*). *Zoonomia; or, the laws of organic life*. Vol. 1. (3rd edn.) London: Johnson.

Darwin, E. (1801*b*). *Zoonomia; or, the laws of organic life*. Vol. 4. (3rd edn.) London: Johnson.

Darwin, E. (1803). *The temple of nature*. London: Johnson.

Darwin, R. W. (1786). New experiments on the ocular spectra of light and colours. *Philosophical Transactions of the Royal Society*, **76**, 313–348.

Davidson, M. L., Fox, M. J., and Dick, A. O. (1973). Effect of eye movements on backward masking and perceived location. *Perception and Psychophysics*, **14**, 110–116.

Delabarre, E. B. (1898). A method of recording eye movements. *American Journal of Psychology*, **9**, 572–574.

Desaguliers, J. T. (1719). *Lectures of experimental philosophy*. London: Mears, Creake, and Sackfield.

Descartes, R. (1637/1902). *La dioptrique*. In C. Adam and P. Tannery (Eds.), *Oeuvres de Descartes*. Vol. 6. (pp. 81–228) Paris: Cerf.

Descartes, R. (1662). *De homine figuris et latinitate*. (Trans. F. Schuyl) Leyden: Leffen and Moyardum.

Descartes, R. (1664/1909). *Traité de l'homme*. In C. Adam and P. Tannery (Eds.), *Oeuvres de Descartes*. Vol. 11. (pp. 119–215) Paris: Cerf.

Descartes, R. (1965). *Discourse on method, optics, geometry, and meteorology*. (Trans. P. J. Olscamp) Indianapolis, IN: Bobbs-Merrill.

Dewhurst, K. (1980). *Thomas Willis's Oxford lectures*. Oxford: Sandford.

Diamant, H. (1984). The Nobel prize award to Robert Bárány—a controversial decision? *Acta Otolaryngologica Supplement*, **406**, 1–4.

Diamond, M. R., Ross, J., and Morrone, M. C. (2000). Extraretinal control of saccadic suppression. *Journal of Neuroscience*, **20**, 3449–3455.

Dichgans, J. and Brandt, T. (1973). Optokinetic motion sickness and pseudo-coriolis effects induced by visual stimuli. *Acta Otolaryngologica*, **76**, 3339–3348.

Dichgans, J. and Brandt, T. (1978). Visual-vestibular interaction: effects on self-motion perception and postural control. In R. Held, H. W. Leibowitz, and H. -L. Teuber (Eds.) *Handbook of sensory physiology. Vol. VIII. Perception* (pp. 755–804). Sringer-Verlag, Berlin.

Diefendorf, A. R. and Dodge, R. (1908). An experimental study of the ocular reactions of the insane from photographic records. *Brain*, **31**, 451–489.

Dierig, S. (1994). Extending the neuron doctrine: Carl Ludwig Schleich (1859–1922) and his reflections on neuroglia at the inception of the neural-network concept in 1894. *Trends in Neurosciences*, **17**, 449–452.

Dirschel, H. and Lange (1956). Über den Frequenzgang der horizontalen Folgebewegungen des menschlichen Auges. *Pflüger's Archiv für die gesamte Physiologie des Menschen und der Tiere*, **262**, 307–333.

Ditchburn, R. W. (1973). *Eye-movements and visual perception*. Oxford: Clarendon Press.

Ditchburn, R. W. and Ginsborg, B. L. (1952). Vision with a stabilized retinal image. *Nature*, **170**, 36–37.

Dodge, R. (1900). Visual perception during eye movement. *Psychological Review*, **7**, 454–465.

Dodge, R. (1903). Five types of eye movement in the horizontal meridian plane of the field of regard. *American Journal of Physiology*, **8**, 307–329.

Dodge, R. (1904). The participation of eye movements and the visual perception of motion. *Psychological Review*, **11**, 1–14.

Dodge, R. (1905). The illusion of clear vision during eye movement. *Psychological Bulletin*, **2**, 193–199.

Dodge, R. (1907). An experimental study of visual fixation. *Psychological Review, Monograph Supplement*, **4**, 1–95.

Dodge, R. (1916). Visual motor functions. *Psychological Bulletin*, **13**, 421–427.

Dodge, R. (1921). A Mirror-recorder for photographing the compensatory movements of the closed eyes. *Journal of Experimental Psychology*, **4**, 165–174.

Dodge, R. (1923). Habituation to rotation. *Journal of Experimental Psychology*, **6**, 1–35.

Dodge, R. (1930). Raymond Dodge. In C. Murchison (Ed.) *A history of psychology in autobiography*. Vol. 1. (pp. 99–121) Worcester, MA: Clark University Press.

Dodge, R. and Cline, T. S. (1901). The angle velocity of eye movements. *Psychological Review*, **8**, 145–157.

Dohlman, G. (1925). Physikalische und physiologische Studien zur Theorie des kalorischen Nystagmus. *Acta Oto-Laryngologica Supplement*, **5**, 1–196.

Dohlman, G. (1935). Towards a method for quantitative measurement of the functional capacity of the vestibular apparatus. *Acta Oto- Laryngologica Supplement*, **23**, 50–62.

Donders, F. C. (1847). Beitrag zur Lehre von den Bewegungen des menschlichen Auges. *Höllandischen Beiträge zu den anatomischen und physiologischen Wissenschaften*, **1**, 104–145.

Donders, F. C. (1864). *On the anomalies of accommodation and refraction of the eye*. (Trans. W. D. Moore) Boston, MA: Milford House.

Dove, H. W. (1841). Die combination der Eindrücke beider Ohren und beider Augen zu einem Eindruck. *Monatsberichte der Berliner preussische Akademie der Wissenschaften*, **41**, 251–252.

Drysdale, A. E. (1975*a*). The visibility of retinal blood vessels. *Vision Research*, **15**, 813–818.

Drysdale, A. E. (1975*b*). The movement after-effect and eye movements. *Vision Research*, **15**, 1171.

Du Laurens, A. (1596/1599/1938). *A discourse of the preservation of the sight: of melancholic diseases; of rheumes, and of old age*. (Trans. R. Surphlet) London: The Shakespeare Association.

Du Laurens, A. (1613). *Toutes les oeuvres de M*$^{E.}$ *André du Laurens*. Paris: Mettayer.

Duchowski, A. T. (2003). *Eye tracking methodology: theory and practice*. London: Springer-Verlag.

Duke-Elder, S. (1932). *Text-book of ophthalmology. Vol. 1. The development, form and function of the visual apparatus*. London: Kimpton.

Duke-Elder, S. (1949). *Text-book of ophthalmology. Vol. IV. The neurology of vision. Motor and optical anomalies*. London: Kimpton.

Duke-Elder, S. and Abrams, D. (1970). *System of ophthalmology, Vol. 5. Ophthalmic optics and refraction*. London: Kimpton.

Duke-Elder, S. and Wybar, K. (1973). *System of ophthalmology, Vol. 6. Ocular motility and strabismus*. London: Kimpton.

Duncker, K. (1929). Über induzierte Bewegung (Ein Beitrag zur Theorie optisch wahrgenommener Bewegung). *Psychologische Forschung*, **12**, 180–259.

Dvorak, V. (1870). Versuche über die Nachbilder von Reizveränderungen. *Sitzungsberichte der Wiener Akademie der Wissenschaften*, **61**, 257–262.

D'Ydewalle, G. and van Rensbergen, J. (Eds.) (1993). *Perception and cognition: advances in eye movement research*. Amsterdam: North-Holland.

D'Ydewalle, G. and van Rensbergen, J. (Eds.) (1994). *Visual and oculomotor functions: advances in eye movement research*. Amsterdam: North-Holland.

Ebenholtz, S. M. (2001). *Oculomotor systems and perception*. Cambridge: Cambridge University Press.

Eccles, J. C. and Gibson, W. C. (1979). *Sherrington. His life and thought*. Berlin: Springer.

Ehrenstein, W. (1925). Versuche über die Beziehungen zwischen Bewegung- und Gestaltwahrnehmung. Erste Abhandlung. *Zeitschrift für Psychologie*, **96**, 305–352.

Emmert, E. (1881). Grössenverhältnisse der Nachbilder. *Klinische Merkblatt der Augenheilkunde*, **19**, 443–450.

Erdmann, B. and Dodge, R. (1898). *Psychologische Untersuchungen über das Lesen auf experimenteller Grundlage*. Halle: Niemeyer.

Evans, C. R. and Marsden, R. P. (1966). A study of the effect of perfect retinal stabilization on some well-known visual illusions, using the after-image as a method of compensating for eye movements. *British Journal of Physiological Optics*, **23**, 242–248.

Exner, S. (1875). Über das Sehen von Bewegungen und die Theorie des zusammengesetzten Auges. *Sitzungsberichte der Wiener Akademie der Wissenschaften*, **72**, 156–190.

Exner, S. (1887). Einige Beobachtungen über Bewegungsnachbilde. *Centralblatt für Physiologie*, **1**, 135–140.

Exner, S. (1894). *Entwurf zu einer physiologischen Erklärung der psychischen Erscheinungen*. Vienna: Deuticke.

Exner, S. (1896). Über autokinetische Empfindungen. *Zeitschrift für Psychologie und Physiologie der Sinnesorgane*, **12**, 313–330.

Fantz, R. L. (1961). The origin of form perception. *Scientific American*, **204**, 66–72.

Faraday, M. (1831). On a peculiar class of optical deception. *Journal of the Royal Institution*, **1**, 205–223.

Farid, M., Murtagh, F., and Starck, J. L. (2002). Computer display control and interaction using eye-gaze. *Journal of the Society for Information Display*, **10**, 289–293.

Fechner, G. T. (1838). Ueber eine Scheibe zur Erzeugung subjectiver Farben. *Annalen der Physik und Chemie*, **45**, 227–232.

Fechner, G. T. (1860). *Elemente der Psychophysik*. Leipzig: Breitkopf and Härtel.

Fick, A. (1854). Die Bewegungen des menschlichen Augapfels. *Zeitschrift für rationelle Medizin*, **4**, 109–128.

Figuier, L. (1866). *Vies des savants illustres*. Paris: Librairie Internationale.

Findlay, J. M. (1981). Local and global influences on saccadic eye movements. In D. F. Fisher, R. A. Monty, and J. W. Senders (Eds.), *Eye movements: cognition and visual perception* (pp. 171–179). Hillsdale, NJ: Lawrence Erlbaum Associates.

Findlay, J. M. (1997). Saccade target selection during visual search. *Vision Research*, **37**, 617–631.

Findlay, J. M. and Gilchrist, I. D. (2003). *Active vision: the psychology of looking and seeing*. Oxford: Oxford University Press.

Findlay, J. M. and Walker, R. (1999). A model of saccade generation based on parallel processing and competitive inhibition. *Behavioral and Brain Sciences*, **22**, 661–721.

Findlay, J. M., Walker, R., and Kentridge, R. W. (Eds.) (1995). *Eye movement research: Mechanisms, processes and applications*. Amsterdam: Elsevier.

Finger, S. and Wade, N. J. (2002). The neuroscience of Helmholtz and the theories of Johannes Müller. Part 2: Sensation and perception. *Journal of the History of the Neurosciences*, **11**, 234–254.

Fink, G. R., Marshall, J. C., Weiss, P. H., and Zilles, K. (2001). The neural basis of vertical and horizontal line bisection judgements: an fMRI study of normal volunteers. *NeuroImage*, **14**, S59–S67.

Flourens, M. P. J. (1824). *Recherches expérimentales sur les propriétés et les fonctions du système nerveux dans les animaux vertébrés*. Paris: Baillière.

Flourens, M. P. J. (1830). Expériences sur les canaux semi-circulaires de l'orielle. *Mémoires de l'Académie Royale des Sciences*, **9**, 455–466.

Flourens, M. P. J. (1842). *Recherches expérimentales sur les propriétés et les fonctions du système nerveux dans les animaux vertébrés*. (2nd edn.) Paris: Baillière.

Ford, A., White, C.T., and Lichtenstein, M. (1959). Analysis of eye movements during free search. *Journal of the Optical Society of America*, **49**, 287–292.

Franklin, B. (1765/1970). Letter to Lord Kames. In A. H. Smyth (Ed.) *The Writings of Benjamin Franklin. Volume IX. 1783–1788*. New York: Haskell House.

Franz, S. I. (1899). After-images. *Psychological Review, Monographs Supplement*, **3**, 1–61.

Fraser, A. C. (1871). *Life and letters of George Berkeley, D.D. formerly Bishop of Cloyne; and an account of his philosophy*. Oxford: The Clarendon Press.

Freher, P. (1688). *Theatrum virorum eruditione clarorum*. Nuremburg: Hofmann.

Fulton, J. F. (Ed.) (1966). *Selected readings in the history of physiology*. (2nd edn.) Springfield, IL: Thomas.

Furman, J. M. and Cass, S. P. (2003). *Vestibular disorders. A case-study approach*. (2nd edn.) New York: Oxford University Press.

Gale, A. G. and Johnson, F. (Eds.) (1984). *Theoretical and applied aspects of eye movement research*. Amsterdam: Elsevier.

Gibson, J. J. (1950). *The perception of the visual world*. Boston, MA: Houghton Mifflin.

Gibson, J. J. (1966). *The senses considered as perceptual systems*. Boston, MA: Houghton Mifflin.

Gibson, J. J. (1979). *The ecological approach to visual perception*. Boston, MA: Houghton Mifflin.

Gilchrist, I. D. and Harvey, M. (2000). Refixation frequency and memory mechanisms in visual search. *Current Biology*, **10**, 1209–1212.

Gitelman, D. R., Parrish, T. B., LaBar, K. S., and Mesulam, M. -M. (2000). Real-time monitoring of eye movements using infrared video-oculography during functional magnetic resonance imaging of the frontal eye fields. *NeuroImage*, **11**, 58–65.

Gogel, W. C. (1977). Independent motion induced in separate portions of the visual field. *Bulletin of the Psychonomic Society*, **10**, 408–410.

Goltz, F. (1870). Ueber die physiologische Bedeutung der Bogengänge des Ohrenlabyrinths. *Archiv für die gesammte Physiologie*, **3**, 172–192.

Goltz, H. C., DeSouza, J. F. X., Menon, R. S., Tweed, D. B., and Vilis, T. (2003). Interaction of retinal image and eye velocity in motion perception. *Neuron*, **39**, 569–576.

Griffith, C. R. (1920). The organic effects of repeated bodily rotation. *Journal of Experimental Psychology*, **3**, 15–47.

Griffith, C. R. (1922). *An historical survey of vestibular equilibration*. Urbana, IL: University of Illinois Press.

Grimes, J. (1996). On the failure to detect changes in scenes across saccades. In K. Atkins (Ed.), *Perception: Vancouver studies in cognitive science*. Vol. 2. (pp. 89–110) New York: Oxford University Press.

Groner, R., Menz, C., Fisher, D. F., and Monty, R. A. (Eds.) (1983). *Eye movements and psychological functions: international views*. Hillsdale, NJ: Erlbaum.

Groner, R., D'Ydewalle, G., and Parham, R. (Eds.) (1990). *From eye to mind: Information acquisition in perception, search, and reading*. Amsterdam: North-Holland.

Guilford, J. P. and Dallenbach, K. M. (1928). A study of the autokinetic sensation. *American Journal of Psychology*, **40**, 83–91.

Guitton, D., Büchtel, H. A., and Douglas, R. M. (1985). Frontal lobe lesions in man cause difficulties in suppressing reflexive glances and in generating goal-directed saccades. *Experimental Brain Research*, **58**, 455–472.

Hainline, L. (1993). Conjugate eye movements of infants. In K. Simons (Ed.), *Early visual development: normal and abnormal* (pp. 47–79). New York: Oxford University Press.

Hainline, L. (1998). Summary and commentary: eye movements, attention, and development. In: J. E. Richards (Ed.), *Cognitive neuroscience of attention: a developmental perspective* (pp. 163–178). Mahwah, NJ: Lawrence Erlbaum Associates.

Hall, T. S. (1972). *Treatise of man. René Descartes*. Cambridge, MA: Harvard University Press.

Hallett, P. E. (1986). Eye movements. In K. R. Boff, L. Kaufman, and J. P. Thomas (Eds.) *Handbook of perception and human performance. Vol 1. Sensory processes and perception* (pp. 10-1–10-112), New York: Wiley.

Harris, J. (1775). *A treatise of optics: Containing elements of the science; in two books*. London: White.

Hartley, D. (1749). *Observations on man, his frame, his duty, and his expectations. In two parts*. London: Richardson.

Hartridge, H. and Thompson, L. C. (1948). Methods of investigating eye movements. *British Journal of Ophthalmology*, **32**, 581–591.

Hayhoe, M. M., Bensinger, D. G., and Ballard, D. H. (1998). Task constraints in visual working memory. *Vision Research*, **38**, 125–137.

Haymaker, W. and Schiller, F. (Eds.) (1970). *The founders of neurology*. (2nd edn.) Springfield, IL: Thomas.

Hebb, D. O. (1949). *The organization of behavior*. New York: Wiley.

Hecht, H. (1993). *Pre-cinema history*. London: Bowker Saur.

Heine, L. (1905). Über Wahrnehmung und Vorstellung von Entfernungsunterschieden. *Albrecht von Graefes Archiv für klinische und experimentelle Opthamologie*, **61**, 484–498.

Heller, D. (1988). On the history of eye movement recording. In G. Lüer and J. Shallo-Hoffmann (Eds.), *Eye movement research. Physiological and psychological aspects* (pp. 37–51). Göttingen: Hogrefe.

Helmholtz, H. (1855). Ueber die Accommodation des Auges. *Archiv für Ophthalmologie*, **1**, 1–74.

Helmholtz, H. (1864). The Croonian Lecture. On the normal motions of the human eye in relation to binocular vision. *Proceedings of the Royal Society of London*, **13**, 186–199.

Helmholtz, H. (1867*a*). *Handbuch der physiologischen Optik*. In G. Karsten (Ed.), *Allgemeine Encyklopädie der Physik*. Vol. 9. Leipzig: Voss.

Helmholtz, H. (1867*b*). *Optique physiologique*. (Trans. L. É. Javal and N. T. Klein) Paris: Masson.

Helmholtz, H. (1873). *Popular lectures on scientific subjects*. (Trans. E. Atkinson) London: Longmans, Green.

Helmholtz, H. (1924*a*). *Helmholtz's treatise on physiological optics*. Vol. 1. (Trans. J. P. C. Southall) New York: Optical Society of America.

Helmholtz, H. (1924*b*). *Helmholtz's treatise on physiological optics*. Vol. 2. (Trans. J. P. C. Southall) New York: Optical Society of America.

Helmholtz, H. (1925). *Helmholtz's treatise on physiological optics*. Vol. 3. (Trans. J. P. C. Southall) New York: Optical Society of America.

Helmholtz, H. (2000). *Helmholtz's treatise on physiological optics*. 3 Vols. (Trans. J. P. C. Southall) Bristol: Thoemmes.

Henn, V. (1984). E. Mach on the analysis of motion sensation. *Human Neurobiology*, **3**, 145–148.

Herbert, S. (Ed.) (2000). *A history of pre-cinema*. Vol. 1. London: Routledge.

Hering, E. (1861). *Vom Ortsinne der Nethaut. Beiträge zur Physiologie*. Part 1. (pp. 1–80). Leipzig: Engelmann.

Hering, E. (1862). *Vom den identischen Nethautstellen. Beiträge zur Physiologie*. Part 2. (pp. 81–170). Leipzig: Engelmann.

Hering, E. (1863). *Vom Horopter. Beiträge zur Physiologie*. Part 3. (pp. 171–224). Leipzig: Engelmann.

Hering, E. (1864*a*). *Allgemeine geometrische Auflösung des Horopterproblems. Von der Bewegungen des menschlichen Auges. Beiträge zur Physiologie*. Part 4. (pp. 225–286). Leipzig: Engelmann.

Hering, E. (1864*b*). *Vom binocularen Tiefsehen. Kritik einer Abhandlung von Helmholtz über den Horopter. Beiträge zur Physiologie*. Part 5. (pp. 287–358). Leipzig: Engelmann.

Hering, E. (1879*a*). Der Raumsinn und die Bewegungen des Auges. In L. Hermann (Ed.), *Handbuch der Physiologie*. Vol. 3. Part 1: *Physiologie des Gesichtssinnes*. (pp. 343–601). Leipzig: Vogel.

Hering, E. (1879*b*). Über Muskelgeräusche des Auges. *Sitzberichte der kaiserlichen Akademie der Wissenschaften in Wien. Mathematisch-naturwissenschaftliche Klasse*, **79**, 137–154.

Hering, E. (1942). *Spatial sense and movements of the eye*. (Trans. C. A. Radde) Baltimore, MA: The American Academy of Optometry.

Herschel, J. F. W. (1833). *A treatise on astronomy*. London: Longman, Rees, Orme, Brown, Green and Longman.

Herz, M. (1786). *Versuch über den Schwindel*. Berlin: Voss.

Higgins, G. C. and Stultz, K. F. (1953). Frequency and amplitude of ocular tremor. *Journal of the Optical Society of America*, **43**, 1136–1140.

Hirsch, A. (Ed.) (1929). *Biographisches Lexikon der hervorragenden Ärzte aller Zeiten und Völker*. Vol. 4. Berlin: Urban and Schwarzenberg.

Hirschberg, J. (1899). Geschichte der Augenheilkunde. In Graefe-Saemisch (Ed.), *Handbuch der gesamten Augenheilkunde*. Vol. 12. Leipzig: Engelmann.

Hirschberg, J. (1908). Geschichte der Augenheilkunde. In Graefe-Saemisch (Ed.), *Handbuch der gesamten Augenheilkunde*. Vol. 13. Leipzig: Engelmann.

Hitzig, E. (1871). Ueber die beim Galvanisiren des Kopfes entstehenden Störungen der Muskelinnervation und der Vorstellung vom Verhalten im Raume. *Archiv für Anatomie, Physiologie und wissenschaftliche Medicin*, 716–771.

Hobbes, T. (1651/1996). Leviathan. In R. Tuck (Ed.), *Hobbes: Leviathan*. Cambridge: Cambridge University Press.

Hobbes, T. (1656/1839–1845). Elements of philosophy. In W. Molesworth (Ed.), *The English works of Thomas Hobbes of Malmesbury*. London: John Bohn.

Hodgson, T. L., Bajwa, A., Owen, A. M., and Kennard, C. (2000). The strategic control of gaze direction in the Tower of London task. *Journal of Cognitive Neuroscience*, **12**, 894–907.

Holland, H. C. (1965). *The spiral after-effect*. Oxford: Pergamon.

Hollingworth, A. and Henderson, J. M. (2002). Accurate visual memory for previously attended objects in natural scenes. *Journal of Experimental Psychology-Human Perception and Performance*, **28**, 113–136.

Holst, E. von (1957). Aktive Leistungen der menschlichen Gesichtswahrnehmung. *Studium Generale*, **10**, 231–243.

Holst, E. von and Mittelstaedt, H. (1950). Das Reafferenzprinzip. *Naturwissenschaften*, **37**, 464–476.

Holt, E. B. (1903). Eye movement and central anaesthesia. *Psychological Monographs*, **4**, 3–45.

Holt-Hansen, K. (1962). Oscillation experienced in perceived figures. *Historisk-filosfiske Meddelelser*, **39**, 1–48.

Home, E. (1794). Some facts relating to the late Mr. John Hunter's preparation for the Croonian Lecture. *Philosophical Transactions of the Royal Society*, **84**, 21–27.

Hooke, R. (1665). *Micrographia: or some physiological descriptions of minute bodies made by magnifying glasses with observations and inquiries thereupon*. London: Martyn and Allestry.

Hooke, R. (1705). *The posthumous works of Robert Hooke. M.D.* London: Waller.

Hopkins, A. A. (1898). *Magic: stage illusions and scientific diversions, including trick photography*. New York: Munn.

Howard, I. P. (1982). *Human visual orientation*. New York: Wiley.

Howard, I. P. (1986). The vestibular system. In K. R. Boff, L. Kaufman, and J. P. Thomas (Eds.), *Handbook of perception and human performance. Vol. 1. Sensory processes and perception* (pp. 11-1–11-30). New York: Wiley.

Howard, I. P. (1996). Alhazen's neglected discoveries of visual phenomena. *Perception*, **25**, 1203–1217.

Howard, I. P. (1999). The Helmholtz-Hering debate in retrospect. *Perception*, **28**, 543–549.

Howard, I. P. (2002). *Seeing in depth. Vol. 1. Basic mechanisms*. Toronto: Porteous.

Howard, I. P. and Rogers, B. J. (1995). *Binocular vision and stereopsis*. New York: Oxford University Press.

Howard, I. P. and Rogers, B. J. (2002). *Seeing in depth. Vol. 2. Depth perception*. Toronto: Porteous.

Howard, I. P. and Templeton, W. B. (1966). *Human spatial orientation*. London: Wiley.

Howard, I. P. and Wade, N. J. (1996) Ptolemy's contributions to the geometry of binocular vision. *Perception*, **25**, 1189–1202.

Hueck, A. (1838). *Die Achsendrehung des Auges*. Dorpat: Kluge.

Hueck, A. F. (1840). Über den Grenzen des Sehvermögens. *Müller's Archiv für Anatomie und Physiologie*, 82–94.

Huey, E. B. (1898). Preliminary experiments in the physiology and psychology of reading. *American Journal of Psychology*, **9**, 575–586.

Huey, E. B. (1900). On the psychology and physiology of reading. Part I: *American Journal of Psychology*, **11**, 283–302.

Huey, E. B. (1901). On the psychology and physiology of reading. Part II: *American Journal of Psychology*, **12**, 292–312.

Huey, E. B. (1908). *The psychology and pedagogy of reading*. New York: Macmillan.

Humboldt, A. von (1850). *Kosmos. Entwurf einer physischen Weltbeschreibung*. Vol. 3. Stuttgart: Cotta.

Hume, D. (1748/1902). An enquiry concerning human understanding. In L. A. Selby-Bigge (Ed.), *Hume's enquiries*. (2nd edn.) (pp. 5–175) Oxford: Clarendon Press.

Hunter, J. (1786). *Observations on certain parts of the animal oeconomy*. London: Published by the author.

Hyönä, J., Munoz, D., Heide, W., and Radach, R. (Eds.) (2002). *The brain's eye: neurobiological and clinical aspects of oculomotor research*. Amsterdam: Elsevier.

Hyönä, J., Radach, R., and Deubel, H. (Eds.) (2002) *The mind's eye: cognitive and applied aspects of eye movement research*. Amsterdam: Elsevier.

Ilg, U. J. and Hoffmann, K. P. (1993). Motion perception during saccades. *Vision Research*, **33**, 211–220.

Irwin, D. E. (1991). Information integration across saccadic eye-movements. *Cognitive Psychology*, **23**, 420–456.

Irwin, D. E. (1992). Visual memory within and across fixations. In K. Rayner (Ed.), *Eye movements and visual cognition: scene perception and reading* (pp. 146–165). New York: Springer-Verlag.

Irwin, D. E. (1993). Perceiving an integrated visual world. In D. E. Meyer and S. Kornblum (Eds.), *Attention and performance XIV: synergies in experimental psychology, artificial intelligence and cognitive neuroscience* (pp. 121–142). Cambridge, MA: MIT Press.

Irwin, D. E. and Zelinsky, G. J. (2002). Eye movements and scene perception: memory for things observed. *Perception and Psychophysics*, **64**, 882–895.

Irwin, D. E., Yantis, S., and Jonides, J. (1983). Evidence against visual integration across saccadic eye-movements. *Perception and Psychophysics*, **34**, 49–57.

Itti, L. and Koch, C. (2000). A saliency-based search mechanism for overt and covert shifts of visual attention. *Vision Research*, **40**, 1489–1506.

Jackson, J. H. and Paton, L. (1909). On some abnormalities of ocular movements. *Lancet*, **176**, 900–905.

Jacobson, E. (1930a). Electrical measurements of neuromuscular states during mental activities. Part I: Imagination of movement involving skeletal muscle. *American Journal of Physiology*, **91**, 567–608.

Jacobson, E. (1930b). Electrical measurements of neuromuscular states during mental activities. Part III: Visual imagination and recollection. *American Journal of Physiology*, **95**, 694–702.

James, W. (1882). The sense of dizziness in deaf-mutes. *American Journal of Otology*, **4**, 239–254.

James, W. (1890). *The principles of psychology*. Vol. 2. New York: Holt.

Javal, L. É. (1878*a*). Essai sur la physiologie de la lecture. *Annales d'Oculistique*, **79**, 97–117.

Javal, L. É. (1878*b*). Essai sur la physiologie de la lecture. *Annales d'Oculistique*, **80**, 135–147.

Javal, L. É. (1878*c*). Essai sur la physiologie de la lecture. *Annales d'Oculistique*, **80**, 240–274.

Javal, L. É. (1879*a*). Essai sur la physiologie de la lecture. *Annales d'Oculistique*, **81**, 61–73.

Javal, L. É. (1879*b*). Essai sur la physiologie de la lecture. *Annales d'Oculistique*, **81**, 157–162.

Javal, L. É. (1879*c*). Essai sur la physiologie de la lecture. *Annales d'Oculistique*, **82**, 72–81.

Javal, L. É. (1879*d*). Essai sur la physiologie de la lecture. *Annales d'Oculistique*, **82**, 159–170.

Javal, L. É. (1879*e*). Essai sur la physiologie de la lecture. *Annales d'Oculistique*, **82**, 242–253.

Javal, L. É. (1904). *Physiologie de la Lecture et de l'Écriture*. Paris: Alcan.

Javal, L. É. (1906). *Physiologie de la Lecture et de l'Écriture*. (2nd edn.) Paris: Alcan.

Javal, L. É. (1907). *Die Physiologie des Lesens und Schreibens*. (Trans. F. Haass) Leipzig: Engelmann.

Jeannerod, M., Gerin, P., and Rougier, J. (1966). Enregistrement bidimensional des mouvements et des pauses oculaires, a propros d'une nouvelle methode. *Review of Oto-Neuro-Ophthalmology*, **38**, 51–53.

Johansson, R. S., Westling, G. R., Backstrom, A., and Flanagan, J. R. (2001). Eye–hand coordination in object manipulation. *Journal of Neuroscience*, **21**, 6917–6932.

John, H. J. (1959). *Jan Evangelista Purkyně. Czech scientist and patriot. 1787–1869*. Philadelphia, PA: American Philosophical Society.

Johnson, M. H., Dziurawiec, S., Ellis, H., and Morton, J. (1991). Newborns' preferential tracking of face-like stimuli and its subsequent decline. *Cognition*, **40**, 1–19.

Johnson, S. P., Amso, D., and Slemmer, J. A. (2003). Development of object concepts in infancy: evidence for learning in an eye-tracking paradigm. *Proceedings of the National Academy of Science*, **100**, 10568–10573.

Jones, B. (1871). *The Royal Institution: its founder and its first professors*. London: Longmans, Green.

Jouvet, M. (2001). *The paradox of sleep: the story of dreaming*. (Trans. L. Garey) Cambridge, MA: MIT Press.

Judd, C. H. (1899). A study of geometrical illusions. *Psychological Review*, **6**, 241–261.

Judd, C. H. (1905*a*). The Müller-Lyer illusion. *Psychological Monographs*, **7**, 55–81.

Judd, C. H. (1905*b*). Movement and consciousness. *Psychological Monographs*, **7**, 199–226.

Judd, C. H. (1932). Charles H. Judd. In C. Murchison (Ed.), *A history of psychology in autobiography*. Vol. 2. (pp. 207–235) Worcester, MA: Clark University Press.

Judd, C. H. and Buswell, G. T. (1922). *Silent reading: a study of the various types*. Chicago, IL: University of Chicago Press.

Judd, C. H. and Courten, H. C. (1905). The Zöllner illusion. *Psychological Monographs*, **7**, 112–139.

Judd, C. H., McAllister, C. N., and Steele, W. M. (1905). General introduction to a series of studies of eye movements by means of kinetoscopic photographs. *Psychological Monographs*, **7**, 1–16.

Julesz, B. (1960). Binocular depth perception and computer-generated patterns. *Bell System Technical Journal*, **39**, 1125–1162.

Jurin, J. (1738). An essay on distinct and indistinct vision. In R. Smith (Ed.), *A compleat system of opticks in four books* (pp. 115–171). Cambridge: Published by the author.

Karn, K. S. and Hayhoe, M. M. (2000). Memory representations guide targeting eye movements in a natural task. *Visual Cognition*, **7**, 673–703.

Kepler, J. (1604). *Ad Vitellionem paralipomena*. Frankfurt: Marinium and Aubrii.

Kepler, J. (1611). *Dioptrice*. Augsburg: Franci.

Kim, J. (2004). A simple pupil-independent method for recording eye movements in rodents using video. *Journal of Neuroscience Methods*, **138**, 165–171.

King-Hele, D. (1999). *Erasmus Darwin: A life of unequalled achievement*. London: De La Mer.

King-Hele, D. (Ed.) (2002). *Charles Darwin's the life of Erasmus Darwin*, Cambridge: Cambridge University Press.

Kleiner, A. (1878). Physiologisch-optische Beobachtungen. *Archiv für die gesammte Physiolologie des Menschen und der Tiere*, **18**, 542–573.

Koelbing, H. M. (1967). *Renaissance der Augenheilkunde 1540–1630*. Bern: Huber.

Koenigsberger, L. (1902). *Hermann von Helmholtz*. Vol. 1. Vieweg: Braunschweig.

Köhler, W. (1942). *Dynamics in psychology*. London: Faber and Faber.

Kornhuber, H. H. (1974). Introduction. In H. H. Kornhuber (Ed.) *Handbook of sensory physiology, volume VI/1. Vestibular system. Part 1: Basic mechanisms.* (pp. 3–14). New York: Springer.

Kreidl, A. (1891). Beiträge zur Physiologie des Ohrenlabyrinthes auf Grund von Versuchen an Taubstummen. *Archiv für die gesammte Physiologie*, **51**, 119–150.

Krieger, G., Rentschler, I., Hauske, G., Schill, K., and Zetzsche, C. (2000). Object and scene analysis by saccadic eye-movements: an investigation with higher-order statistics. *Spatial Vision*, **13**, 201–214.

Kruta, V. (1964). *M.-J.-P. Flourens, J.-E. Purkyne et les débuts de la physiologie de la posture et de l'équilibre.* Paris: Alençonnaise.

Kruta, V. (1969). *J. E. Purkyně [1787–1869] physiologist. A short account of his contributions to the progress of physiology with a bibliography of his works.* Prague: Czechoslovak Academy of Sciences.

Küchle, H. J. (1982). In memoriam Aurel von Szily. Das Leben und Wirken eines grossen Ophthalmologen. *Historia Ophthalmologica Internationalis*, **2**, 231–261.

Kuntze, J. E. (1892). *Gustav Theodor Fechner (Dr. Mises). Ein deutsches Gelehrtenleben.* Leipzig: Breitkopf and Härtel.

La Hire, P. de (1685). Dissertation sur la conformation de l'oeil. *Journal des Sçavans*, **13**, 335–363.

La Hire, P. de (1694). Dissertation sur les differens accidens de la vue. In *Mémoires de Mathématique et de Physique.* (pp. 233–302) Paris: Anisson.

Lamansky, S. (1869). Bestimmung der Winkelgeschwindigkeit der Blickbewegung, respective Augenbewegung. *Archiv für die gesammten Physiologie des Menschen und der Tiere*, **2**, 418–422.

Lamare, M. (1892). Des mouvements des yeux dans la lecture. *Bulletins et Mémoires de la Société Française d'Ophthalmologie*, **10**, 354–364.

Land, M. F. (1993). *Eye–head coordination during driving.* Paper presented at the IEEE Systems, Man and Cybernetics, Le Touquet.

Land, M. F. and Hayhoe, M. M. (2001). In what ways do eye movements contribute to everyday activities? *Vision Research*, **41**, 3559–3565.

Land, M. F. and Lee, D. N. (1994). Where we look when we steer. *Nature*, **369**, 742–744.

Land, M. F. and McLeod, P. (2000). From eye movements to actions: how batsmen hit the ball. *Nature Neuroscience*, **3**, 1340–1345.

Land, M. F., Mennie, N., and Rusted, J. (1999). The roles of vision and eye movements in the control of activities of daily living. *Perception*, **28**, 1311–1328.

Landolt, E. (1879). *A manual of examination of the eyes.* (Trans. S. M. Burnett) London: Bailliere, Tindall, and Cox.

Landolt, E. (1891). Nouvelles récherches sur la physiologie des mouvements des yeux. *Archives d'Ophthalmologie*, **11**, 385–395.

Langenbeck, M. A. (1849). *Klinische Beiträge aus dem Gebiet Chirugie und Ophthalmologie.* Göttingen: Dieter.

Lavater, J. C. (1799). *Essays on physiognomy, designed to promote the knowledge and love of mankind.* Vol. 4. (Trans. H. Hunter) London: John Murray, Hunter, and Holloway.

Le Clerc, G., Count of Buffon. (1866). *Natural history, general and particular: containing the history and theory of the earth, a general history of man, the brute creation, vegetables, minerals, &c. &c.*, Vol. 1. (Trans. W. Smellie) London: Thomas Kelly.

Leigh, R. J. and Zee, D. S. (1999). *The neurology of eye movements*. (3rd edn.) New York: Oxford University Press.

Lejeune, A. (Ed.) (1956). *L'optique de Claude Ptolémée dans la version latine d'après l'arabe de l'Émir Eugène de Sicile*. Louvain: Université de Louvain.

Lesky, E. (1965). *Die Wiener medizinische Schule im 19. Jahrhundert*. Graz: Böhlaus.

Levi, D. M. and Schor, C. M. (1984). Spatial and velocity tuning of processes underlying induced motion. *Vision Research*, **24**, 1189–1196.

Levy, J. (1972). Autokinetic illusion: a systematic review of theories, measures and independent variables. *Psychological Bulletin*, **78**, 457–474.

Lindberg, D. C. (1968). The theory of pinhole images from antiquity to the thirteenth century. *Archive for History of Exact Sciences*, **5**, 154–176.

Lindberg, D. C. (Ed. and trans.)(1970). *John Pecham and the science of optics*. Madison, WI: University of Wisconsin Press.

Lindberg, D. C. (1976). *Theories of vision from Al-Kindi to Kepler*. Chicago: University of Chicago Press.

Lindberg, D. C. (1983). *Roger Bacon's philosophy of nature*. Oxford: Clarendon.

Listing, J. B. (1845). *Beiträge zur physiologischen Optik*. Göttingen: Vanderhoeck & Ruprecht.

Locke, J. (1690/1997). An essay concerning human understanding. In R. Woolhouse (Ed.), *John Locke: an essay concerning human understanding*. St. Ives: Penguin.

Lord, M. P. and Wright, W. D. (1948). Eye movements during monocular fixation. *Nature*, **162**, 25.

Lucretius, T. C. (1975). *De Rerum Natura*. (Trans. W. H. D. Rouse) Cambridge, MA: Harvard University Press.

Luer, G. and Lass, U. (Eds.) (1987). *Fourth European Conference on Eye Movements: proceedings*. Gottingen: Hogrefe and Huber.

Luer, G., Lass, U., and Shallo-Hoffman (Eds.) (1988). *Fourth European Conference on Eye Movements: proceedings volume 2: Eye movement research: physiological aspects*. Gottingen: Hogrefe and Huber.

MacDougall, H. G. (2003). Human eye-movement response to maintained surface galvanic vestibular stimulation. Doctoral dissertation, University of Sydney.

Mach, E. (1873). Physikalische Versuche über den Gleichgewichtssinn des Menschen. *Sitzungsberichte der Wiener Akademie der Wissenschaften*, **68**, 124–140.

Mach, E. (1874). Physikalische Versuche über den Gleichgewichtssinn des Menschen. *Sitzungsberichte der Wiener Akademie der Wissenschaften*, **69**, 121–135.

Mach, E. (1875). *Grundlinien der Lehre von den Bewegungsempfindungen*. Leipzig: Engelmann.

Mach, E. (1886). *Beiträge zur Analyse der Empfindungen*. Jena: Fischer.

Mach, E. (1897). *The analysis of the sensations and the relation of the physical to the psychical*. (Trans. C. M. Williams) New York: Open Court.

Mach, E. (1926). *The principles of physical optics. An historical and philosophical treatment*. (Trans. J. S. Anderson and A. F. A. Young) London: Methuen.

Mack, A. (1986). Perceptual aspects of motion in the frontal plane. In K. R. Boff, L. Kaufman, and J. P. Thomas (Eds.), *Handbook of perception and human performance. Vol 1. Sensory processes and perception* (pp. 17-1–17-38), New York: Wiley.

MacKay, D. M. (1970). Elevation of visual threshold by displacement of visual images. *Nature*, **225**, 90–92.

MacKinnon, G. E., Forde, J., and Piggins, D. J. (1969). Stabilized images, steadily fixated figures and prolonged after-images. *Canadian Journal of Psychology*, **23**, 184–195.

Mackworth, N. H. and Morandi, A. J. (1967). The gaze selects informative details within pictures. *Perception and Psychophysics*, **2**, 547–552.

Mackworth, N. H. and Thomas, E. L. (1962). Head-mounted eye-movement camera. *Journal of the Optical Society of America*, **52**, 713–716.

Magnus, H. (1901). *Die Augenheilkunde der Alten*. Breslau: Kern.

Malebranche, N. (1699/1742). Reflections on light and colours, and on the generation of fire. *The philosophical history and memoirs of the Royal Academy of Sciences at Paris*. Vol. 1. (Trans. J. Martyn and E. Chambers) (pp. 32–46). London: Knapton and Nourse.

Mannoni, L. (2000). *The great art of light and shadow. Archaeology of the cinema*. (Trans. R. Crangle) Exeter: University of Exeter Press.

Mariotte, E. (1668). A new discovery touching vision. *Philosophical Transactions of the Royal Society*, **3**, 668–669.

Mariotte, E. (1683). An account of two letters of Mr. Perrault and Mr. Mariotte, concerning vision. *Philosophical Transactions of the Royal Society*, **13**, 266–267.

Marr, D. (1982). *Vision: a computational investigation into the human representation and processing of visual information*. San Francisco, CA: Freeman.

Marx, E. and Trendelenburg, W. (1911). Uber die Genauigkeit der Einstellung des Auges beim Fixieren. *Zeitschrift fur Psychologie und Physiologie der Sinnesorgane—Abt 2: Zeitschrift fur Sinnesphysiologie*, **45**, 87.

Matin, E. (1974). Saccadic suppression: a review and an analysis. *Psychological Bulletin*, **81**, 899–917.

Matin, L. (1972). Eye movements and perceived visual direction. In D. Jameson and L. M. Hurvich (Eds.), *Handbook of sensory physiology, vol. VII/4, Visual Psychophysics* (pp. 331–380) Berlin: Springer.

May, M. T. (1968). *Galen. On the usefulness of the parts of the body*. Ithaca, NY: Cornell University Press.

McAllister, C. N. (1905). The fixation of points in the visual field. *Psychological Monographs*, **7**, 17–53.

McConkie, G. W. and Currie, C. B. (1996). Visual stability across saccades while viewing complex pictures. *Journal of Experimental Psychology: Human Perception and Performance*, **22**, 563–581.

McConkie, G. W. and Loschky, L. C. (2002). Perception onset time during fixations in free viewing. *Behavior Research Methods, Instruments & Computers*, **34**, 481–490.

McConkic, G. W. and Rayncr, K. (1976). Identifying the span of the effective stimulus in reading: literature review and theories of reading. In H. Singer and R. B. Ruddell (Eds.), *Theoretical models and processes of reading* (pp. 137–162). Newark, NJ: International Reading Association.

McConkie, G. W. and Zola, D. (1979). Is visual information integrated across successive fixations in reading? *Perception and Psychophysics*, **25**, 221–224.

McMurray, B., Spivey, M., and Aslin, R. (2000). The perception of consonants by adults and infants: categorical or categorised? In K. M. Crosswhite and L. S. Magnuson (Eds.), *University of Rochester working papers in the language sciences*. Vol. 1. pp. 215–256.

Ménière, P. (1861). Mémoire sur des lésions de l'oreille interne donnant lieu à des symptoms de congestion cérébrale apoplectiforme. *Gazette médicale de Paris*, **16**, 597–601.

Mersenne, M. (1651). *L'optique et la catoptrique*. Paris: Langlois.

Merton, P. A. (1961). The accuracy of directing the eyes and hand in the dark. *Journal of Physiology*, **156**, 555–577.

Meyerhof, M. (1928). *The book of the ten treatises on the eye, ascribed to Hunain ibn Is-Hâq* (809–877 AD). Cairo: Government Press.

Meyers, I. L. (1929). Electronystagmography. A graphic study of the action currents in nystagmus. *Archives of Neurology and Psychiatry Chicago*, **21**, 901–918.

Millodot, M. (1968). Influence of accommodation on the viewing of an optical illusion. *Quarterly Journal of Experimental Psychology*, **20**, 329–335.

Molesworth, W. (Ed.) (1839). *The English works of Thomas Hobbes*, Vol. 1. London: Bohn.

Monty, R. A. and Senders, J. W. (Eds.) (1976). *Eye movements and psychological processes*. Hillsdale, NJ: Erlbaum.

Moore, S. T., Curthoys, I. S., and McCoy, S. G. (1991). VTM: An image processing system for measuring ocular torsion. *Computer Methods and Programs in Biomedicine*, **35**, 219–230.

Moore, S. T., Haslwanter, T., Curthoys, I. S., and Smith, S. T. (1996). A geometric basis for measurement of three-dimensional eye position using image processing. *Vision Research*, **36**, 445–459.

Moore, T., Tolias, A. S., and Schiller, P. H. (1998). Visual representations during saccadic eye movements. *Proceedings of the National Academy of Sciences*, **95**, 8981–8984.

Morgan, M. J. and Thompson, P. (1974). Apparent motion and the Pulfrich effect. *Perception*, **4**, 3–18.

Mowrer, O. H., Ruch, R. C., and Miller, N. E. (1936). The corneoretinal potential difference as the basis of the galvanometric method of recording eye movements. *American Journal of Physiology*, **114**, 423.

Müller, H. (1855). Über die entoptische Wahrnehmung der Netzhautfässe, insbesonder als Beweissmittel für die Lichtperception durch die nach hintern gelegenen Netzhautelemente. *Verhandlungen der physikalische-medicinische Gesellschaft zu Würzburg*, **5**, 411–447.

Müller, J. (1826*a*). *Zur vergleichenden Physiologie des Gesichtssinnes des Menschen und der Thiere, nebst einen Versuch über die Bewegung der Augen und über den menschlichen Blick*. Leipzig: Cnobloch.

Müller, J. (1826*b*). *Über die phantastischen Gesichtserscheinungen*. Coblenz: Hölscher.

Müller, J. (1840). Handbuch der Physiologie des Menschen für Vorlesungen. Vol: 2. Coblenz: Hölscher.

Müller, J. (1843). *Elements of physiology*. Vol. 2. (2nd edn.) (Trans. W. Baly) London: Taylor and Walton.

Müller, J. (2003). *Müller's elements of physiology*. Bristol: Thoemmes.

Munsterberg, H. (1913). *Psychology and industrial efficiency*. Boston, MA: Houghton Mifflin.

Murchison, C. (Ed.) (1930). *A history of psychology in autobiography. Vol.* 1. Worcester, MA: Clark University Press.

Murchison, C. (Ed.) (1932). *A history of psychology in autobiography*. Vol. 2. Worcester, MA: Clark University Press.

Nagel, W. A. (1896). Über kompensatorische Raddrehungen der Augen. *Zeitschrift für Psychologie und Physiologie der Sinnesorgane*, **12**, 331–354.

Newhall, S. M. (1928). Instruments for observing ocular movements. *American Journal of Psychology*, **40**, 628–629.

Newton, I. (1691/1829). Letter to John Locke. In Lord King (Ed.), *The life of John Locke, with extracts from his correspondence, journals and common-place books*. London: Henry Colburn.

Newton, I. (1704). *Opticks: or, a treatise of the reflections, refractions, inflections and colours of light*. London: Smith and Walford.

Noorden, G. K. von (1996). *Binocular vision and ocular motility*. (5th edn.) St. Louis: Mosby.

Norn, M. and Jensen, O. E. (2004). Marius Tscherning (1854–1939): his life and work in optical physiology. *Acta Ophthalmologica Scandinavica*, **82**, 501–508.

Nuttin, J. (1961). *Psychology in Belgium*. Louvain: Studia Psychologica.

O'Leary, De L. (1949). *How Greek science passed to the Arabs*. London: Routledge.

Ockham, W. (1323/1974). *Ockham's theory of terms: part 1 of Summa Logicae*. (Trans. M. J. Loux) Notre Dame: University of Notre Dame Press.

Ogle, K. N., Mussey, F., and Prangen, A. H. (1949). Fixation disparity and the fusional processes in binocular single vision. *American Journal of Ophthalmology*, **32**, 1069–1087.

Ono, H. (1981). On Wells' 1792 law of visual direction. *Perception and Psychophysics*, **30**, 403–406.

Oppel, J. J. (1856). Neue Beobachtungen und Versuche über eine eigentümliche, noch wenig bekannte Reaktionsthätigkeit des menschlichen Auges. *Annalen der Physik und Chemie*, **99**, 540–561.

O'Regan, J. K. (1992). Solving the real mysteries of visual-perception—the world as an outside memory. *Canadian Journal of Psychology-Revue Canadienne de Psychologie*, **46**, 461–488.

O'Regan, J. K. and Levy-Schoen, A. (Eds.) (1987). *Eye movements: from physiology to cognition*. Amsterdam: Elsevier.

O'Regan, J. K. and Noë, A. (2001). A sensorimotor account of vision and visual consciousness. *Behavioral and Brain Sciences*, **24**, 939–973; discussion 973–1031.

O'Regan, J. K., Deubel, H., Clark, J. J., and Rensink, R. A. (2000). Picture changes during blinks: looking without seeing and seeing without looking. *Visual Cognition*, **7**, 191–211.

Orschansky, J. (1899). Eine Methode die Augenbewegungen direct zu untersuchen. *Centralblatt für Physiologie*, **12**, 785–790.

Pagel, J. (1901). *Biographisches Lexikon hervorragender Ärzte des neunzehnten Jahrhunderts*. Berlin: Urban & Schwarzenberg.

Paré, A. (1951). *The apologie and treatise of Ambroise Paré containing the voyages made into divers places with many of his writings upon surgery*. (G. Keynes Ed.) London: Falcon Educational Books.

Park, D. (1997). *The fire within the eye*. Princeton: Princeton University Press.

Parkhurst, D. J. and Niebur, E. (2003). Scene content selected by active vision. *Spatial Vision*, **16**, 125–154.

Parkhurst, D. J., Law, K., and Niebur, E. (2002). Modeling the role of salience in the allocation of overt visual attention. *Vision Research*, **42**, 107–123.

Pasnau, R. (Ed.) (2002). *The Cambridge translations of medieval philosophical texts. Volume 3: Mind and knowledge*. Cambridge: Cambridge University Press.

Pastore, N. (1971). *Selective history of theories of visual perception: 1650–1950*. New York: Oxford University Press.

Peckham, R. H. (1934). Foveal projection during ductions. *Archives of Ophthalmology*, **12**, 562–566.

Pecquet, A. (1668). Answer to Mr. Mariotte . . . *Philosophical Transactions of the Royal Society*, **3**, 669–671.

Pelz, J. B. and Canosa, R. (2001). Oculomotor behavior and perceptual strategies in complex tasks. *Vision Research*, **41**, 3587–3596.

Pettigrew, T. J. (1840*a*). *Medical portrait gallery*. Vol. 3. London: Whittaker.

Pettigrew, T. J. (1840*b*). *Medical portrait gallery*. Vol. 4. London: Whittaker.

Plateau, J. (1829). *Dissertation sur quelques propriétés des impressions produites par la lumière sur l'organe de la vue*. Liége.

Plateau, J. (1833). Des illusions sur lesquelles se fonde le petit appareil appelé récemment Phénakisticope. *Annales de Chimie et de Physique de Paris*, **53**, 304–308.

Plateau, J. (1836). Notice sur l'anorthoscope. *Bulletins de l'Académie Royale des Sciences et Belles-Lettres de Bruxelles*, **3**, 7–10.

Plateau, J. (1849). Quatrième note sur de nouvelles applications curieurses de la persistence des impressions de la rétine. *Bulletins de l'Académie Royale des Sciences, des Lettres et des Beaux-Arts de Bruxelles*, **16**, 254–260.

Plateau, J. (1850). Vierte Notiz über neue, sonderbare Anwendungen des Verweilens der Eindrücke auf die Netzhaut. *Annalen der Physik und Chemie*, **80**, 287–292.

Plateau, J. (1878). Bibliographie analytique des principaux phénomènes de la vision, depuis les temps anciens jusqu'a la fin du XVIIIe siècle. Première section. Persistance des impressions sur la rétine. *Mémoires de l'Académie Royale de Belgique*, **42**, 1–59.

Platter, F. (1583). *De corporis humani structura et usu*. Basel: König.

Pollatsek, A. and Rayner, K. (1992). What is integrated across fixations? In K. Rayner (Ed.), *Eye movements and visual cognition: scene perception and reading* (pp. 166–191) New York: Springer Verlag.

Pollatsek, A. and Rayner, K. (2002). Simple rotary motion is integrated across fixations. *Perception and Psychophysics*, **64**, 1120–1129.

Polyak, S. L. (1942). *The retina*. Chicago, IL: University of Chicago Press.

Polyak, S. L. (1957). *The vertebrate visual system*. Chicago, IL: University of Chicago Press.

Porterfield, W. (1737). An essay concerning the motions of our eyes. Part I: Of their external motions. *Edinburgh Medical Essays and Observations*, **3**, 160–263.

Porterfield, W. (1738). An essay concerning the motions of our eyes. Part II: Of their internal motions. *Edinburgh Medical Essays and Observations*, **4**, 124–294.

Porterfield, W. (1759*a*). *A treatise on the eye, the manner and phænomena of vision*. Vol. 1. Edinburgh, Hamilton and Balfour.

Porterfield, W. (1759*b*). *A treatise on the eye, the manner and phænomena of vision*. Vol. 2. Edinburgh, Hamilton and Balfour.

Post, R. B. and Leibowitz, H. W. (1985). A revised analysis of the role of efference in motion perception. *Perception*, **14**, 631–643.

Pritchard, R. M. (1958). Visual illusions viewed as stabilized retinal images. *Quarterly Journal of Experimental Psychology*, **10**, 77–81.

Pritchard, R. M. (1961). Stabilized images on the retina. *Scientific American*, **204**(5), 1–8.

Psotníčková, J. (1955). *Jan Evangelista Purkyně*. Prague: Orbis.

Pulfrich, C. (1922). Die Stereoskopie im Dienste der isochromen und heterochromen Photometrie. *Naturwissenschaften*, **10**, 553–564.

Purkinje, J. (1820). Beyträge zur näheren Kenntniss des Schwindels aus heautognostischen Daten. *Medicinische Jahrbücher des kaiserlich-königlichen öesterreichischen Staates*, **6**, 79–125.

Purkinje, J. (1823*a*). *Beobachtungen und Versuche zur Physiologie der Sinne. Beiträge zur Kenntniss des Sehens in subjectiver Hindicht*. Prague: Calve.
Purkinje, J (1823*b*). *De examine physiologico organi visus et systematis cutanei*. Breslau: University of Breslau.
Purkinje, J. (1825). *Beobachtungen und Versuche zur Physiologie der Sinne. Neue Beiträge zur Kenntniss des Sehens in subjectiver Hinsicht*. Berlin: Reimer.
Purkinje, J. (1826). Flourens De physiologia systemis nervorum. *Kritisches Repertorium für die gesammte Heilkunde*, **11**, 101–123.
Purkinje, J. (1827). Ueber die physiologische Bedeutung des Schwindels und die Beziehung desselben zu den neuesten Versuchen über die Hirnfunctionen. *Magazin für die gesammte Heilkunde*, **23**, 284–310.
Purkinje, J. (1846). Wachen, Schlaf, Traum und verwandte Zustände. In R. Wagner (Ed.), *Handwörterbuch der Physiologie*. Vol. 3. (pp. 412–480) Braunschweig: Vieweg.
Purkinje, J. (1918). *Opera omnia*. Vol. 1. (K. J. Lhotak Ed.) Prague: Society of Czech Physicians.
Radach, R., Kennedy, A., and Rayner, K. (Eds.) (2002). *Eye movements and information processing during reading: special issue of the European Journal of Cognitive Psychology*. Hove: Psychology Press.
Radach, R., Kennedy, A., and Rayner, K. (Eds.) (2004). *Eye movements and information processing during reading*. New York: Psychology Press.
Rao, R. P. N., Zelinsky, G. J., Hayhoe, M. M., and Ballard, D. H. (1996). Modelling saccade targeting in visual search. In D. Touretzky, M. Mozer, and M. Hasselmo (Eds.), *Advances in neural information processing systems*. Vol. 8. (pp. 830–836). Cambridge, MA: MIT Press.
Ratliff, F. (1952). The role of physiological nystagmus in monocular acuity. *Journal of Experimental Psychology*, **43**, 163–172.
Ratliff, F. (1971). On the objective study of subjective phenomena: the Purkyně Tree. In V. Kruta (Ed.), *Jan Evangelista Purkyně 1787–1869. Centenary symposium*. (pp. 77–92) Brno: Universita Jana Evangelisty Purkyně.
Ratliff, F. and Riggs, L. A. (1950). Involuntary motions of the eye during monocular fixation. *Journal of Experimental Psychology*, **40**, 687–701.
Rayner, K. (1978). Foveal and parafoveal cues in reading. In J. Requin (Ed.), *Attention and performance*. Vol. 7. (pp. 149–162) Hillsdale, NJ: Lawrence Erlbaum Associates.
Rayner, K. (Ed.) (1983). *Eye movements in reading: perceptual and language processes*. New York: Academic Press.
Rayner, K. (1992). *Eye movements and visual cognition: scene perception and reading*. New York: Springer.
Rayner, K. (1998). Eye movements in reading and information processing: 20 years of research. *Psychological Bulletin*, **124**, 372–422.
Rayner, K. and Pollatsek, A. (1983). Is visual information integrated across saccades? *Perception and Psychophysics*, **34**, 39–48.
Rayner, K. and Pollatsek, A. (1992). Eye-movements and scene perception. *Canadian Journal of Psychology-Revue Canadienne de Psychologie*, **46**, 342–376.
Rayner, K., McConkie, G. W., and Zola, D. (1980). Integrating information across eye movements. *Cognitive Psychology*, **12**, 206–226.
Reid, T. (1764). *An inquiry into the human mind, on the principles of common sense*. Edinburgh: Millar, Kincaid and Bell.
Reinagel, P. and Zador, A. M. (1999). Natural scene statistics at the centre of gaze. *Network-Computation in Neural Systems*, **10**, 341–350.

Rensink, R. A. (2000*a*). Seeing, sensing, and scrutinizing. *Vision Research*, **40**, 1469–1487.

Rensink, R. A. (2000*b*). The dynamic representation of scenes. *Visual Cognition*, **7**, 17–42.

Rensink, R. A. (2002). Change detection. *Annual Review of Psychology*, **53**, 245–277.

Rensink, R. A., O'Regan, J. K., and Clark, J. J. (1995). Image flicker is as good as saccades in making large scene changes invisible. *Perception*, **24** (suppl.), 26–27.

Rensink, R. A., O'Regan, J. K., and Clark, J. J. (1997). To see or not to see: the need for attention to perceive changes in scenes. *Psychological Science*, **8**, 368–373.

Rensink, R. A., O'Regan, J. K., and Clark, J. J. (2000). On the failure to detect changes in scenes across brief interruptions. *Visual Cognition*, **7**, 127–145.

Riggs, L. A., Ratliff, F., Cornsweet, J. C., and Cornsweet, T. N. (1953). The disappearance of steadily fixated visual test objects. *Journal of the Optical Society of America*, **43**, 495–501.

Ritter, J. W. (1801). Versuche und Bemerkungen über den Galvanismus der Voltaischen Batterie. *Annalen der Physik*, **7**, 431–484.

Robinson, D. A. (1963). A method of measuring eye movement using a scleral search coil in a magnetic field. *IEEE Transactions on Bio-Medical Electronics*, **BME-10**, 137–145.

Robinson, J. O. (1972). *The psychology of visual illusion*. London: Hutchinson University Library.

Robinson, N. H. (1980). *The Royal Society catalogue of portraits*. London: The Royal Society.

Rogers, B. J. and Graham, M. E. (1979) Motion parallax as an independent cue for depth perception. *Perception*, **8**, 125–134.

Roget, P. M. (1825). Explanation of an optical deception in the appearance of the spokes of a wheel seen through vertical apertures. *Philosophical Transactions of the Royal Society*, **115**, 131–140.

Rohault, J. (1671). *Traité de physique*. Paris: Savreux.

Rohault, J. (1723). *Rohault's system of natural philosophy*. (Trans. J. Clarke) London: Knapton.

Rosander, K. and von Hofsten, C. (2004). Infants' emerging ability to represent occluded object motion. *Cognition*, **91**, 1–22.

Ross, H. E. and Murray, D. J. (1978). *E. H. Weber: The sense of touch*. London: Academic Press.

Ross, W. D. (Ed.) (1927). *The works of Aristotle*. Vol. 7. Oxford: Clarendon.

Ross, W. D. (Ed.) (1931). *The works of Aristotle*. Vol. 3. Oxford: Clarendon.

Ruete, C. G. T. (1845). *Lehrbuch der Ophthalmologie für Aerzte und Studirende*. Braunschweig: Vieweg.

Ruete, C. G. T. (1853). *Lehrbuch der Ophthalmologie*. (2nd edn.) Leipzig: Vieweg.

Ruete, C. G. T. (1857). *Lehrbuch der Ophthalmologie für Aerzte und Studirende*. (2nd edn.) Braunschweig: Vieweg.

Runes, D. D. (1959). *Pictorial history of philosophy*. New York: Philosophical Library.

Sabra, A. I. (1989). (Trans. and ed.) *The Optics of Ibn Al-Haytham. Books I–III. On direct vision*. London: The Warburg Institute.

Salapatek, P. and Kessen, W. (1966). Visual scanning of triangles in the human newborn. *Journal of Experimental Child Psychology*, **3**, 155–167.

Scheiner, C. (1619). *Oculus, hoc est fundamentum opticum.* Innsbruck: Agricola.

Scheiner, C. (1630). *Rosa ursina.* Bracciani: Phaeum.

Schmid, R. and Zambarbieri, D. (Eds.) (1991). *Oculomotor control and cognitive processes: normal and pathological aspects.* Amsterdam: North-Holland.

Schmitz, E.-H. (1983). *Handbuch zur Geschichte der Optik.* Vol. 3. Bonn: Wayerborgh.

Schnell, T., Kwon, Y., Merchant, S., and Etherington, T. (2004). Improved flight technical performance in flight decks equipped with synthetic vision information system displays. *International Journal of Aviation Psychology,* **14**, 79–102.

Schott, E. (1922). Über die Registrierung des Nystagmus und anderer Augenbewegungen vermittels des Seitengalvenometers. *Deutsches Archiv für Klinische Medizin,* **140**, 79–90.

Schweizer, G. (1857). Über das Sternschwanken. Part I: *Bulletin de la Société Impériale des Naturalistes de Moscou,* **30**, 440–457.

Schweizer, G. (1858). Über das Sternschwanken. Part II: *Bulletin de la Société Impériale des Naturalistes de Moscou,* **31**, 477–500.

Seidman, S. H., Leigh, R. J., and Thomas, C. W. (1992). Eye movements during motion aftereffect. *Vision Research,* **32**, 167–171.

Sekuler, R. W. and Ganz, L. (1963). Aftereffect of seen motion with a stabilized retinal image. *Science,* **139**, 419–420.

Senders, J. W., Fisher, D. F., and Monty, R. A. (Eds.) (1978). *Eye movements and the higher psychological functions.* Hillsdale, NJ: Erlbaum.

Shackel, B. (1960). Review of the past and present in oculography. *Medical electronics proceedings of the second international conference* (p. 57). London: Hiffe.

Sharpe, C. R. (1972). The visibility and fading of thin lines visualized by their controlled movement across the retina. *Journal of Physiology,* **222**, 113–134.

Shastid, T. H. (1917). History of ophthalmology. In C. A. Wood (Ed.), *The American encyclopedia and dictionary of ophthalmology.* Vol. 11. (pp. 8524–8904) Chicago, IL: Cleveland Press.

Shebilske, W. L. (1977). Visuomotor coordination in visual direction and position constancies. In W. Epstein (Ed.), *Stability and constancy in visual perception* (pp. 23–69). New York: Wiley.

Sherrington, C. S. (1900). The muscular sense. In Schäfer A. E. (Ed.), *Text-book of physiology.* Vol. 2. (pp. 1002–1025) Edinburgh, Pentland.

Sherrington, C. S. (1906/2000). The integrative action of the nervous system. In N. J. Wade (Ed.), *The emergence of neuroscience in the nineteenth century.* Vol. 8. London: Routledge/Thoemmes.

Sherrington, C. S. (1918). Observations on the sensual role of the proprioceptive nerve-supply of the extrinsic ocular muscles. *Brain,* **41**, 332–343.

Siegel, R. E. (1970). *Galen on sense perception.* Basel: Karger.

Singer, C. (1956). *Galen on anatomical procedures.* London: Oxford University Press.

Skolnick, A. (1940). The role of eye movements in the autokinetic phenomenon. *Journal of Experimental Psychology,* **26**, 373–393.

Smeets, J. B. J., Hayhoe, M. M., and Ballard, D. H. (1996). Goal-directed arm movements change eye-head coordination. *Experimental Brain Research,* **109**, 434–440.

Smith, A. M. (1996). *Ptolemy's theory of visual perception: An English translation of the* Optics *with introduction and commentary.* Philadelphia, PA: The American Philosophical Society.

Smith, A. M. (1998). Ptolemy, Alhazen, and Kepler and the problem of optical images. *Arabic Sciences and Philosophy*, **8**, 9–44.

Smith, R. (1738). *A compleat system of opticks in four books*. Cambridge: Published by the author.

Smith, R. (2004). *A compleat system of opticks in four books*. Bristol, Thoemmes Continuum.

Smith, W. M. and Warter, P. J. Jr. (1960). Eye movement and stimulus movement: new photoelectric electromechanical system for recording and measuring tracking motions of the eye. *Journal of the Optical Society of America*, **50**, 245–250.

Sperling, G. (1960). The information available in brief visual presentations. *Psychological Monographs*, **74**, 1–29.

Sperling, G. (1967). Successive approximations to a model for short-term memory. *Acta Psychologica*, **27**, 285–292.

Stampfer, S. (1833). *Die stroboskopischen Scheiben; oder, die optischen Zauberscheiben, deren Theorie und wissenschaftliche Anwendung, erklärt von dem Erfinder S. Stampfer*. Vienna: Trentsensky & Vieweg.

Steinman, R. M. and Collewijn, H. (1980). Binocular retinal image motion during active head rotation. *Vision Research*, **20**, 415–429.

Stewart, D. (1800). *Account of the life and writings of Thomas Reid, D.D. F.R.S.Edin.* Edinburgh: Bell and Bradfute.

Stratton, G. M. (1902). Eye-movements and the aesthetics of visual form. *Philosophische Studien*, **20**, 336–359.

Stratton, G. M. (1906). Symmetry, linear illusions and the movements of the eye. *Psychological Review*, **13**, 82–96.

Stratton, G. M. (1917). *Theophrastus and the Greek physiological psychology before Aristotle*. New York: Macmillan.

Swanston, M. T. and Wade, N. J. (1981). Consistency of response during steady visual stimulation. *Perception*, **10**, 339–349.

Swanston, M. T. and Wade, N. J. (1992). Motion over the retina and the motion aftereffect. *Perception*, **21**, 569–582.

Szily, A. von (1905). Bewegungsnachbild und Bewegungskontrast. *Zeitschrift für Psychologie und Physiologie der Sinnesorgane*, **38**, 81–154.

Szily, A. von (1908). Zum Studium des Bewegungs nachbildes. *Zeitschrift für Psychologie und Physiologie der Sinnesorgane*, **42**, 109–114.

T. J. (1794). Letter to the editor. *The Gentleman's Magazine and Historical Chronicle*, **64**, 1093.

Tatler, B. W. and Trościanko, T. (2002). Last but not least: a rare glimpse of the eye in motion. *Perception*, **31**, 1403–1406.

Tatler, B. W. and Wade, N. J. (2003). On nystagmus, saccades and fixations. *Perception*, **32**, 167–184.

Tatler, B. W., Baddeley, R. J., and Gilchrist, I. D. (2005). Visual correlates of eye movements: effects of scale and time. *Vision Research*, **45**, 643–659.

Tatler, B. W., Gilchrist, I. D., and Land, M. F. (2005). Visual memory for objects in natural scenes: from fixations to object files. *Quarterly Journal of Experimental Psychology Section A-Human Experimental Psychology*, In press.

Taylor, E. A. (1937). *Controlled reading*. Chicago, IL: University of Chicago Press.

Taylor, W. C. (1846). *The national portrait gallery of illustrious and eminent personages*. Vol. 2. London: Jackson.

Theeuwes, J. and Burger, R. (1998). Attentional control during visual search: the effect of irrelevant singletons. *Journal of Experimental Psychology-Human Perception and Performance*, **24**, 1342–1353.

Thomas, E. L. (1968). Movements of the eye. *Scientific American*, **219**(2), 88–95.

Thompson, S. P. (1880). Optical illusions of motion. *Brain*, **3**, 289–298.

Thorwald, J. (1962). *Science and secrets of early medicine*. (Trans. R. and C. Winston) London: Thames and Hudson.

Titchener, E. B. (1901). *Experimental psychology. A manual of laboratory practice*. Vol. 1. New York: Macmillan.

Toglia, J. O. (1973). Electronystagmography. *Diseases of the Nervous System*, **34**, 379–383.

Torok, N., Guillemin, V., and Barnothy, J. M. (1951). Photoelectric nystagmography. *Annals of Otology, Rhinology and Laryngology*, **60**, 917.

Troxler, D. (1804). Ueber das Verschwinden gegebener Gegenstände innerhalb unseres Gesichtskreises. *Ophthalmologische Bibliothek*, **2**, 1–53.

Tschermak, A. (1931). Optische Raumsinn. In A. Bethe, G. Bergmann, G. Embden, and A. Ellinger (Eds.), *Handbuch der normalen und pathologischen Physiologie*. Vol. XII/2. (pp. 834–1000) Berlin: Springer.

Tschermak-Seysenegg, A. (1939). Über Parallaktoskopie. *Archiv für die gesamte Physiologie*, **241**, 454–469.

Tscherning, M. (1898). *Optique physiologique*. Paris: Carré and Naud.

Tscherning, M. (1900). *Physiologic optics*. (Trans. C. Weiland) Philadelphia, PA: Keystone.

Turner, R. S. (1994). *In the eye's mind. Vision and the Helmholtz-Hering controversy*. Princeton, NJ: Princeton University Press.

Uenoyama, K., Uenoyama, N., and Iinuma, I. (1964). Vector-electroculography and its clinical applications. *British Journal of Ophthalmology*, **48**, 318–330.

Uglow, J. (2002). *The lunar men: the friends who made the future*. London: Faber.

Underwood, G. (Ed.) (1998). *Eye guidance in reading and scene perception*. Oxford: Elsevier.

Underwood, G. (Ed.) (2005). *Cognitive processes in eye guidance*. Oxford: Oxford University Press.

Venezky, R. L. (1977). Research on reading processes. A historical perspective. *American Psychologist*, **32**, 339–345.

Verheijen, F. J. (1961). A simple after image method demonstrating the involuntary multi-directional eye movements during fixation. *Journal of Modern Optics*, **8**, 309–312.

Vernon, M. D. (1931). *The experimental study of reading*. Cambridge: Cambridge University Press.

Verriest, G. (1990). Life, eye disease and work of Joseph Plateau. *Documenta Ophthalmologica*, **74**, 9–20.

Vesalius, A. (1543). *De humani corporis fabrica*. Basel: Oporini.

Vieth, G. U. A. (1818). Ueber die Richtung der Augen. *Annalen der Physik*, **28**, 233–253.

Volkmann, A. W. (1836). *Neue Beiträge zur Physiologie des Gesichtssinnes*. Leipzig: Breitkopf and Härtel.

Volkmann, A. W. (1846). Sehen. In R. Wagner (Ed.), *Handwörterbuch der Physiologie*. Vol. 3. Part 1 (pp. 265–351). Braunschweig: Vieweg.

Volkmann, A. W. (1859). Das Tachistoscop, ein Instrument, welches bei Untersuchung des momentanen Sehens den Gebrauch des elektischen Funkens ersetz. *Berichte über die Verhandlungen der königlichen sächsischen Akademie der Wissenschaften mathematische-naturwissenschaftliche Klasse*, **2**, 90–98.

Volkmann, F. C. (1976). Saccadic suppression: a brief review. In R. A. Monty and J. W. Senders (Eds.), *Eye movements and psychological processes* (pp. 73–83). Hillsdale, NJ: Lawrence Erlbaum Associates.

Wade, N. (1982). *The art and science of visual illusions*. London: Routledge and Kegan Paul.

Wade, N. J. (1977). Distortions and disappearances of geometrical patterns. *Perception*, **6**, 407–433.

Wade, N. J. (1978). Why do patterned afterimages fluctuate in visibility? *Psychological Bulletin*, **85**, 338–352.

Wade, N. J. (1983). (Ed.) *Brewster and Wheatstone on vision*. London: Academic Press.

Wade, N. J. (1987). On the late invention of the stereoscope. *Perception*, **16**, 785–818.

Wade, N. J. (1995). *Psychologists in word and image*. Cambridge, MA: MIT Press.

Wade, N. J. (1998). *A natural history of vision*. Cambridge, MA: MIT Press.

Wade, N. J. (2000*a*). Porterfield and Wells on the motions of our eyes. *Perception*, **29**, 221–239.

Wade, N. J. (2000*b*). William Charles Wells (1757–1817) and vestibular research before Purkinje and Flourens. *Journal of Vestibular Research*, **10**, 127–37.

Wade, N. J. (2000c). An upright man. *Perception*, **29**, 253–257.

Wade, N. J. (2002). Erasmus Darwin (1731–1802). *Perception*, **31**, 643–650.

Wade, N. J. (2003*a*). *Destined for distinguished oblivion: the scientific vision of William Charles Wells (1757–1817)*. New York: Kluwer/Plenum.

Wade, N. J. (2003*b*). The search for a sixth sense: the cases for vestibular, muscle, and temperature senses. *Journal of the History of the Neurosciences*, **12**, 175–202.

Wade, N. J. (2004*a*). Philosophical instruments and toys: optical devices extending the art of seeing. *Journal of the History of the Neurosciences*, **13**, 102–124.

Wade, N. J. (2004*b*). Visual neuroscience before the neuron. *Perception*, **33**, 869–889.

Wade, N. J. and Brožek, J. (2001). *Purkinje's vision. the dawning of neuroscience*. Mahwah, NJ: Lawrence Erlbaum Associates.

Wade, N. J. and Heller, D. (1997). Scopes of perception: the experimental manipulation of space and time. *Psychological Research*, **60**, 227–237.

Wade, N. J. and Swanston, M. T. (2001). *Visual perception: an introduction*. (2nd edn.) Hove, East Sussex: Psychology Press.

Wade, N. J. and Verstraten, F. A. J. (1998). Introduction and historical overview. In G. Mather, F. Verstraten, and S. Anstis (Eds.), *The motion after-effect: a modern perspective* (pp. 1–23). Cambridge, MA: MIT Press.

Wade, N. J., Norrsell, U., and Presly, A. (2005). Cox's chair: 'a moral and a medical mean in the treatment of maniacs'. *History of Psychiatry*, **16**, 73–88.

Wade, N. J., Spillmann, L., and Swanston, M. T. (1996). Visual motion aftereffects: critical adaptation and test conditions. *Vision Research*, **36**, 2167–2175.

Wade, N. J., Swanston, M. T., Howard, I. P., Ono, H., and Shen, X. (1991). Induced rotary motion and ocular torsion. *Vision Research*, **31**, 1979–1983.

Wade, N. J., Tatler, B. W., and Heller, D. (2003). Dodge-ing the issue: Dodge, Javal, Hering and the measurement of saccades in eye movement research. *Perception*, **32**, 793–804.

Walker, J. (1923). Alexander Crum Brown. *Journal of the Chemical Society*, **123**, 3422–3431.

Walker, R., Walker, D. G., Husain, M., and Kennard, C. (2000). Control of voluntary and reflexive saccades. *Experimental Brain Research*, **130**, 540–544.

Wardrop, J. (1808). *Essays on the morbid anatomy of the human eye*. Vol. 1. Edinburgh: Archibald Constable.

Weber, E. H. (1834). *De pulsu, resorptione, auditu et tactu*. Leipzig: Koehler.

Weber, E. H. (1846). Der Tastsinn und das Gemeingefühl. In R. Wagner (Ed.), *Handwörterbuch der Physiologie*. Vol. 3. (pp. 481–588) Braunschweig: Vieweg.

Weisstein, N. (1972). Metacontrast. In D. Jameson and L. M. Hurvich (Eds.), *Handbook of sensory physiology, Vol. VII/4, Visual psychophysics* (pp. 233–272) Berlin: Springer.

Wells, L. S. (1906). *The journal of a voyage from Charlestown, S.C., to London, undertaken during the American Revolution*. (W. G. Aikman Ed.), New York: New York Historical Society.

Wells, W. C. (1792). *An essay upon single vision with two eyes: together with experiments and observations on several other subjects in optics*. London: Cadell.

Wells, W. C. (1794*a*). Reply to Dr. Darwin on vision. *The Gentleman's Magazine and Historical Chronicle*, **64**, 794–797.

Wells, W. C. (1794*b*). Reply to Dr. Darwin on vision. *The Gentleman's Magazine and Historical Chronicle*, **64**, 905–907.

Wells, W. C. (1814). *An essay on dew and several appearances connected with it*. London: Taylor and Hessey.

Welsh, D. (1825). *Account of the life and writings of Thomas Brown, M.D.* Edinburgh: Tait.

Wendt, G. R. (1951). Vestibular functions. In S. S. Steves (Ed.), *Handbook of experimental psychology*. (pp. 1191–1223) New York: Wiley.

Wertheimer, M. (1912). Experimentelle Studien über das Sehen von Bewegung. *Zeitschrift für Psychologie*, **61**, 161–265.

Westheimer, G. (1973). Saccadic eye movements. In V. Zikmund (Ed.), *The oculomotor system and brain functions* (pp. 59–77). Sevenoaks, Kent: Butterworth.

Wheatstone, C. (1832). Appendix to D. Brewster: on the undulations excited in the retina by the action of luminous points and lines. *Report of the British Association for the Advancement of Science. Transactions of the Sections. Oxford Meeting*. pp. 550–551.

Wheatstone, C. (1838). Contributions to the physiology of vision—part the first. On some remarkable, and hitherto unobserved, phenomena of binocular vision. *Philosophical Transactions of the Royal Society*, **128**, 371–394.

Wheatstone, C. (1852). Contributions to the physiology of vision—part the second. On some remarkable, and hitherto unobserved, phenomena of binocular vision. *Philosophical Transactions of the Royal Society of London*, **142**, 1–17.

Wheeless, L. L., Boynton, R. M., and Cohen, G. H. (1966). Eye movement responses to step and pulse-step stimuli. *Journal of the Optical Society of America*, **56**, 956–960.

Whytt, R. (1765). *Observations on the nature, causes, and cure of those disorders which have commonly been called nervous hypochondriac, or hysteric*. Edinburgh: Becket, Du Hondt, and Balfour.

Wilkes, A. L. and Wade, N. J. (1997). Bain on neural networks. *Brain and Cognition*, **33**, 295–305.

Wilkie, R. M. and Wann, J. P. (2003). Eye-movements aid the control of locomotion. *Journal of Vision*, **3**, 677–684.

Willcox, W. B. (1978). *The papers of Benjamin Franklin*. Vol. 21. New Haven: Yale University Press.

Willis, T. (1672). *De anima brutorum*. London: Wells & Scott.

Wohlgemuth, A. (1911). On the after-effect of seen movement. *British Journal of Psychology. Monograph Supplement*, **1**, 1–117.

Wood, R. W. (1895). The 'haunted swing' illusion. *Psychological Review*, **2**, 277–278.

Wood, W. (1880). *Portraits of the one hundred greatest men in history*. Vol. 4. London: Sampson Low, Marston, Searle, and Rivington.

Woodworth, R. S. (1923). *Psychology*. London: Methuen.

Woodworth, R. S. (1938). *Experimental psychology*. New York: Holt.

Wundt, W. (1862). *Beiträge zur Theorie der Sinneswahrnehmung*. Leipzig: Winter.

Wundt, W. (1896). *Grundriss der Psychologie*. Leipzig: Engelmann.

Wundt, W. (1897). *Outlines of psychology*. (Trans. C. H. Judd) Leipzig: Engelmann.

Wundt, W. (1898). Die geometrisch-optischen Täuschungen. *Abhandlungen der Sachsischen Akademie der Wissenschaften*, **24**, 53–178.

Yarbus, A. L. (1967). *Eye movements and vision*. New York: Plenum Press.

Young, L. R. and Sheena, D. (1975*a*). Eye-movement measurement techniques. *American Psychologist*, **30**, 315–330.

Young, L. R. and Sheena, D. (1975*b*). Survey of eye movement recording methods. *Behavior Research Methods and Instrumentation*, **7**, 397–429.

Young, L. R., Henn, V., and Scherberger, H. (2001). (Trans. and ed.) *Fundamentals of the theory of movement perception by Dr. Ernst Mach*. New York: Kluwer/Plenum.

Young, T. (1793). Observations on vision. *Philosophical Transactions of the Royal Society*, **83**, 169–181.

Young, T. (1801). On the mechanism of the eye. *Philosophical Transactions of the Royal Society*, **91**, 23–88.

Young, T. (1894). *Oeuvres Ophthalmologique de Thomas Young* (Trans. M. H. E. Tscherning). Copenhagen: Höst.

Zelinsky, G. J., Rao, R. P. N., Hayhoe, M. M., and Ballard, D. H. (1997). Eye movements reveal the spatiotemporal dynamics of visual search. *Psychological Science*, **8**, 448–453.

NAME INDEX

Numbers in **boldface** indicate pages that contain portraits. Numbers in roman are for entries in the text, quotes and figure legends.

SUBJECT INDEX